GENDER AND SCIENTIFIC DISCOURSE IN EARLY MODERN CULTURE

Literary and Scientific Cultures of Early Modernity

Series editors:

This series provides a forum for groundbreaking work on the relations between literary and scientific discourses in Europe, during a period when both fields were in a crucial moment of historical formation. We welcome proposals for books that address the many overlaps between modes of imaginative writing typical of the sixteenth and seventeenth centuries – poetics, rhetoric, prose narrative, dramatic production, utopia – and the vocabularies, conceptual models, and intellectual methods of newly emergent "scientific" fields such as medicine, astronomy, astrology, alchemy, psychology, mapping, mathematics, or natural history. In order to reflect the nature of intellectual inquiry during the period, the series is interdisciplinary in orientation and publishes monographs, edited collections, and selected critical editions of primary texts relevant to an understanding of the mutual implication of literary and scientific epistemologies.

Gender and Scientific Discourse in Early Modern Culture

Edited by
KATHLEEN P. LONG
Cornell University, USA

ASHGATE

Published by

Ashgate Publishing Limited
Wey Court East
Union Road
Farnham
Surrey, GU9 7PT
England

Ashgate Publishing Company
Suite 420
101 Cherry Street
Burlington
VT 05401-4405
USA

www.ashgate.com

British Library Cataloguing in Publication Data

Gender and scientific discourse in early modern culture. – (Literary and scientific cultures of early modernity)

1. Women in science – Europe – History. 2. Women in science – Europe – History – Sources. 3. Women in medicine – Europe – History. 4. Women in medicine – Europe – History – Sources. 5. Alchemy – Europe – History. 6. Alchemy – Europe – History – Sources. 7. Midwifery – Europe – History. 8. Midwifery – Europe – History – Sources. 9. Medical literature – Europe – History. 10. Literature and science – Europe – History. I. Series II. Long, Kathleen P., 1957–

809.9'3356'0903-dc22

Library of Congress Cataloging-in-Publication Data

Gender and scientific discourse in early modern European culture / edited by Kathleen Perry Long.

p. cm.— (Literary and scientific cultures of early modernity)

Includes bibliographical references.

ISBN 978-0-7546-6971-5 (hardback: alk. paper) — ISBN 978-0-7546-9763-3 (Ebook)

1. Women in science—Europe—History. 2. Women in medicine—Europe—History. 3. Alchemy—Europe—History. 4. Midwifery—Europe—History. I. Long, Kathleen P., 1957–

Q130.G444 2010

305.43'5094—dc22

2010018927

ISBN: 9780754669715 (hbk)
ISBN: 9780754697633 (ebk)

FSC Mixed Sources
Product group from well-managed forests and other controlled sources
www.fsc.org Cert no. SA-COC-1565
© 1996 Forest Stewardship Council

Printed and bound in Great Britain by
MPG Books Group, UK

Contents

List of Illustrations

List of Contributors

Jayne Elisabeth Archer, PhD, is Lecturer in Medieval and Renaissance Literature in the Department of English and Creative Writing at Aberystwyth University. She is an Associate Fellow of the Centre for the Study of the Renaissance, University of Warwick. She is General Editor of *John Nichols's The Progresses and Public Processions of Queen Elizabeth I: A New Edition of the Early Modern Sources*, 5 vols (Oxford University Press, forthcoming) and coeditor of two essay collections: *The Progresses, Pageants, and Entertainments of Queen Elizabeth I* (Oxford University Press, 2007) and *The Intellectual and Cultural World of the Early Modern Inns of Court* (Manchester University Press, forthcoming). She is currently editing *Volume 3: The Verse Treatises* for the Oxford University Press *Works of Fulke Greville.* She has published articles on Elizabethan and Jacobean masques, early modern women's receipt books, and alchemy in early modern literature, and is currently working on a book-length study of the relationship between housewifery and natural philosophy in early modern England.

Penny Bayer has a PhD from the University of Warwick, England, for a thesis on "Women's alchemical literature in Italy, France, the Swiss Cantons, and England, 1560–1616, and its diffusion to 1660." She is author of various articles and essays based on this research: "Jeanne du Port, alchemist daughter of Joseph du Chesne," *Rosenholmeren: Notiitser og Meddelelser fra Renaessancestudier ved Aarhus Universitet*; "Alchemy and female culture 1560–1616," Proceedings of the Graduate Conference, Centre for British and Comparative Cultural Studies, University of Warwick, 2001; "Lady Margaret Clifford's Alchemical Receipt Book and the John Dee Circle," *Ambix*, November 2005; and "From kitchen hearth to learned Paracelsianism: women and alchemy in the Renaissance," in *"Mystical Metal of Gold": Essays on Alchemy and Renaissance Culture.*

Alain Ekorong obtained both his Master's and his PhD from the University of Oregon, where he taught French and Francophone cultures to graduate and undergraduate students for 6 years, and where he was also an adjunct assistant professor. He has taught at Depauw University in Greencastle, Indiana. A specialist of the French Renaissance, his research focuses on exploring this period from marginal spaces, especially mysticism and colonial metaphors.

Dorothea Heitsch, PhD, formerly Associate Professor of French at Shippensburg University and currently lecturer in French in the Department of Romance Languages at the University of North Carolina-Chapel Hill, is the author of *Practising Reform in Montaigne's* Essais (2000) and of articles on Montaigne, Marie de Gournay, Antoine de la Sale, Léon l'Hébreu, and Hélisenne de Crenne. She has coauthored, with Jean-François Vallée, *Printed Voices: The Renaissance Culture of Dialogue* (2004) and she is finishing a book manuscript on literature and medicine.

Kathleen P. Long, PhD, is Professor of French at Cornell University. She has published several books, including *Hermaphrodites in Renaissance Europe* (Ashgate, 2006), and several edited volumes, including *Religious Differences in France* (Truman State Press, 2006), as well as a number of articles on sexuality and gender in early modern France. Her current project is a study of the representation of human bodies in alchemical treatises.

Simone Pinet, PhD, is Associate Professor of Spanish and Medieval Studies at Cornell University. She teaches undergraduate and graduate courses in medieval and Renaissance Spanish literature and culture; the approach in these courses tends to be interdisciplinary, addressing literary cultures, theories of space, poetics, books of chivalry and prose fiction in general, theories of fiction, cartography, and critical theory. Her books include: *El baladro del sabio Merlín: Notas para la historia y caracterización del personaje en España*. México: JGH, 1997. Bibliotheca Litterarum Humaniorum, Krinein, no. 2; *Archipelagoes: Insularity and Fiction in Medieval and Early Modern Spain* (University of Minnesota Press, 2010); *The Task of the Cleric: Three Studies on the 'Libro de Alexandre'* (in progress); and *Courting the Alhambra: Cross-Disciplinary Approaches to the Hall of Justice,* coedited with Cynthia Robinson (Brill: Leiden, 2009). She has also published numerous articles on medieval and Golden Age Spanish literature and culture.

Meredith K. Ray, PhD, is Associate Professor of Italian at the University of Delaware and the author of *Writing Gender in Women's Letter Collections of the Italian Renaissance* (University of Toronto Press, 2009). She has published articles on gender and epistolary writing, convent culture in early modern Venice, and the Renaissance *querelle des femmes*. She coedited the *Lettere familiari* of Arcangela Tarabotti (Rosenberg & Sellier, 2005) and has received grants from the Fulbright Foundation, the American Association of University Women, the Penn Humanities Forum Mellon Research Seminar, the National Endowment for the Humanities, and the Renaissance Society of America.

Kirk D. Read, PhD, is Associate Professor of French and Chair of the Humanities Division at Bates College in Lewiston, Maine. He has published on questions of sex, gender, and sexuality in early modern France, concentrating on how literary expression is informed by medical, historical, and political discourses. Recent work has focused on midwives' accounts of birthing as compared with lyric, popular, and satirical renderings in writers such as Catherine des Roches, Pierre Boaistuau, André Thevet, and Agrippa d'Aubigné. His current book-length project, *Birthing Bodies: Inscribing Reproduction in Early Modern France*, explores the currency of the birthing body across these genres and disciplines in early modern France. Kirk Read teaches a range of courses in both language and literature ranging from women writers of the 17th century, to the literature and film of francophone North Africa, to a course on Tintin and *bande dessiné*.

Bridgette Sheridan, PhD, is Assistant Professor of History at Framingham State College. She was the guest editor and contributor for *New England Journal of History: Special Issue on Gender,* Fall 2008. She has also published numerous articles and gender, sexuality, and childbirth, including: "From a Manly Knowledge to a Man's Helpmeet: Changing Conceptions of Midwives' Roles in Seventeenth-Century France," in an edited collection of essays from *Creating Women: Notions of Femininity from 1350 to 1700 Conference*, "Elite and Vernacular Medicine: The Practices and Epistemologies of Midwives and Medical Men, 1550–1700," (with Cynthia Klestinec) in *Attending to Early Modern Women—and Men*, and "Midwives and Physicians," in *The Greenwood Encyclopedia of Love, Courtship, and Sexuality through History*.

Elliott M. Simon, PhD, is Professor of English at the University of Haifa. He is author of *The Myth of Sisyphus: Renaissance Theories of Human Perfectibility* (Fairleigh Dickinson University Press, 2007) and *The Problem Play in British Drama, 1890–1914*, as well as editor of a volume on *The Jewish Self-Portrait in European and American Literature* (1996). He has also authored a number of articles on a wide range of subjects, including Renaissance Neoplatonism.

Sean Teuton, PhD, is Associate Professor of English and American Indian Studies at the University of Wisconsin, Madison. His publications include the book, *Red Land, Red Power: Grounding Knowledge in the American Indian Novel* (Duke University Press, 2008), and numerous articles on Native American literature and culture (as well as pedagogical issues relative to Native American Studies), for example: "In Open Daring: Risk and Vulnerability in the Poetry of Simon J. Ortiz," in *A Spring Wind: The Work of Simon J. Ortiz*, and "The Callout: Writing American Indian Politics." *Reasoning Together: Native Critics in Dialogue*, "Internationalism and the American Indian Scholar: Native Studies and the Challenge of Pan-Indigenism," *Identity Politics Reconsidered*, and "Placing the Ancestors: Postmodernism, 'Realism,' and American Indian Identity in James Welch's Winter in the Blood," *American Indian Quarterly* 25.4 (2001). He is at work on a second book on human rights and Native diplomacy entitled, *Cities of Refuge: American Indian Literary Internationalism*, a project that has received the Woodrow Wilson National Fellowship and the Katrin H. Lamon Fellowship from the School of American Research.

Acknowledgments

The idea for this collection of essays on alchemy and other forms of early modern science began with a seminar on "Alchemy and Abjection" that I taught many years ago at the Society for the Humanities at Cornell University. The atmosphere at the Society gave me room to rethink early modern science, beyond the Jungian and history of science models already circulating. The students in that seminar, Sean Teuton among others, inspired me to think differently about alchemy in particular, with their perceptive analyses of the highly elaborate rhetoric of the treatises they encountered over the course of the semester.

As is evident from the list of contributors, the work of many minds and hands went into this collection. I would like to thank my patient contributors, many of whom revised and polished their work over and over again, to make this collection of essays more of a harmonious whole. This project would never have come to fruition without the tireless support and wise advice of Erika Gaffney, our editor. Anything that is excellent in this project is due to her inspiration, as well as the hard work of the contributors; any errors are my own.

But the support of many others helped to refine our work, and I can only name a few here. Michael Giordano encouraged me from the very beginning of the long evolution of this collection. Gary Ferguson, David LaGuardia, and Larry Kritzman have given me advice on my work and on the collection, as well as opportunities to present portions of this material and receive feedback from others at the University of Delaware and at Dartmouth College. Marilyn Migiel read portions of the manuscript and gave valuable advice and kept me motivated throughout the process. I also thank our anonymous reader, who gave detailed guidance for reworking a number of the essays. My frequent exchanges with Leah DeVun have helped me to refine my understanding of medieval and early modern alchemy; she has been a valued interlocutor during this entire process. The Rare Book and Manuscript Division of the Cornell University Library has provided valuable resources for the research that went into this project; many of our images come from this collection. I am grateful to the entire staff of this collection for the help they extended to me as I undertook research on this topic. I thank Katherine Reagan in particular for the help she gave in navigating the collection. Last but not least my thanks go to my ever-patient and helpful tech support, Douglas Long, without whom this work would never have seen the light of day.

Introduction
Gender and Scientific Discourse in Early Modern Culture

Kathleen P. Long

This collection proposes an exploration of the relationship of women and questions of gender to the scientific domain in early modern Europe, particularly but not exclusively continental Europe. The essays in this volume present new views of this relationship by scrutinizing two very different fields: alchemy, where the existence of women practitioners has gone largely unacknowledged until quite recently, and obstetrics, a field in which women lost considerable ground as practitioners over the course of the seventeenth century.[1] Alchemy, in the wake of the pioneering work of Allen Debus,[2] has been ably rehabilitated as a scientific pursuit by a number of scholars, among them Bruce T. Moran,[3] Didier Kahn,[4] William R. Newman,[5] Tara Nummedal,[6] and Lawrence Principe.[7] The social importance of its more spiritual and philosophical aspects has yet to be thoroughly explored, although the volume

[1] See in particular Lianne McTavish, *Childbirth and the Display of Authority in Early Modern France* (Aldershot, UK: Ashgate, 2005), but also Barbara Ehrenreich and Deirdre English, *Witches, Midwives, and Nurses: A History of Women Healers* (New York: The Feminist Press, 1973), Jean Donnison, *Midwives and Medical Men* (New York: Schocken Books, 1977), Jacques Gélis, *La sage-femme ou le médecin: une nouvelle conception de la vie* (Paris: Fayard, 1988), Wendy Perkins, *Midwifery and Medicine in Early Modern France: Louise Bourgeois* (Exeter: University of Exeter Press, 1996).

[2] For example, *The Chemical Philosophy: Paracelsian Science and Medicine in the Sixteenth and Seventeenth Centuries*, 2 vols (New York: Science History Publications, 1977) and *The French Paracelsians: The Chemical Challenge to Medical and Scientific Tradition in Early Modern France* (Cambridge: Cambridge University Press, 1991).

[3] For example, his *Distilling Knowledge: Alchemy, Chemistry, and the Scientific Revolution* (Cambridge, MA: Harvard University Press, 2005).

[4] Including his magnum opus *Alchimie et Paracelsisme en France (1567–1625)* (Geneva: Droz, 2007).

[5] Prominent among his work is *Promethean Ambitions: Alchemy and the Quest to Perfect Nature* (Chicago: The University of Chicago Press, 2004).

[6] *Alchemy and Authority in the Holy Roman Empire* (Chicago: University of Chicago Press, 2007).

[7] Among his considerable corpus is *Chymists and Chymistry: Studies in the History of Alchemy and Early Modern Chemistry* (Sagamore Beach, MA: Science History Publications, 2007).

edited by Principe moves convincingly in this direction; this collection proposes some further steps in this direction.

Similarly, the social significance of surgeons replacing midwives in the birthing room will be the focus of Bridgette Sheridan's essay on Louise Bourgeois (Boursier) and on Kirk Read's essay on Catherine des Roches. Essays on cultural manifestations of scientific notions, particularly in the form of literary reworkings, demonstrate the broader reception of scientific innovations and traditions. The guiding thread that unites all of the essays in this collection is a very different notion of gender roles than that presented in mainstream university science of the early modern period. Alchemy and midwifery provide an intellectual realm in which women can act as practitioners, scientific investigators in their own right.

Not only did alchemy and midwifery provide women with a context in which they might gather knowledge and practice their skills, these pursuits also, since they were marginalized from the realm of more carefully (officially) controlled disciplines, provided the opportunity to construct theories about the role of the gendered individual in the world at large, theories that did not necessarily conform to official (theological and political) discourses concerning the proper roles of men and women in society. As Meredith Ray points out in her essay on Caterina Sforza's recipe or receipt book, *Experimenti*, and as Jayne Archer points out in her essay on Sarah Wigges' receipt book, alchemical practices create communities of knowledge in which women can communicate and confirm their own discoveries and ideas. In a period in which women are largely excluded from official domains of scientific inquiry, these disciplines offer a means of exchanging knowledge with other women and with men. As in the case of literary salons, women create their own intellectual communities.

But these domains, no doubt at least in part because of their separation from zones of power and authority (except in the case of royal births), also present very different notions of gender and of the feminine than do officially sanctioned discourses. For example, while the University of Paris continues to promote Aristotelian notions of gender, according to which the male alone is the perfected form of humanity, many alchemical treatises portray the conjunction of male and female as necessary to the process of perfecting the individual and nature; this conjunction is most frequently portrayed in the form of the alchemical *rebis*, or double being. The presentation of gender similarity or identification as well as difference confounds the simple hierarchy promoted by Aristotelians. Midwifery, as the example of Louise Bourgeois demonstrates, allows women to take on authority vis-à-vis the lords of state. Granted, this authority was evidently seen as threatening to the assumption of male superiority, and thus was almost constantly under attack. But both midwives' manuals and alchemical treatises provide alternative views of gender roles over a significant period of time. These views seep into other aspects of culture, thus extending their reach.

From the groundbreaking work of Debus, alchemy has been linked to the early development of modern science. Moran and Newman restate this link eloquently, demonstrating how alchemical pursuits, as questionable as their objects might have been, were crucial to the development of forms of experimentation and informed attitudes towards nature present (for better or worse) in much of modern science.[8] This collection will focus on how the period before and during the shift towards empirical science created these intellectual spaces where new ideas could be tried out, old ideas given new twists, and women could participate. The essays in this collection will also explore how this fluidity becomes hardened, notions of gender become more hierarchical, and women are excluded, as male practitioners strive to make science more "respectable."

The ubiquity of alchemy throughout early modern culture, from household recipe books to treatises on secret societies, and on to arcane poetry produced at court and elsewhere, suggests that alchemy is much more than an early form of chemistry. It is this wider purpose of alchemy that links it to such concepts as that of astral magic, discussed by philosophers and alchemists as a means of perfecting nature, particularly the human spirit, as Elliott Simon demonstrates in his essay on Pico, Paracelsus, and Dee. As Lynn Thorndike[9] and Frances Yates[10] made clear in their monumental works, natural magic and experimental science were closely linked in the medieval and early modern periods, as means of exploring the causes and connections between various natural phenomena, as well as means of influencing those phenomena. The belief that all things have particular properties or essences joins these two fields, as well as practical approaches to isolating, intensifying, or mitigating those properties through distillation, fermentation, production of compounds, and other methods. The talismanic practices of Marsilio Ficino's natural magic[11] are echoed in the images of alchemical emblem-books, which serve as a code for specific materials and practices, but also serve a meditative purpose. The joining of these diverse strains brings forth a different sort of alchemy, one that serves as a spiritual or philosophical exercise rather than only a science of physical transformation. In this process, the imagination rather than the intellect serves a central role, as a means of understanding the place of the divine in the world and of seeing that which is not immediately apparent or visible. The imagination leads human beings to perfection, in the feminine form of the *Shechinah*, from the Kabbalah, a divine wisdom superior to the intellect. This view of wisdom, along with the mystical, Gnostic, kabbalistic, and alchemical notion of a male/ female divinity, consonant with the hermaphroditic Adam, the perfect and unfallen form of human existence, passes into western European philosophy via Giovanni Pico della Mirandola, and is echoed in the works of Paracelsus and Dee. Just as alchemy on one level perfects the physical form of things by means of purification, so astral magic works through the imagination to perfect human nature. This perfection can only be achieved by the joining of body and soul, "animal"

[8] See, for example, Newman's chapter on "The Art-Nature Debate and the Issue of Experiment" in *Promethean Ambitions*, pp. 238–89.

[9] Lynn Thorndike, *A History of Magic and Experimental Science* (New York: Columbia University Press, 1923–1958), 6 vol.

[10] For example, Frances Yates, *Giordano Bruno and the Hermetic Tradition* (London: Routledge and Kegan Paul, 1964).

[11] Yates, "Ficino's Natural Magic," in *Giordano Bruno*, pp. 62–83.

and "sidereal" spirits, male and female. The theory of gender presented by Pico, Paracelsus, and Dee is not hierarchical or Aristotelian, but one that recognizes both difference and resemblance between the sexes. The male/ female binary is not effaced, but complicated by the notion that perfection can only be achieved by uniting these two aspects. The opposition of male and female, the fragmentation of human identity into these two roles, is at the root of human imperfection, and the practitioner of astral magic must imagine a reunification of fragments, a resolution of the binaries, in order to see the way to human perfection.

Alain Ekorong, in his essay on "Guillaume Postel, the Shechinah, and the Feminine Principle," emphasizes the revolutionary nature of the introduction of the mystical practices of Kabbalah into the alchemical/scientific arena. In particular, he links the *Shechinah*, considered a feminine principle, to the feminist discourses of Guillaume Postel, a noted translator and editor of Arab astronomical treatises as well as of an Arabic version of Euclid's *Elements*, thus placing scientific practices in a wider cultural context. Postel clearly saw the possibility of world harmony as achievable only through the conjunction of masculine and feminine principles, and even favored the feminine, and women, as superior vehicles for mystical and intellectual illumination, in spite of their inferior status in European society. He also questions the factitious division between masculine and feminine in his works, suggesting that both masculine and feminine principles are present in all of humankind.

Postel's work raises another issue vis-à-vis early modern alchemy and mysticism, one that has been discussed by Leah DeVun in her study of John of Rupescissa,[12] but that merits further exploration: alchemy can be read as a response to, and a way of dealing with, crisis. As Ekorong suggests, Postel very presciently saw the divisions between religions in the post-Reformation era as destructive; he included Judaism and Islam as well as the newly divided Christianity as candidates for some form of reunification, in a move reminiscent of Pico's *900 Theses*. The alchemical *rebis* becomes in this context a very different model for the union of opposites, suggesting that individuals and groups with significant differences can coexist peacefully without relinquishing their distinct identities.

This is the conclusion that Michel de Montaigne seems to be drawing as well in his very alchemical reading "Of a Monstrous Child," which I analyze at the end of my essay on "Odd Bodies: Reviewing Corporeal Difference in Early Modern Alchemy." Comparing the images in Michael Maier's *Atalanta fugiens* to those predominating in anatomical treatises of the sixteenth and early seventeenth centuries, I suggest that alchemy appropriates the clearly gendered (generally masculine) images of these treatises in order to turn them to more ambiguous ends. Alchemical figures mimic the classically inspired Vesalian Man, but with a twist, and alchemical treatises offer a very different vision of the human body than that of the classical models of early modern anatomical imagery. Montaigne gives a

---

[12] Leah Devun, *Prophecy, Alchemy, and the End of Time: John of Rupescissa in the Late Middle Ages* (New York: Columbia University Press, 2009), particularly chapter 3, "John of Rupescissa's Vision of the End," pp. 32–51.

similarly doubled body a very political interpretation, hinting at a broader context for the alchemical images. For, while these images are coded as symbols of stages of the alchemical process, they also resonate with other forms of knowledge familiar to their early modern audience: not only anatomy, but also religion and political theory. Christ, in alchemical treatises, does represent a stage of perfection, but he is also Christ, and early modern audiences would recognize the religious aspect of many alchemical images, as well as their alchemical purpose. Thus, the *rebis* represents the stage of conjunction, but also resonates with very active debates in that period concerning gender roles and gender ambiguity. What I am suggesting is that the alchemical code can work both ways: the royal, religious, and medical metaphors can represent alchemical materials and processes, but they can also become a means of expressing certain beliefs and opinions that might not be easily expressed in a more direct fashion.

In a very different context, Sean Teuton presents alchemy as a repository for notions of the effacement of difference, which allow the possibility of thinking beyond racial and gender differences, of at least pretending to transcend them, while manipulating their more typical representations to serve various ideological ends, such as the justification of conquest and the discrediting of imperial rivals. The *America* series, a collection of accounts of the discovery, exploration, and conquest of the western hemisphere by Europeans, gathered and voluminously illustrated by Theodor de Bry, his son, and son-in-law, present the cultural other as monstrous, often resembling the strange forms of humanity that appear in alchemical emblem-books. Michael Maier's *Atalanta fugiens*, probably illustrated by Matthäus Merian, a son-in-law of Theodor de Bry, is a superb example of such an emblem-book, displaying gender ambiguity and other forms of difference as objects of contemplation. Both the *America*, based as it is on imaginative recreations of scenes from the so-called "New World," and the *Atalanta* seem to express basic fears and desires lurking in the European imagination, fears of being swallowed up (or of swallowing oneself), fears of and desires for reversal of social roles, fears of the essential ambiguity of individual identity. The *Atlanta fugiens* offers a series of images that resolve the other into the same; in fact, as in the work of Pico, perfection is attained by uniting seeming opposites into a harmonious whole. Such assimilation seems only to work in one direction: monstrous images in the *America* of Tupinamba cannibals eating Europeans suggests that absorption of the European same by the American other is too profoundly disturbing. Thus, while alchemical works can be seen as inculcating a more nuanced understanding of difference, they can also be read as a justification of the brutal assimilation of the other by means of conquest. The confusion of gender that arises with some frequency in the *America*'s depiction of the indigenous people of the western hemisphere merely confirms the monstrosity of the cultural other, with its effeminate men, even hermaphrodites, and violent and ugly women. This seeming confusion of gender roles is seconded by the blurring of lines between species as some native Americans are depicted as hairy and animalistic. This association of blurring of gender difference with animal appearance and even monstrosity is echoed in literary works invoking the "New World," as Simone Pinet's essay suggests. The *America* and *Atalanta* engravings, when compared, reveal some of the possible political implications of alchemical theories of gender and difference, and these implications can be read as both revolutionary and profoundly conservative (in the sense of preservation of traditional gender and power hierarchies).

Pinet, in her essay on "The Animal Within," also traces the intersection between the literary and scientific domains, this time in the context of medieval and early modern Spain. Early modern Spanish chivalric romance combines the imagined monsters of the New World with more typically medieval European monsters (it should be noted that a number of place-names in the Western Hemisphere come from the names of monsters in Spanish literature – Patagonia and California being striking examples). This should serve as a reminder that early modern science was still entangled in its medieval roots. Her focus on monsters as the result of deviant desire in the *Amadis* reflects attitudes in a number of medical treatises of the period, but also speaks volumes about the politics of early modern Spain. Pinet points out that monsters reveal not only the problematic boundary between animal and human, but also between male and female. In the *Primaléon*, however, feminine beauty and sweet rhetoric (also associated with the feminine) become means for resolving the divide between monstrous and human, thus underscoring both the potential of the civilizing process to render the animal or monstrous human, but also conversely revealing the potential for monstrosity or some form of radical alterity in all humans. The *Primaléon*, very possibly authored by a woman, distances the monstrous from gestation and birth, thus reversing the trend apparent in most medical treatises of the period. Women become part of the ennobling process, helping to restore order to disorderly Nature, rather than being key contributors to disorder. In short, Pinet presents the chivalric novels of the period of Isabella as responses to the misogyny of medical treatises, a revision of gender roles and the association of the feminine with the monstrous towards a conceptualization of women's role in constructing social order and power.

While the monstrous patrols the boundaries of gender roles, both in medical treatises focusing on teratology and in literary works that feature monstrous forms, even if those works also seem to call those boundaries into question, alchemical bodies offer striking alternatives to the long-standing gender hierarchy. In the hermetic works of the early modern period, gender ambiguity becomes crystallized in one figure, that of the alchemical hermaphrodite, or *rebis*, or double being, which plays a central role in most representations of the process. Most frequently portrayed as male on one side and female on the other, with two heads, one clearly designated as masculine by means of short hair, and the other feminine, with long hair, the *rebis* symbolizes the stage of conjunction in the alchemical process. Conjunction itself is represented as the union of opposites, in which the properties of those opposites are united to create a perfected being. This being is then destroyed by calcination, eerily portrayed by Merian as a form of death by "slow fire," an Inquisitional torture in the early modern period, or by putrefaction. Distillation might be used to further purify the compound; the essence distilled from it is then used to revive the material in some way. This process is always portrayed in a gendered way, with the masculine and feminine principles joining in a sexual union. The *rebis* thus formed does not subsume one principle into the other; rather, both are joined and yet maintain their separate identities or properties, as suggested by the two heads and the body divided into two sexes.

This insistent and unconventional gendering of the *rebis* does more than serve as a code for various alchemical processes; it provides a language and a set of images that play with established gender roles. Ambroise Paré's discussion of hermaphrodites is fairly typical of the medical and legal response to intersexed individuals in the early modern period. He divides them into four categories, mostly male, mostly female, neuter, and double, but then insists that the double hermaphrodites (that is, having both male and female characteristics in more or less equal measure in the same body) must choose which sex they will be.[13] To put it simply, the *rebis* not only evades that choice, but suggests that the ideal being transcends simple gender divisions. Not only is the feminine revalorized, as it is in the Kabbalah in the form of the *Schechinah*, but it is reintegrated into a larger, human, whole that is not so easily designated as masculine or feminine, but encompasses both identities in a fluid process of transformation. The *rebis* is already presented in alchemical imagery of the late Middle Ages, and is presented in some as "Mercurial" and others as "diabolical."[14] The medieval alchemical hermaphrodite is a complex figure, as Leah DeVun has demonstrated, that encompasses a series of opposing qualities, human and divine as well as male and female. It is the perfect solution to a number of challenges faced by alchemists:

> For alchemists pondering the philosopher's stone, the metaphor of the hermaphrodite was an attractive solution. Ovid's stories of metamorphosis mirrored the alchemists' goal in metal transmutation – the change of one thing into another – and the hybrid nature of the hermaphrodite provided a useful model for the hybrid philosophers' stone. The metamorphosis of two individuals into a single creature of biform sex was particularly useful to characterize the sexed elemental qualities with which alchemists believed they worked, as well as the biform quality of the alchemical product. The hermaphrodite also satisfied the need to solve the linguistic puzzle of the "rebis," or "two thing." Moreover, the image fit readily within the conventional vocabulary of sexual reproduction used in scholastic natural philosophy.[15]

Medieval alchemy saw the hermaphrodite as a useful metaphor for the alchemical process; in true scholastic manner, this metaphor could be read *in bono* or *in malo*, either as a symbol of the divine or of the diabolical.

---

[13] Ambroise Paré, *Des Monstres et prodiges*, Jean Céard, ed. (Geneva: Droz, 1971), pp. 24–5.

[14] See Barbara Obrist, *Les Débuts de l'imagerie alchimique (XIVe–XVe siècles)* (Paris: Le Sycomore, 1982), pp. 152–65.

[15] Leah DeVun, "The Jesus Hermaphrodite: Science and Sex Difference in Premodern Europe," *Journal of the History of Ideas*, 69/2 (April 2008): 193–218 (215).

What changes between the Middle Ages and the early modern period is the rediscovery and revalorization of the *Corpus Hermeticum*, translated and commented upon by Ficino.[16] The *Corpus* privileges a double-gendered deity as the source of all creation.[17] After this revival of Hermes Trismegistus in the late fifteenth century, the diabolical aspect of the hermaphroditic *rebis* seems to be effaced from the alchemical corpus, and its place as a means to perfection in the alchemical process seems assured.

From these more theoretical representations of gender, relative to alchemical treatises and historical narrative, the collection moves on to a more precise question: what is at stake when women participate in scientific enterprises and discourses? In what contexts do women engage in scientific inquiry, how might that engagement be limited, and how do women bypass or overcome these limitations? Three articles in this collection present an overview of continental European women engaged in alchemical practices. This collection neglects Germany, since the work of Tara Nummedal on Anna Maria Zieglerin,[18] as well as her book on *Alchemy and Authority in the Holy Roman Empire*, cited above, already provide a fair amount of information on that region. Meredith Ray's essay on the alchemical receipt or recipe book of Caterina Sforza shows how this pursuit played a significant role in the life of this powerful woman, and how it was intricately woven into her efforts to maintain or regain her power. At the same time, exchanges of letters between Sforza and others show how alchemy was practiced through networks of men and women sharing information. Women are not merely the audience for a number of alchemical works (particularly the receipt books), but they are actively producing them – and scholars are becoming increasingly aware of how widespread these practices were among elite women. As Ray points out, popular medicine, frequently practiced by women, involved early forms of organic chemistry, particularly distillation, the production of elixirs, and the production of compounds. Sforza also seems to have been involved in studying metallurgy in her role as regent, responsible for the financial well-being of her state. It is clear from her book of *Experimenti* and from her correspondence that she was actively engaged in experimentation. The practicality of her pursuits is not unusual for women of her period. But what is most striking is that a woman of this stature would be engaged in these pursuits, which thus become more than an artisan's way of making a living. Intellectual and scientific curiosity clearly provides other motivations for elite women in this period.

Penny Bayer presents a number of alchemical manuscripts from France and the Swiss cantons, ascribed to or prominently referencing women alchemists. These manuscripts do raise the question of authorial identity, as the term "philosopher's daughter" was used to designate the soul, but may also have been used as code

---

[16] Yates, "Ficino's *Pimander* and the *Asclepius*," in *Giordano Bruno*, pp. 20–43.

[17] From *The Theological and Philosophical Works of Hermes Trismegistus, Christian Neoplatonist*, John David Chambers, trans. (Edinburgh: T. & T. Clark, 1882), pp. 4–6.

[18] Nummedal, Tara, "Alchemical Reproduction and the Career of Anna Maria Zieglerin," *Ambix* 49 (2001): 56–68.

for the identity of a woman alchemist. Certainly the frequent use of pseudonyms blurs authorial identity for many alchemical treatises; this practice might well have permitted women to participate in alchemical inquiry undisturbed, but could also have served to marginalize them from the most active and public discussions of this art. In fact, recent research, including Jayne Archer's essay in this volume, suggests that the participation of women in alchemical practices was more widespread than previously recognized, in part because this participation was largely a private, unpublished activity, nonetheless creating significant networks among women as well as among women and men, as they shared recipes for perfumes and medicines, ideas about spiritual perfection, and references to useful or particularly enlightening books. That this activity had a spiritual as well as practical dimension suggests that officially sanctioned theological versions of spirituality might not have been as satisfying to women as more privately elaborated forms. Also, excluded from universities, women developed their own ways of acquiring and sharing knowledge. Objects of inquiry and doctrine in these public domains, women become subjects of inquiry in the context of alchemical practices. A Madame de la Martinville is treated as a respected practitioner of the art by Théodore de Mayenne, a member of Joseph du Chesne's circle – du Chesne himself being one of the foremost French Paracelsians of his time.[19] These French women alchemists in du Chesne's circle focus primarily on the more elevated pursuits: the transformation of base metals into gold, making medicine, and spiritual and philosophical inquiries. Manuscripts ascribed to Madame de la Martinville reveal a woman engaged in chemistry experiments who references a broad range of learned alchemical treatises, including Paracelsus, Arnold de Villanova, and Bernard Trevisan. She is quite aware of the metaphorical aspect of alchemy as well as its practical potential, and is conversant with the allegorical images used to designate the stages of the alchemical process (as well as various aspects of each stage). She is apparently practicing chymistry as well as spiritual alchemy. If anything, the woman designated as Quercitan's daughter is even more learned, having read Aristotle, the *Turba philosophorum*, and the *Book of Morienus*. While many male alchemists sought to appropriate the female procreative role, from Paracelsus on, she seeks to claim both the masculine and feminine roles in creating a resurrected alchemical body. The manuscripts written by Madame de la Martinville and Quercitan's Daughter are different enough in style and terminology that they most likely are the work of two different authors. Madame de la Martinville's language uses a full range of symbolic imagery; Quercitan's Daughter uses a more limited range of symbols, focusing more on experiments. Insertions and annotations in several of the manuscripts indicate a strong resistance to the notion of women practitioners, a resistance that persists today, in that women practitioners are not mentioned in general histories of alchemy.

Jayne Archer's essay on the receipt book of Sarah Wigges suggests how alchemical thought may have filtered into a broader section of women's culture and become a part of their everyday life, with the Philosopher's Stone sharing

[19] Debus, *French Paracelsians*, pp. 51–9.

space with medical recipes and sugar-craft. This receipt book suggests not only that women may have practiced alchemy in greater numbers than scholars have previously suspected, but also that alchemy was a much more widespread and open practice, not merely a marginal occult discourse, but a part of everyday life for a number of people, perhaps even ordinary in some respects. Some early modern texts suggest that the conjunction of housekeeping and alchemy – or "chymistry" as Principe prefers to call it, to mitigate the contrast between alchemy and modern chemistry – was fairly common. Arguments are made in support of the view of alchemy as "women's work," a common metaphor for the alchemical process, particularly the stage of *solution* or dissolution, compared to washing. A tradition of books on housekeeping includes discussion of the importance of medical knowledge for women, particularly knowledge of how to make and dispense medicines. Receipt books demonstrate a wide range of skills required of women, and often reveal a considerable amount of erudition. Sarah Wigges' manuscript reveals a sharing of this knowledge among women, with recipes passed down from her mother-in-law, among others. This manuscript and others reveal that women also received advice from men they knew and from male authors, in this case Andreas Libavius, Boethius, Nicholas Culpeper, and Paracelsus, among others. Women's experience in distilling essences and making compounds made them skilled practitioners of "chemical medicine." These practices were also linked to the notion of perfectability of all things: the essences were generally considered to be the purer or more perfect form of something. Focusing on women practitioners of chymistry also radically transforms our understanding of early modern science as a pursuit that existed in the context of practical, everyday experimentation and often with utilitarian ends, rather than as an isolated and abstract debate among elite men.

As Dorothea Heitsch demonstrates, Marie de Gournay reinvents herself in this context of alchemical practices. Not only does she follow in the footsteps of previous women practitioners, performing her own experiments, but she uses the philosophical aspect of alchemy in order to situate herself as an intellectual woman who transcends the stereotypical gender roles of the period. The freedom that alchemy granted to women practitioners also allows her to define herself as a woman writer, one who uses mixed gender identities to construct a newer, transmuted self freed from the constraints of a misogynist society. While clear references to her own practical experiments are evident in her works, suggesting that she was continually involved in this practice, metaphorical references found throughout her works suggest that alchemy offered her an intellectual framework that supported her unconventional approach both to writing and to the status of women. What Gournay's work suggests, and this is true for the alchemical pursuits of a number of women, is that alchemy served both as a source for practical experiments to enhance physical well-being and a philosophical framework within which one could reimagine and reinvent oneself and the world. This returns us to the association that both Yates and Thorndike have made between magical thinking, alchemical thought, and early modern science.

Private alchemical pursuits might have provided a space for the freeplay of women's intellectual interests, but where women practiced a profession openly, their status was subject to increasingly stringent limitations by male authority figures. So, as alchemy is opening up new avenues for women, midwifery is being shut off as a profession, and the power over childbirth being transferred to men. In this context, Bridgette Sheridan traces the increased marginalization of midwives in the seventeenth century. Whereas before this period, birth was almost exclusively a female domain, by the late sixteenth and early seventeenth centuries male practitioners, both physicians and surgeons, increasingly claimed authority over pregnancy and birth, first regulating midwives and then taking over their roles. By the late seventeenth century, there was a clear preference for male birthing experts, even among artisan women. This marginalization of midwives was reinforced by the power struggle between physicians and surgeons. Surgeons sought to enhance their status by linking their practices to the new empirical forms of medicine, often by means of treatises vaunting both their erudition and their practical experience. They also sought to broaden their clientele, and thus began to push midwives out of the profession. By means of newly created regulations, both physicians and surgeons gained control over midwives. Sheridan focuses particularly on the polemical attacks of Jacques and Charles Guillemeau, father and son surgeons, against Louise Bourgeois, as well as her defense of her status, as examples of these new limitations on women's work. Jacques Guillemeau was an apprentice of Ambroise Paré, thus already at a young age in an elevated status in his profession. But he enhanced the status of this profession even more by his learning; he had studied with physicians and could read and write Latin. As a woman, Louise Bourgeois was excluded from most of these avenues to success: university education, apprenticeship, and training with experts linked to and protected by political authorities. While she did not have any of these initial aids to success, Bourgeois did rise to preeminence in her field, becoming the midwife to Marie de Medicis in 1601. She had apparently made connections at court. She also enhanced the status of midwives by publishing a manual as well as accounts of her experiences at court. She was unusual among midwives because of her use and creation of written works, in the form of treatises on childbirth.

In the early seventeenth century, the role of a surgeon in childbirth was intervention if something went wrong in the birthing process. Midwives had a more continuing relationship with the pregnant mother, and mediated various situations. Guillemeau père and Bourgeois published their manuals in 1609, and neither work expressed a widely divergent view. According to both, midwives had a longstanding role in the birthing process, and surgeons or physicians were to be called in at any sign of trouble.

The ambitious Guillemeau fils was a different matter, desiring to impose himself as the expert in all matters medical. The death of Marie de Bourbon-Montpensier, sister-in-law of Louis XIII, a week after childbirth, fueled the confrontation between Charles Guillemeau and Bourgeois. The autopsy report, prepared by five physicians and five surgeons, implied that Bourgeois had failed in her duties. She published a defense of herself, but in the end Guillemeau's attacks on her competence ended her career at court. This effacement of women's role in the birthing process became more and more general over the course of the seventeenth century.

We have seen how women, already excluded from academic disciplines, were pushed out of professions and practices of knowledge that they had occupied up until the seventeenth century. We have also seen how women created their own networks of knowledge, in the absence of any institutional acceptance, and how those networks included men and tapped into more institutionally accepted forms of knowledge, as well as more marginal forms. The subversion and critique of masculinist structures of knowledge extended into the wider cultural sphere. Discourses of alchemy, childbirth, and monstrosity, all present in the works discussed in the first five essays of this collection, allow literary authors to redefine or reimagine women's roles in society and their place in the world.

As Kirk Read points out in his essay on "Touching and Telling: Gendered Variations on a Gynecological Theme," nowhere is gender, and the divide between men's and women's perspectives on a subject, more evident than in the practice of obstetrics in the early modern world, for obvious reasons. The appropriation of obstetrics and childbirth from midwives by male surgeons over the course of the seventeenth century underscores the differences between men's and women's approaches to scientific knowledge. For example, the poet Catherine des Roches retells the story of Agnodice, the first woman doctor according to an account by Hyginus, as a recreation of intellectual community by, of, and for women, a community destroyed by patriarchy's refusal to grant women access to intellectual pursuits in any officially sanctioned manner. The joy and pride women experience in the community they have created with Agnodice's guidance contrasts sharply with Jacques Guillemeau's account of the male surgeon groping pregnant women's bodies, shamefully and in the dark. Where men dare not look, women may intervene without shame. This contrast renders the insistence upon male surgeons' control of the birthing process by practitioners such as Guillemeau absurd. The proclamation by Catherine des Roches of the importance of intellectual communities of women is echoed by the sense of community evoked by women's receipt books, in which other women's ideas are cited openly, and the participation in alchemical thought delineated by Jayne Archer and Penny Bayer in their essays.

Indeed, what this collection proposes to its readers is the picture of an early modern scientific culture very different from that presented until very recently by the history of science. For, in the shadow of a university, church, and state-based culture run by, for, and primarily about men, lived alternative cultures that perceived gender in a range of ways and that created communities of intellectual women sharing ideas with each other as well as with men. What this picture suggests is that other ways of understanding social order and the relations between men and women always already existed, only covered over by the discourse of institutions intent on protecting themselves and the social hierarchies they thrived upon from alternative world views.

Chapter 1
Pico, Paracelsus, and Dee: The Magical Measure of Human Perfectibility

Elliott M. Simon

Astral magic may be considered one of the most poignant creative modes of the imagination through which human excellence is conceived as an attribute of celestial powers believed to animate the world. Perceived as planetary influences, astral magic, as it relates to Renaissance theories of human perfectibility, positions the study of human nature epistemologically and ontologically as an eternal process of becoming. Through astral magic what is believed to be true as an intellectually constructed theory of causality is more important than what may be known through actual physical experience. Although the methods of the astral magician in alchemy and astrology may appear empirically faulty, the imagination validates the magician's faith that all material being could potentially assume its perfected condition.[1] Even the miraculous can be explained in terms of mysteries inherent in natural causes that are believed to emanate from the divine in a process of creating a perfected order of being.

This perfected order aspires to eliminate all conventional dualities of abstract idealism and concrete actuality, celestial and earthly forms, cultural and natural conditions, mental and physical powers, and male and female gender oppositions.[2]

---

[1] In *Asclepius* (16), Hermes Trismegistus asserts that "Spirit supplies and invigorates all things in the world; like an instrument or a mechanism it is subject to the will of the supreme god," in the *Hermetica*, trans. Brian P. Copenhaver (Cambridge: Cambridge University Press, 1992), p. 76. On the *via imaginativa* present in astral magic as a subjective and transitive experience, see Daniel P. Walker, *Spiritual and Demonic Magic, from Ficino to Campanella* (University Park: Pennsylvania State University Press, 1958, reprint with introduction by Brian P. Copenhaver, 2003), pp. 76–82.

[2] In contemporary feminists terms this essential union of "the two" into "the one" is found in Nancy C.M. Hartsock's (and others') female construction of the self. "The female construction of the self in relation to others leads . . . toward opposition to dualisms of any sort, valuation of concrete, everyday life, [a] sense of a variety of connectedness, and continuities both with other persons and with the natural world. If material life structures consciousness, women's relationally defined existence, bodily experience of boundary challenges, and activities of transforming both physical objects and human beings must be expected to result in a world-view to which dichotomies are foreign." Nancy C.M. Hartsock, "The Feminist Standpoint: Developing the Ground for a Specifically Feminist Historical

Such a union or synthesis of binary oppositions is essential to the quest for a perfected psychological and social wholeness. This quest for wholeness is found in Renaissance humanist syncretism in philosophy and theology based on the unity of all being in God and faith in the existence of a singular and universal Truth within all speculative thought. It is also predicated on the biblical assertion that the human being—both the Hermaphrodite Adam (Genesis 1:26–28) and the divinely undifferentiated Adam and Eve before the Fall (Genesis 2:21–25)—was originally created in the "image and likeness" of God. Such a perfected *anthropos* as the bodily and spiritually united male and female symbolizes the great expectations that God was presumed to have for His human creation to whom He gave dominion over the earth.[3] In Plato's version of the "Myth of the Androgyne" (hermaphrodite), the conflict of heavenly and earthly dominion was solved by Zeus who divided this half-male half-female creature into separate beings to weaken its powers. However, the gods took pity on these differentiated inadequate creatures and offered them the potential restoration of their original condition as a reunion with their particular other half through the "alchemy" of love.[4]

For Giovanni Pico della Mirandola (1463–1494), the positive aspects of astral magic are refashioned in his syncretic study of Neoplatonism and Kabbalah concerned with the perfectibility of human nature and the modalities of intellectual enlightenment. For Philippus Aureolus Theophrastus Bombastus von Hohenheim (called Paracelsus, 1493–1541), astral magic is essential in his medical practice in which the binary oppositions within human nature are united into an essential whole that insures the physical and spiritual well being of the individual. For John Dee (1527–1608), astral magic and mathematics are both scientific and artistic modes used to perfect one's understanding of natural philosophy and its occult signification. In their theories of human perfectibility and the valorization of the

Materialism," in *The Feminist Standpoint Theory Reader: Intellectual and Political Controversies*, ed. Sandra Harding (New York: Routledge, 2004), pp. 45, 49, and 53n.26.

[3] The biblical figure of the "hermaphrodite" is found in Genesis 1:26–7: "And God said: 'Let us make man [singular] in our image, after our likeness; and let them [plural] have dominion . . . And God created man in His [singular] own image, in the image of God created He him [singular]; male and female created He them [plural]." Although Moses Maimonides (1135–1204) and other biblical exegetes argue that there can be no "image" of God since God has no imaginable form, the figure of the hermaphrodite Adam, in *Midrash Rabbah-Genesis* VIII: 1, was interpreted symbolically as a unity of One whose psychological and reproductive potentialities joined together male and female to achieve a union of the two separate spirits. In the Christian Gnostic's *Nag Hamadi Text*, "The Apocalypse of Adam," the Adam and Eve androgyne (male and female) was a creature whose divine powers and perfect knowledge were greater than the eternal angels (a perfect *anthropos* also called *Adamas*). Out of jealousy, the angel Sama'el separated Adam and Eve, and that superior knowledge and power was lost.

[4] For Plato's "myth of the androgyne," translated as hermaphrodite, and the origin of love, see: *Symposium* 189d–191d, in *The Collected Dialogues of Plato*, ed. Edith Hamilton and Huntington Cairns, Bollingen Series LXXI (New York: Bollingen Foundation and Pantheon Books, 1961), pp. 542–44.

imagination, intuition, reason, subjectivity, and empirical objectivity must be reconciled within the astral magician's creative process to unite the inferior human spirit with superior celestial spirits.

In the period from Francesco Petrarch (1304–1374) to Tommaso Campanella (1568–1639) the privileged status of the imagination as a rational faculty of the mind mediating between the earthly and celestial worlds is a controversial issue in both moral and natural philosophy. For Petrarch in *De Ignorantia* (1368), the imagination must be governed by piety, defined as obedience to the moral authority of Holy Scripture. However, in order to manifest the intellectual tenets of "the Good" the imagination must also be open to the erudition of classical philosophy, metaphysics, and poetic eloquence.[5] Through the imagination, the moral discipline of Scripture and the intellectual application of philosophical principles are endowed with aesthetic qualities that subjectively unite the Good and the Beautiful. In *Secretum*, Francesca's imaginary dialogue with St. Augustine, the intellectual rigors of doctrinal piety must be reconciled with the subjective emotional desires for earthly love.[6] In *Il Canzoniere*, Petrarch imagines that his love for Laura, the female embodiment of virtuous beauty, is in conflict with the poet-lover's male *cupiditas*. The transformations of his conflicted self-projections of love upon Laura reach their apotheosis in his imagination, which unites his love for the beautiful lady with his adoration of the *Vergine Bella*, the Virgin Mary, within the context of his poetry. Only through his imagination can Petrarch approximate a sense of potential excellence and redemptive wholeness for himself as he resolves his ambiguous masculine and feminine perceptions of love by elevating them to the angelic beauty of his beloved and the celestial beauty of the Virgin.

Coluccio Salutati (1331–1406) in *De laboribus Herculis* (*The Labors of Hercules*) argues that human perfectibility through the acquisition of "enlightened knowledge" is dependent on uniting one's self with the primary feminine creative power of all nine Muses, not through the agency of reason but through the imagination.[7] Clio serves the desire for fame; Euterpe facilitates the enjoyment

---

[5] "If Thou dost not wish to grant me more, let it be my portion at least to be a good man ... Whenever I have made a sober use of learning, I have sought in it nothing but to become good ... I desire to be both, I confess, since human longing is boundless and insatiable until it comes to rest in Thee, above Whom there is no place to which it could still rise. I desire to be both good and learned." Francesco Petrarch, *De ignorantia* [*On his own ignorance and that of many others*], trans. Hans Nachod, in *The Renaissance Philosophy of Man*, ed. Ernst Cassirer, Paul O. Kristeller, and John H. Randall, Jr. (Chicago: The University of Chicago Press, Phoenix Books, 1948), pp. 62–3.

[6] Francesco Petrarch, *Secretum*, trans. Davy Carozza and H. James Shey (New York: Peter Lang, 1989).

[7] Whereas Salutati conventionally treats the intellect as a male faculty that which inspires the intellect to achieve any positive goal in its quest for perfectibility is distinctly embodied in the feminine figures of the Muses. For Coluccio Salutati's "doctrine *perfectionem*," see *De laboribus Herculis*, ed. Berthold L. Ullman (Zürich: Artemis Verlag, 1951, in two volumes) I: 9, pp. 43–4. Also see: Ernesto Grassi *Renaissance Humanism: Studies in Philosophy and Poetics* (Binghamton, NY: Medieval & Renaissance Texts & Studies, vol. 51, 1988), pp. 33–6.

of one's studies, which are inspired by Melpomene. Knowledge based on sense perception is identified with the power of Thalia, and the crucial preservation of all that is perceived falls into the domain of Polyhymnia. Whereas most humanists base their quest for knowledge upon the use of reason, Salutati emphasizes the importance of "finding similarities" (*similitudines*) through the imagination as an "ingenious" (*ingenium*) cognitive power attributed to Erato.[8] Similitude reveals hitherto unappreciated relations between different aspects of nature and illuminates their significance. Salutati's concept of *ingenium* transforms the limited light of masculine rationality into the greater enlightenment of the imagination symbolized by the diverse feminine powers of the Muses. Such enlightenment aspires to understand the manifestations of the divine working through celestial powers in the world. Terpsichore and Urania join the earthly world with their perfected celestial image, and under the guidance of Calliope, the temporal world with its God(s), its male and female creatures, social institutions, and historical narrative can achieve a universal and coherent wholeness.

In *De immortalitate animae* (1516), Pietro Pomponazzi (1462–1525) argues that the process of knowing cannot exist without the imagination. Just as the intellect is inseparable from matter, it is impossible for the intellect to be separated from the imagination, irrespective of the gender of the scientist, for both are convertible.[9] Pomponazzi places the human being totally within the physical world, and defends astrology as a rational, physical science. The celestial qualities of the planets and stars illuminate the effective relationship between the heavenly and the human as literal or symbolic manifestations of the otherwise ineffable divine causality in the world. In other words, God is manifest in all natural phenomena, and one's faith in those manifestations can be configured by the imagination as the influences of celestial bodies on the physical world. The problem for Pomponazzi is that whereas the emanations of God constitute good astral magic, human superstitions and perverse interpretations of celestial influences may produce a demonic magic in which the true significance of astral configurations is lost. Therefore, the primary task of the astral magician must be to assert the pious intentions to which his/her imagination is directed as a prelude to a justification of celestial speculations.

[8] Erato, the Muse of lyric poetry and mime (from the Greek *Eratō*, *Eros*, or *erasthai*, to love), works similarly to Moses de Leon's conception of *Binah*, the celestial *siferah* of divine understanding in whose womb the seeds of divine wisdom are implanted by *Hokhmah*, divine wisdom, and from whom the rest of the Kabbalist's *siferot* are created. See: Moses de Leon, *The Zohar*, Pritzker Edition, Vol. 1:15a–b, trans. Daniel C. Matt (Stanford: Stanford University Press, 2004), pp. 110–12.

[9] Based on Aristotle's *De anima* 1.12 [I.1, 403a 8–9], Pomponazzi argues that "Knowing is either imagination or not without imagination," and "there is no knowing without some phantasm—which experience also proves." Pietro Pomponazzi (1516), *De immortalitate animae*, IV, trans. William H. Hay II, rev. John H. Randall, Jr., in *The Renaissance Philosophy of Man* (Chicago: The University of Chicago Press, Phoenix Books), 287, pp. 292–3. Pomponazzi of Mantua taught at the University of Padua. On the significance of natural philosophy taught in northern Italian universities, see: S.J. Tester, *A History of Western Astrology* (Suffolk, UK: The Boydell Press, 1987, reprint 1999), pp. 215–6.

For the prognosticator Girolamo Cardano (1501–1576), the pious astrologer knows that the stars are open to various interpretations about the natural causes that animate life:

> we, who cultivate true piety, observe nothing superstitious in the stars, but natural causes. All men alike are tormented by heat, cold, and pain. Similarly, we cannot deny that the bodies and minds of princes are bent to good and evil effect, violently or gently, [by the stars].[10]

The occult philosopher Henry Cornelius Agrippa (1486–1535) believes that the magician could purify his enlightened imagination through faith to conceive a more perfect understanding of God's creation. Through astral magic vivified by the imagination the "religious *magus*" had the power to perform miracles.[11] Taking this idealization of imaginative speculation to a greater extreme, the Hermeticist Giordano Bruno (1548–1600) asserts that by creating correspondences between celestial and earthly bodies, his magician hero, Nolan, could empower human beings to aspire to their moral and intellectual perfectibility transcending their natural and rational abilities.

> the man [Nolan] who has surmounted the air, penetrated the sky, wandered among the stars, passed beyond the borders of the world, [who has] effaced the imaginary walls of the first [earthly elements], eighth [identified with Saturn and the intelligence and reason of the golden age], ninth [wisdom, law, and pure intellect], tenth [identified with the *Primum Mobile*] spheres, and many more you could add according to the tattlings of empty mathematicians and the blind visions of vulgar philosophers. Thus by the light of his senses and reason [and imagination], he opened those cloisters of truth, which it is possible for us to open with the key of most diligent inquiry; he laid bare covered and veiled nature, gave eyes to moles and light to the blind, who could not fix their gaze and see their image reflected in the many mirrors which surround them on every side.[12]

The Dominican Tommaso Campanella (1568–1639) created *Hoh*, his fictional embodiment of metaphysics, as the philosopher-king standing at the summit of his educationally designed *City of the Sun* (1623). *Hoh* uses its intellect and imaginative powers of magic to envision the sublime epiphany of "*natura spirituale*" and "*natura*

---

[10] Girolamo Cardano, *Libelli duo* (1538), cited in Anthony Grafton, *Cardano's Cosmos: The Worlds and Works of a Renaissance Astrologer* (Cambridge, MA: Harvard University Press, 1999), p. 68.

[11] Henry Cornelius Agrippa, *De occulta philosophia*, III, 1–4, in *Three Books of Occult Philosophy*, trans. J[ames] F[rench] (London, 1651), pp. 215–7, 253–4, and 357–8. Also see: Charles G. Nauert Jr., *Agrippa and the Crisis of the Renaissance* (Urbana: University of Illinois Press, 1965).

[12] Giordano Bruno, *Le Cena De Le Ceneri* [*The Ash Wednesday Supper*, 1584], ed. and trans. Edward A. Gosselin and Lawrence S. Lerner (Toronto, Buffalo, and London: University of Toronto Press, Renaissance Society of America Reprint Texts 4, 1977, reprint 1995), p. 90.

corporale" united in a perfect "*concordia harmonica*." Astral magic in *The City of the Sun* follows, to a large extent, Marsilio Ficino's *De vita coelitùs comparanda* and the well known syncretism of magic, music-spirit theory, philosophy, theology, and occult sciences in *Picatrix*, in which the imagination configures all earthly and celestial analogical relationships. Campanella argues that if the *Picatrix* provides a revelation of ancient secrets, it is intended only for the wise person to use only for the good.[13] In *Astrologicorum Libri VI* (Six *Books on Astrological Matters*, 1629), Campanella argues that astral magic can neither overthrow divine providence nor completely impact upon human free will. Nevertheless, he believes that: "when God wishes to make a perfect Holy Man, He may use the stars and elements for tempering the body rightly for the reception of the soul, and thus make animal spirits subtle and pure."[14] Campanella and Giordano Bruno got into serious trouble with the Catholic Church when they attributed this magical-creative process to their astral magicians, even when expressed as theoretical potentialities of the imagination to inspire the moral refashioning of human nature.

In *De vita coelitùs comparanda* (1489/1490) Marsilio Ficino (1433–1499) argues:

> Now in the soul we locate the imagination, the reason, and the understanding.
>
> Our imagination is able to be so disposed, composed, and conformed especially to Mars or to the Sun (either on account of the quality and motion of our spirit or through election or through both) that it might instantly be a proper receptacle for Martial or Phoebean influence. Similarly, our reason (either through the imagination and the spirit together, or through deliberation, or through both) by imitation is so able to adapt itself to Jupiter on account of its dignity and nearness to him that it can receive Jupiter and the rewards of Jupiter much more than the imagination or spirit could, just as on this same principle the imagination and the spirit can capture celestial things much more readily than do inferior things and materials.[15]

---

13 Tommaso Campanella (1623), *The City of the Sun*, in *Ideal Commonwealths*, ed. Henry Morley (New York: Colonial Press, 1901), pp. 144, 151–2, 174–6. Campanella's theories of astral magic also incorporate Ficino's sources, Iamblichus, Proclus, and Prophyry as well as the *Corpus Hermeticum* and *Asclepius* often in contradiction to Ficino's theses. He also relied heavily on Antonio Persio's *Trattato dell'ingegno dell'huomo* (1576), and Bernardino Telesio's *De rerum natura* (1587).

14 Tommaso Campanella, *Astrologicorum Libri VI. In quibus Astrologia, omni superstitione Arabum & Iudæorum eliminata, physiologicè tratatur, secundùm S. Scripturas, & doctrinam S. Thomæ, & Alberti, & summorum Theologorum; Ita ut absque suspicione mala in Ecclesia Dei multa cum utilitate legi possint*, Lugduni. [*Six Books of Astrological matters, in which Astrology, purged of all superstitions of the Arabs and Jews, is treated physiologically, in accordance with the Holy Scriptures and the doctrine of St. Thomas* (*Aquinas*) *and Albert* (*Albertus Magnus*) *and the greatest theologians; so that they may, without suspicion of evil, be read in the Church of God with useful benefit*, Lyons, 1629], p. 5.

15 *De vita coelitùs comparanda* 22: 18–27, in *Three Books on Life*, ed. and trans. Carol V. Kaske and John R. Clark (Tempe, AZ: Medieval & Renaissance Texts & Studies, The Renaissance Society of America, 1998), p. 365.

Ficino was skeptical about the veracity of judicial astrology as an influence on human free will except as physical indicator of one's predisposition to receive celestial influences.[16] He believed that *providentia* (the mind subject to providence), *fatum* (the soul, imagination, and sensibility subject to fate), and *natura* (the particular body subject to the general laws of nature) constituted the threefold order of existence. The human being's intention to know God and himself, to "obtain life from the heavens," empowered the individual to aspire to higher forms of truth and reality beyond sensual perception. Through the interaction of phantasm and feeling, the mind could ascend to a greater consciousness of a higher state of being.[17] In *De vita coelitùs comparanda* (2: 87–94), Ficino argues that:

> the cosmos is animate just like any animate thing, and more effectively so, not only Platonic arguments but also the testimony of Arabic astrologers thoroughly proves. In the same works, the Arabic writers also prove that by an application of our spirit to the spirit of the cosmos, achieved by physical science and our affect [perhaps astral magic and the imagination], celestial goods pass to our soul and body. This happens from down here through our spirit within us which is a mediator, strengthened then by the spirit of the cosmos, and from above by the way of the rays of the stars acting favorably on our spirit, which not only is similar to the rays by nature but also then makes itself more like celestial things (255).[18]

In Ficino's version of a Platonic-Neoplatonic universe in which imperfect forms are recreated or made capable of apprehending themselves as perfected ideas (reflections of God's ineffable model of Creation), astral magic must eliminate all binary oppositions of pure and impure substance, good and evil qualities, and male and female forms to achieve this higher state of being.

---

[16] Ficino identifies his defense of astrological images with his commentaries on Plotinus' *Ennead* 4.3.11 and 4.4.30–42. However his rejection of the deterministic properties of judicial astrology in favor of the separation of divine providence and human free will seem to follow Albertus Magnus' thesis in *De Spiritu & Respiratione*, in *Opera Omnia*, XI, ed. Borgnet (Paris: Louis Vivès, 1890), p. 213. Also see: St. Thomas Aquinas' argument in *Contra Gentiles*, III, civ–cvi; and Lorenzo Valla's *Dialogue on Free Will*, trans. Charles E. Trinkaus, Jr., in *Renaissance Philosophy of Man*, pp. 163, 167, and 169.

[17] On Ficino's theory of *providentia*, *fatum*, and *natura*, see: Ernst Cassirer, *The Individual and the Cosmos in Renaissance Philosophy*, trans. Mario Domandi (Mineola, NY: Dover Publications, 2000), p. 114. On Ficino's distinctions between *intentiones*, the imagination, and phantasy derived from sense-impressions, see: Paul O. Kristeller, *The Philosophy of Marsilio Ficino*, trans. Virginia Conant (New York: Columbia University Press, 1943), pp. 235, 369f. Also see: Daniel P. Walker, pp. 6–10; and Tester, *A History of Western Astrology*, p. 207.

[18] On the attributes of the Sun, the Moon, Mercury, Venus, Mars, Saturn, and Jupiter, see: *De vita coelitùs comparanda* 2: 30–81, pp. 251–5; and 9:52–156, pp. 293–7. Also see: Daniel P. Walker, p. 15.

Giovanni Pico della Mirandola believed that the divine spirit operated in the natural world as the universal cause of all motion and life, which justified the human aspiration for perfectibility through the agency of the *spiritus mundi* made accessible through the imagination. Both Ficino and Pico aspire to elevate the human intellect from the imperfect world of the senses to a purely spiritual, albeit philosophical, *gnosis*. However, in *Disputationes Adversus Astrologiam Divinatricem* (1496), Pico questions whether human beings could legitimately discover the divine processes of perfectibility within natural elements and celestial bodies, and then combine them into a beatific vision of "the good life."[19] How could the "Ficinian imagination" enhance the power of reason to access these higher powers, and how could astral magic as a "*phantastic* art" perfect the nature of human beings? Could beautiful words and songs attract the influence of the Sun; could emotion and imagination capture the power of Mars; could discursive reason aspire to the excellence of Jupiter; and could intellectual contemplation and divine intuition achieve the perfection of Saturn? Pico was particularly critical of the arbitrary divisions of the zodiac into houses and the inadequate measurements used to create celestial tables, natal charts, and other astral signs that rendered divinatory astrology uncertain and lead to contrary interpretations of the rational principles of causality (III.7).[20] To what extent was the sublime knowledge of divine processes embodied in astral powers frustrated by the realization that every endeavor to imagine a magical process of perfectibility was rendered imperfect?[21]

---

[19] *Disputationes Adversus Astrologiam Divinatricem*, (1493–4, first edition 1496), III. iv, ed. Eugene Garin (Florence: Vallechi, 1952), pp. 194, 208, and 218. Pico attempted to clarify his conception of the rightful place of the fallen human being in the physical world, while at the same time arguing that the excellence of human intelligence could make him a creative partner with God. See: Daniel P. Walker, pp. 54–9.

[20] The astrologer's interpretation of signs was inadequate because he could not make truly accurate measurements, which Pico considered impossible (III.19). He observes: *Ex hac autem tam varia tamque multiplici opinionum varietate quam incerta reddatur astrologia divinatrix facile est perspicere.* [From this variety of opinions, it can be easily perceived how uncertain divinatory astrology must become.] *Disputationes Adversus Astrologiam Divinatricem* (VIII.2). In "Book IX," he attacks the accuracy of astrological tables, which are unsupported by observations. In "Books X and XI," he attempts to prove that the *rationes* of the astrologer are not true for neither he nor his contemporaries have any idea based on *experimentum* (experience) of what is actually up in the celestial spheres.

[21] Pico's criticism of the astrologer's inadequate observations of celestial bodies and conflicted significance of celestial influences on humans anticipates the more profound assault on astrology and astral magic made by the followers of Nicolaus Copernicus' (1473–1543) theory of heliocentricity. As Thomas Digges (d. 1595) noted in his revised *Prognosticon* (1576), the finite geocentric universe changes radically, in terms of planetary alignments, proximity, and the effectiveness of celestial rays, in the Copernican vision of a heliocentric organization of the planets in an infinite universe. See: Francis R. Johnson, *Astronomical Thought in Renaissance England: A Study of English Scientific Writings from 1500–1645* (Baltimore: Johns Hopkins Press, 1963), pp. 164ff; Charles Webster, *From Paracelsus to Newton: Magic and the Making of Modern Science*, (Cambridge: Cambridge University Press, 1982), p. 11.

In the *Oration: on the Dignity of Man*, Pico argues that God created human beings with an indeterminate nature capable of aspiring to an angelic identity or degenerating into bestiality. He imagines that God told Adam about his "indeterminate nature":

> We have made thee neither of heaven nor of earth, neither mortal nor immortal, so that with freedom of choice and with honor, as though the maker and molder of thyself, thou mayst fashion thyself in whatever shape thou shalt prefer. Thou shalt have the power to degenerate into the lower forms of life, which are brutish. Thou shalt have the power, out of thy soul's judgment, to be reborn into the higher forms, which are divine.[22]

In Pico's vision, the Hermaphrodite Adam was not created as a half-male half-female creature, but as one possessing the binary opposition of "angelic" and "bestial"—referring to angels and beasts of the field that had already been created (Genesis 1:14–25). Whereas the angelic, embodied in fixed stars and planets, has no need for free will and the bestial is fixated by its instinctual nature, the human is differentiated from them by its free will. Although celestial spirits could inspire the intellect in forms appealing to an intuitive consciousness of an angelic excellence, the human being's free will working through its own inventions could only approximate that excellence as a process of perfectibility rather than an actual realization of a perfected individual. The human spirit was not capable of performing these sense-perceptions or realizing these philosophical speculations based on reason without the help of the imagination working psychologically and subjectively to strengthen the inferior body and make it more akin to the soul.[23] In other words, the magic of astrological determinism could not trespass on either human free will or divine providence.

Nevertheless, what Pico considered truly magical was not the actual transformation of being, but rather the creative work of the imagination that could receive the true *spiritus* or "channels of influences" that passed from heaven to earth manifesting the divine signification of all natural beings.[24] Pico considered astral magic closely related to Jewish Kabbalah, Gnostic mysticism, and Orphic incantations as imaginative modes of interpreting the hidden qualities of the divine presence in nature. In *Conclusiones Orphicæ*, he asserts that: "In natural magic

---

[22] *Oration: On the Dignity of Man*, trans. Elizabeth L. Forbes, in *The Renaissance Philosophy of Man*, (Chicago: The University of Chicago Press, Phoenix Books, 1948), pp. 224–5.

[23] *Disputationes Adversus Astrologiam Divinatricem*, III.iv, p. 218.

[24] Similar to Marsilio Ficino's study and translation of the *Corpus Hermeticum*, Pico's syncretism of Platonism, Neoplatonism, Pythagoreanism, Jewish Kabbalah, Persian magic, Chaldean astrology, and Greek, Roman, and Egyptian occultism evidenced his attempt to regain an archetypal configuration of wisdom to reconnect the human being with his divine essence. The essential spirits (*daemons*) are planetary elements and Ariel bodies that have souls, and transmit celestial influences to the human spirit. Both Ficino and Pico argued that the hierarchy of *daemons* might be analogous to the Christian hierarchy of angels.

nothing is more effectual than the Hymns of Orpheus, if there be applied to them the suitable music, and disposition of the soul, and the other circumstances known to the wise."[25] For Pico, "suitable music" signifies the influence of *harmonia* on the associative powers of the imagination to find, or even create, the unifying affinities of all being in nature. His interest in astral magic as a "non-mechanical science" focuses on the Neoplatonic ascent of the soul as a philosophical and religious experience transformed into a mystical experience. Through his study of kabbalistic literature Pico found correspondences between Ptolemy's planetary spheres, with their mythic-magical identities and affinities, and the Kabbalists' conception of *sefirot* representing the divine attributes of God in the cosmos to which the human soul must aspire.[26] He was particularly attracted to Moses de Leon's (d. 1305) *Sefer ha-Zohar* (*Book of Splendour*, 1280–86?) with its speculations on the secret meanings of every word in the *Torah*, which created a dynamic process of transforming the "word" into a mystical communion with God. He was also influenced by R. Menahem Recanti's *Commentary on the Pentateuch* (ca. 1250–ca. 1310) and by the works of R. Abraham Abulafia (1240–1292?). Recanti's speculations on the symbolism of the *sefirot* and Abulafia's analysis of Divine Names, theory of language, and *gemateria* provided Pico with a complex hermeneutic system for interpreting divine wisdom embodied in the feminine form of the *Shekhinah* and "her" influence on human perfectibility.

In the early *Sefer ha-Bahir* and *Sefer Yetzirah*, following the Gnostic typology linking God the Father/Husband with the *Shekhinah* the Daughter/Bride, Kabbalists argue that the Divine Presence or Holy Spirit is embodied in the *Shekhinah* as a manifestation of divine wisdom.[27] In *Sefer Yetzirah* (3: 1–9), the letters *alef*, *mem*,

---

25 *Opera Omnia* (Basel, 1572) I, p. 106.

26 Pico began his study of Kabbalah with Elia Del Medigo in Padua in 1480, but most of his knowledge came from his Hebrew teacher and translator of numerous kabbalistic texts, Samuel ben Nissim Abulfaraj, who converted to Christianity, and took the name, Guglielmo Rasmondo Moncada also known as Flavius Mithridates. Pico was not interested in Kabbalah as a Jewish interpretation of the Bible, but in Christianizing kabbalistic ideas, as illustrated in *Heptaplus* (1489), to find new ways of certifying Christian belief. See: Brian P. Copenhaver and Charles B. Schmitt, *Renaissance Philosophy*, A History of Western Philosophy: 3 (New York and Oxford: Oxford University Press, 1992), pp. 171–5. The order of the *sefirot* is: 1) *Malkhut* (kingdom/sovereignty), 2) *Yesod* (righteousness or foundation of the world), 3) *Hod* (majesty), 4) *Nezah* (lasting endurance), 5) *Tiferet* (beauty, compassion), 6) *Gevurah* (power, judgment), 7) *Hesed* (divine love), 8) *Binah* (divine understanding), 9) *Hokhmah* (divine wisdom), and 10) *Keter* (the supreme crown). See: Moshe Idel (*Kabbalah: New Perspectives*, New Haven and London: Yale University Press, 1988), pp. 46–7.

27 R. Abraham ha-Levi Berukhim (a disciple of Isaac Luria), R. Hayyim Vital, R. Levi Isaac, R. Solomon ha-Levi Alkalbez, and R. Joseph Karo profess visions of the *Shekhinah* as a beautiful woman. See: Gershom Scholem, *Kabbalah* (New York: New York Times Book Co., 1974/1987), pp. 6, 17, 22, and 35; and Moshe Idel (1988), pp. 39, 80–81. Christians interpreted the feminine *Shekhinah* in connection with their veneration of the Virgin Mary and her role in the incarnation of God in Jesus. Gershom Scholem (1974/1987), pp. 283, 293, and 302.

and *shin* are identified as the "Three Mother Letters" of the 22 Foundation Letters of the Hebrew alphabet through which God created the world. In terms of their placement within the hierarchy of the *sefirot*, the letter *shin* (symbolizing fire/light) is placed in the first triad between *Hokhmah* (divine wisdom) and *Binah* (divine understanding); the letter *alef* (symbolizing breath/life) is placed in the second triad between *Hesed* (divine love) and *Gevurah* (divine judgment); and *mem* (water/generation) is placed in the fourth triad between *Netzah* (endurance) and *Hod* (splendor) constituting the figure of the *Supernal Human*.[28] In the Kabbalists' cosmological system, each of the ten *sefirot* has an important symbolic identity, and the most important of these symbols are the *Knesset Yisrael* (the community of Israel) and the *Shekhinah* linked to the eighth *sefirah*, *Binah*, and the ninth *sefirah*, *Hokhmah*.[29] The imagination, open to the celestial influence of the feminine *Shekhinah*, will guide human beings to their ultimate sphere of perfectibility in the domain of *Yesod* (righteousness) and *Tiferet* (beauty and compassion). In the kabbalistic interpretation of the "fall of Adam" as a prophetic paradigm, the Hebrew letters of Adam's name, *alef*, *dalet*, and *mem* symbolize Adam as the "first unitary human being" whose disobedience and exile from Eden necessitates the rise of the House of David that will rebuild the Temple and restore the *Shekhinah* to Israel. The destruction of the Temple necessitates the coming of the Messiah, who will reunite the holy spirit with humanity, which the Jews anticipate, but which St. Paul identifies with Jesus as "the last man" (Romans 5:17).[30] For Pico, Kabbalah not only proves that Jesus is the Messiah, but that the Trinitarian God/Son/Holy Spirit provides the ideal paradigm for human perfectibility through the human being's communion with God through the divine agency of the *Shekhinah*.

The kabbalistic interpretation of "Adam's fall" also justifies the doctrine of the *Du-parzufim*, which R. Moses de Leon, in his book *Ha-nefesh Ha-hakhamah* (*The Wise [Rational] Soul*) uses to illuminate the double-faceted nature of the primordial human being.[31] The binary God/male and Divine Spirit/female referring

---

[28] *Sefer Yetzirah: The Book of Creation in Theory and Practice*, revised edition, ed. Aryeh Kaplan (San Francisco: Weiser Books, 1997), pp. 139–55.

[29] The early Kabbalists also identified the *Shekhinah* with *Knesset Yisrael* as a paradigm of God's relation with His "chosen people" and their adherence to the divine ethical attributes revealed in the *Torah*. "The Kingdom of Heaven, which is realized in time in the historical *Knesset Yisrael*, represents therefore the latter's meta-historical aspect as well. The supernal *Knesset Yisrael* is the mother (*matrona*), the bride, and also the daughter of the "king," and they appear in numerous midrashic parables on the relationship between God and the Jewish people." Gershom Scholem (1974/1987), pp. 111–2.

[30] "For if by one man's offence death reigned by one; much more they which receive abundance of grace and of the gift of righteousness shall reign in life by one, Jesus Christ." Also see: *Romans* 5:18–21. On the exile of the *Shekhinah* in relations to Adam's "fall," see: Gershom Scholem (1974/1987), pp. 162–7, 194–5; and Moshe Idel (1988), p. 166.

[31] For a detailed explication of the *du-parzufim*, see: Gershom Scholem (1974/1987), pp. 140–44; and Moshe Idel (1988), pp. 128–36. For Moses de Leon's theory of the *du-parzufim* and his contribution to the composition of the *Zohar*, see: Gershom Scholem, *Major Trends in Jewish Mysticism* (New York: Schocken Books, 1961), pp. 186–204; and *Elements of the Kabbalah and Its Symbolism* (Jerusalem: Keter Publishing, 1976), p. 294.

to spiritual nature of *Tiferet* and *Shekhinah* are embodied in the divine image of the Hermaphrodite Adam. The division of the Hermaphrodite Adam is justified by the God's judgment "as if" He is making a kabbalistic *tikkun* (repair) of his own work: "It is not good that the man should be alone; I will make him a help meet [mate] for him" (Genesis 2:18). They are separated into Adam and Eve at Creation, and differentiated from the divine image as physical forms with the Fall. Such binary relationships are incorporated into Ficino's upper and lower faculties of the soul; the opposition of the soul (male) to the body (female) in negative terms results from Adam and Eve's act of disobedience. In the *Zohar*, the greatness of the male is not an inherent quality but is acquired through his union with the female partner.

> Great is the Lord and highly to be praised, in the city of our God, in the mountain of his holiness. When is the Lord called "great"? When *Knesset Yisrael* is to be found with him, as it is written, 'In the city of our God is he great.' 'In the city of our God' means 'with the city of our God' . . . and we learn that a king without a queen is not a [real] king and is neither great nor praised. Thus, so long as the male is without a female, all his excellency is removed from him and his is not in the category of Adam, and moreover he is not worthy of being blessed.[32]

The kabbalistic gender symbolism for the feminine representing the human soul aspiring to a relationship with the masculine intellect of God can be inverted such that the masculine *Zaddik* (the righteous human being) aspires to a union with the divine potency of the *Shekhinah* in the feminine role.

R. Ezra of Gerona (1160–1238) argues that the mystical union of the human soul with the *Shekhineh* in the eighth *sefirah* (*Binah*-understanding) and ninth *sefirah* (*Hokhmah*-divine wisdom) constitutes a process of ecstatic epistemological enlightenment similar to Plotinus' ascent of the soul and the prophetic powers of astral magic in which binary oppositions are erased in favor of a divine similitude of moral righteousness and psychic wholeness.

> The righteous causes his unblemished and pure soul to ascend [until she reaches] the supernal holy soul [universal soul] [and] she [the human soul] unites with her [the supernal soul] and knows future things. And this is the manner [in which] the prophet acted, as the evil inclination did not have any dominion over him, to separate him from the supernal soul. Thus the soul of the prophet is united with the supernal soul in a complete union.[33]

---

32 Cited in Moshe Idel (1988), p. 223. Such a conception of human perfectibility is analogous to the Platonic reunion of the two halves (male and female) of the Hermaphrodite as an integral whole (*Symposium* 193c).

33 Cited in Moshe Idel (1988), p. 42. On the relationship between Plotinus and R. Ezra of Gerona, see: E.R. Dodds, *Pagan and Christian in an Age of Anxiety* (Cambridge: Cambridge University Press, 1965), pp. 93–6; and Menahem Stern, *Greek and Latin Authors on Jews and Judaism*, in two volumes (Jerusalem: Israel Academy of Sciences and Humanities, 1980) II: pp. 206–16.

Similarly, in his *Commentary on Pentateuch*, R. Menahem Recanti wrote:

> When the pious and men of deeds [engaged in a state of mental] concentration, and were involved in supernal mysteries, they imagined, by the power of their thought, as if these things were engraved before them [before their eyes], and when they linked their souls to the supernal soul [Neoplatonic universal soul], these things increased and expanded and revealed themselves . . . as when he cleaved his soul to the supernal soul, these awesome things were engraved in his heart.[34]

In both theurgic operations, the free application of the imagination to sacred texts is essential to kabbalistic hermeneutics. For Pico, the imagination has the power to find correspondences between Plotinus' Neoplatonic concept of the One, the Divine Intellect, and the World Soul and the mythical attributes of Uranus ("everything excellent above all other things"), Saturn ("intellectual nature, which alone is capable of understanding and contemplation"), and Jupiter (the "active life").[35] Through the imagination both the philosophical Idea and the astral-mythological identifications can be refashioned in terms of the Christian God, the Angelic Mind, and the Rational Soul, and the kabbalistic conception of God, the Divine Attributes of *Sefirot* (particularly *Keter*, *Hokhmah*, and *Binah*) and the *Shekhinah*. For Pico, the *Shekhinah* functions in the feminine role of the creative imagination, with powers akin to those God's "Mother Letters" of the alphabet creating its own enlightened *gnosis* to access the Angelic Mind. Working on the intellective and sensitive faculties of the soul through the imagination, the *Shekhinah* inspires the human aspirant to refashion a particular physical experience to make it more universal and spiritual as a perfected perception of Divine Wisdom.

In addition to using Kabbalah as a hermeneutic system involving the free play of the imagination, Pico was also interested in R. Abraham Abulafia's theory of language and his method of reciting and refashioning Divine Names in combinations of the letters of the Hebrew alphabet with their numerical value.[36] The ultimate mystical meaning of letters and words is based on a free associative combination of letters (each considered a divine name itself) that enables a new symbolic language to emerge. His process of encoding and decoding letters, following

---

[34] R. Menachem Recanti, *Commentary on the Pentateuch*, fol. 38b, cited in Moshe Idel (1988), p. 43.

[35] See: Giovanni Pico della Mirandola (1486), *Commentary on a Poem of Platonic Love* [by Girolamo Benivieni], "Chapter Eight," trans. Douglas Carmichael (New York and London: University Press of America, 1986) "Book One," pp. 18–9. For Pico's application of the imagination to his conception of angelic and human love, see: "Book Three," pp. 61–9.

[36] For Abraham Abulafia's theory of language, see: Moshe Idel, *Language, Torah, and Hermeneutics in Abraham Abulafia*, trans. Menahem Kallus (Albany: State University of New York Press, 1989) "Chapter 1," pp. 1–28. On *gematria* as a hermeneutic system for attributing meaning to a word or group of words according to the numerical values of the letters, see: Gershom Scholem (1974/1987), pp. 337–43.

the mathematical rules of *gematria* and his geometric symbols (especially the circle), enables the Kabbalist to use his imagination to reconstruct his perceptions of physical and intellectual realities into a more profound spiritual relationship with God. Abulafia uses his formulations of words and numbers to illuminate the psychological relationship between the intellect and the imagination in his mystical exegesis of the "hidden wisdom" of the *Torah*. For the uninformed, the biblical text maintains its history and divine commandments as a sacred revelation. However, for those who followed Abulafia's magical-mystical theory of language, a superior wisdom based on the inner logic of the word and its supernal allegorical-spiritualistic interpretation provides an illumination of the perfectibility of the human being's body and soul.

Pico used the Kabbalists' belief that Hebrew is a "sacred language" that could invoke the divine spirit, but in his attempt to Christianize kabbalistic practice, he united Hebrew and other ancient languages to interpret a more universal significance for divine and philosophical ideas through the symbolism of word/images. The greater reality of human perfectibility to which he aspired was not a mutable material form, but a creation of the imagination. Pico seems to be following Aristotle's observation that:

> Now for the thinking soul images take the place of direct perception; and when it asserts or denies that they are good or bad, it avoids or pursues them. Hence the soul never thinks without a mental image (*De Anima* III.7.431a).

Through the associative powers of the imagination, words "imaged" the transcendent essence of the things they symbolized and revealed a hidden wisdom that was not evident in conventional denotations. Pico argues that whereas kabbalistic interpretations of Scripture confirm Christian revelation, kabbalistic practice could reveal other forms of truth about the nature of existence seemingly hidden from rational inquiry.[37] However, the success of kabbalistic interpretation is also dependent upon the moral intention of its practitioner to use his revelation to affect the *tikkun olam*, the human being's primary task to strive for the perfection of the imperfect world.[38] As Moshe Idel observed:

> Following the Lurianic pattern . . . 'The soul of the King Messiah cleaves to the tree of life [and] he is the master of all the treasures of his Father, and he performs restorations [*tikkunim*] in all aspects [of the divine powers] and [all levels of] existence . . . by virtue of his adherence to the tree of life everything he

[37] Giovanni Pico della Mirandola, *Opera Omnia*, I, p. 105. "*Nulla potest esse operatio Magica alicuius efficaciae, nisi annexum habeat opus Cabalae explicitum vel implicitum.*"

[38] Gershom Scholem (1961) identifies the concept of *Tikkun* as having several meanings: "the restoration of the cosmic harmony" (pp. 233, 287, and 305); "the striving for perfection" (pp. 246, 327); "restoring the scattered lights of God to their rightful place" (pp. 269–73); "a system of practical theosophy" (pp. 273–8); a process of "restoration" from evil to good (p. 283); to "eliminate the stigma of sin" (p. 315); to salvage holiness (p. 316); and to aid in the construction of a messianic world (p. 319).

> does is a restoration.' Cleaving and adhering are strikingly presented as enabling the Messiah to play a restorative role on all levels of reality, the theurgical goal being achieved only after the accomplishment of the mystical experience.[39]

This remarkable anthropomorphic conception of the human being restoring the perfection of God in the world and of God's Creation needing such restitution borders on Christian heresy. For Pico this role belongs to Jesus Christ, but the implication of kabbalistic theories of *tikkun* indicate that every enlightened astral magician, mystic, or philosopher, as an anticipation or imitation of the Messiah, is a participant in this great process of worldly perfectibility.[40] Pico believed, within the limitations of Christian doctrine, that the mystical link between the human being, the feminine *Shekhinah*, and the unity of God illuminated by the Kabbalah represents the true astral magic by which celestial (heavenly) powers invest a real "dignity" in human beings.[41]

Paracelsus also believed in the correlation between astral magic, Kabbalah, and the idealistic practice of medicine.

> If we would know the inner nature of man by his outer nature; if we would understand his inner heaven by his outward aspect; if we would know the inner nature of trees, herbs, roots, stones by their outward aspect, we must pursue our exploration of nature on the foundation of the cabala. For the cabala opens up

[39] Moshe Idel (1989), p. 57. The "tree of life" refers both to the tree of immortality in the Garden of Eden, untouched by Adam (*Genesis* 2:9, 3:22–3) and to the *Torah* (*Proverbs* 3:18, "She is the tree of life to them that lay hold upon her, And happy is everyone that holdeth her fast."). Isaac Luria (1534–1572) believed in the unification of the *Sefirot* and in mental exercises concentrating on certain divine names and their combination, and especially by means of *kavvanah*, the mystical reflection, or meditation on the act of prayer and the fulfillment of religious precepts. He was a remarkable innovator in kabbalistic teachings. His pious life gave the impression that he was truly possessed by the Holy Spirit, linking the ideal of the righteous man (*Zaddik*) to the idea of the Messiah. See: Gershom Scholem (1974/1987), pp. 420–22.

[40] Using the kabbalist's practice of letter substitutions and word reformulations, Pico could place the *Shin* of the three "mother letters" in the middle of the Tetragrammaton (*yod*, *heh*, *vav*, *heh*) and create a new word, *Yod*, *heh*, *shin*, *vav*, *heh* (*Yehehshu'eh*), Jesus, as the revealed name of God.

[41] Pico's kabbalistic studies were particularly influential on Johann Reuchlin (1455–1522) and Henry Cornelius Agrippa. For Johann Reuchlin's interest in Pico and his defense of Jewish Kabbalah and *humanista* against Johann Pfefferkorn and the scholastic theologians of Cologne, see: Erika Rummel, *The Case Against Johann Reuchlin: Religious and Social Controversy in Sixteenth-Century Germany* (Toronto and London: University of Toronto Press, 2002). In *De arte cabalistica* [On the Art of the Kabbalah] (Hague, 1517), Reuchlin is particularly interested in showing the affinity between his kabbalistic texts and Pythagorean philosophy.

> access to the occult, to the mysteries; it enables us to read sealed epistles and books, and likewise the inner nature of men.[42]

Paracelsus believed that such "shadowy similitude," "mirror images," and "enigmas" of astral signs and symbols and kabbalistic interpretations revealed the mysterious hand of God intervening in human affairs. Any serious work dealing with magic, alchemy, astrology, and religion must involve the "veiling" of Truth that might impact adversely on one's deeply felt belief systems. Celestial powers interpreted through kabbalistic methods constitute a symbolic codex of human perfectibility based on faith, apprehended by intuition, and rendered into forms by the imagination that become accessible to the astral magician aspiring to a spiritual understanding of nature rather than a mere physical transformation of matter.[43] For Paracelsus, the imagination and intuition elevate intellectual inquiry regarding the mysteries of divine processes into a revelation of nature's unseen and perhaps otherwise ineffable dimensions that are inaccessible to reason.

> From the 'imagination,' and its objects, the child receives its reason. And just as heaven infuses the child with its motion, its good and evil qualities, sometimes strongly, sometimes weakly, so the imagination of man—like the stars—has a course, and makes the child's reason turn to higher or lower things.[44]

---

42 Paracelsus, *Selected Writings*, ed. Jolande Jacobi, Bollingen Series XXII (Princeton: Princeton University Press, 1951/1979), p. 133. Paracelsus warns that only if the practitioner "seeks the kingdom of God" will the revelations of Kabbalah and astral magic be truly manifest. "The art of the cabala is beholden to God, it is in alliance with Him, and it is founded on the words of Christ. But if you do not follow the true doctrine of the cabala, but slip into geomancy, you will be led by that spirit which tells you nothing but lies (p. 134)." Both Pico and Paracelsus interpreted the Hebrew and Christian Kabbalah as analogies to the Eleusinian, Orphic, Dionysian, and Hermetic mysteries.

43 Johann Reuchlin also assumed that the magician could use natural and spiritual magic to perfect his understanding of divinity within the inferior earthly existence. The spiritual magician must first transform his baser human instincts into more edifying attributes analogous to the astrologer's progression from earthly elements within the lunar sphere, through the planetary spheres (Mercury, Venus, Sol, Mars, Jupiter, and Saturn), to the angelic sphere, and finally to the *Primum Mobile*. The discovery of the divine within the human serves as an intuitive apprehension of the good life and its spiritual perfection. In *De arte cabalistica*, Reuchlin argues that natural magic in its cruder physical operation and kabbalistic magic in its more contemplative manifestation lead to the purer forms of spiritual magic akin to the wisdom of the angels.

44 "The imagination of a pregnant woman is so strong that it can influence the seed [the child in the womb] and change the fruit, so that its nature is thereby deeply and solidly shaped and forged … The child requires no stars or planets: its mother is its stars and its planets" (Paracelsus, *Selected Writings*, p. 32). Human desires are also attributed to the imagination. "God left man free to propagate his kind … planted the seed in all its reality and specificity deep in the imagination of man … If a man has the will, the desire arises in his imagination and the desire generates the seed" (p. 33).

In *De Vita Longa*, Paracelsus defined astral magic as an "artful and indispensable science" that "reveals its highest powers through faith." Whereas alchemy is an art that carries something that has not been completed to its end by making its impurities and imperfections pure and perfect through fire, astral magic works in harmony with the psychic powers of the imagination to elevate human nature to a transcendent state of completion. "Magic has power to experience and fathom things which are inaccessible to human reason. For magic is a great secret wisdom, just as reason is a great public folly."[45] Astral magic provides a comprehensible explanation of the dynamics of alleged divine inspiration underlying all forms of creativity and ingenious inventions that denoted human excellence.

> In the stars all skills are arts, all crafts are hidden, and also all wisdom, all reason, as well as foolishness and what belongs to it; for there is nothing in man that does not flow into him from the light of nature. . . . If there had been no Venus, music would never have been invented, and if no Mars, neither would the crafts ever have been invented. Thus the stars teach us all the arts that exist on earth; and if the stars were not active in us, and if we had been compelled to discover everything in ourselves, no art would ever have come into being.[46]

Because all human skills and arts come from God, the true astral magician is holy in that he believes that God, rather than demonic spirits, inspired his magical arts. Paracelsus' magician possesses an imaginative power that transcends human reason, but not his natural humanity. He believes in divine immanence and strives to use his astral magic to illuminate that "Godly light in nature."[47]

For Paracelsus, astral magic is an art through which the physician aspires to heal the body through the invocation of celestial influences and restore an essential

---

[45] Paracelsus, *Selected Writings*, p. 137. Also see pp. 139, 141–2. "The great virtues that lie hidden in nature would never have been revealed if alchemy had not uncovered them and made them visible" (p. 144). Only the ultimate secrets regarding why nature was created constitutes divine mystery and is forbidden to man's arts.

[46] Paracelsus, *Selected Writings*, pp. 128–9. Through alchemy and astrology, one can discover the secrets of the innate disposition of all being in terms of the stars and human nature. Paracelsus' connections between classical gods, planets, and the inventions of significant crafts are consistent with numerous Medieval and Renaissance writers whose demystified versions of "ancient gods" transformed them into symbols of the creative inspiration necessary for all-important human inventions.

[47] Paracelsus identifies the "wise men of the East" (Matthew 2:1) as *magi* (astral magicians) who follow the "star" that announces the birth of a savior also identified as shepherds who are led by an "angel" to worship the baby Jesus. The biblical star infused with the divine spirit, similar to all natural forms that possess a divine essence, is analogous to an angelic being. The wise men as shepherds or magicians are those whose intuitive wisdom make them receptive to such a divine revelation and worthy to be present at the divine convocation of the Nativity.

physical and spiritual wholeness to human beings.[48] He believed that at Creation, the human being was created from primordial matter, which he identified as *limbus*.

> He who knows the nature of the *limbus* knows also what man is . . . How *limbus* is heaven and earth, the upper and lower sphere of the cosmos, the four elements and everything they comprise; therefore, it is just to identify it with the microcosm, for it too is the whole world . . . Consider how great and noble man was created, and what greatness must be attributed to his structure! No brain can fully encompass the structure of man's body and the extent of his virtues; he can be understood only as an image of the macrocosm, of the Great Creature.[49]

The *compositio humana* of natural elements (humors and celestial bodies) contributes to Paracelsus' image of the Hermaphrodite Adam as the Vitruvian Man, not the gender but the species, symbolizing the primary unity of "divine Oneness formed of a great diversity."

> Just as in heaven there is a Saturn of fiery nature, so on earth there is one of earthly nature; and just as there is a sun in the water, so is there one in heaven. . . . What is the difference between the sun, moon, Mercury, Saturn, and Jupiter in heaven, and the same planets in man? The difference is only one of form.[50]

Assuming that all physical matter possesses spiritual properties and potentialities, astral magic is the re-creative art that attempts to reveal the mysterious correspondences between divinity and nature. As the human being "emerged from

[48] Both astrology and medicine are arts in which the observation of natural phenomena requires hypotheses to explain and interpret those phenomena. Whereas medical hypotheses can be physically verified through experiments on the body, psychological hypotheses are more complex and speculative, and spiritual hypotheses can only be verified through the imagination rather than through mechanical processes. On the challenge of astrology to the empiricism and mechanics of natural philosophy, see: Charles Webster, *From Paracelsus to Newton: Magic and the Making of Modern Science*, p. 11. Similar to Paracelsus, Newton advocated the recovery of ancient Egyptian, Chaldean, and esoteric practices of occult sciences to aid in his investigations and understanding of the natural universe.

[49] Paracelsus, *Selected Writings*, p. 21. The four elements of creation—earth, air, fire, and water—the "trinity" of mercury, sulfur, and salt—the "celestial spirits of the sun, moon, stars, and planets," and the human being's four humors—choleric, melancholy, phlegm, and sanguine were all united (pp. 19–21). Based on John 1:1 and 1:14, and Genesis 1:26–31, Paracelsus believed that God created human beings in order to give His spirit a dwelling place in the flesh, and that God created the natural world as a manifestation of His own essence. Human nature is differentiated from animal nature in that it is endowed with the spirit of the divine wisdom and art: "For the light of nature is in us, and this light is God" (*Selected Writings*, pp. 38–9, 44, 127). Paracelsus seems to be paraphrasing John 1:3–4: "All things were made by him; and without him was not any thing made that was made. In him was life; and the life was the light of men."

[50] Paracelsus, *Selected Writings*, pp. 38, 61. Similarly: "In the stars there dwell reason, wisdom, ruse, strife, weapons, just as they do in us men" (p. 152).

the first matrix, the maternal womb of the Great Word," it acquired its human identity as both an "animal body," composed of the elements of earth and water, and a "sidereal body," composed of spirit and motion, fire and air.[51]

For Paracelsus, the binary oppositions of "animal body" and "sidereal body," body and soul, female and male must be resolved by the astral magician-physician performing that kabbalistic *tikkun* of repairing the damage of such separations to achieve a perfected wholeness. Although God wills man to be man, and woman to be woman, He also wills that both should be one essential human kind. "There may be two of them, and yet only one; two kinds of flesh, and yet only one." Man originates in the "Great World" and is inseparably bound to it; woman is created from man and cannot be separated from him. Neither the male nor the female is perfect alone, but only together can they be perfected as a whole human being.

> A man without a woman is not whole, only with a woman is he whole. Because woman was created from earth and he too is of earth, both are of earth and form together one whole. . . . Similarly man and [medical and spiritual] remedy derive from the same substance, and both together form a whole, that is to say, a whole man. . . . In this sense, the disease desires its wife, that is, the medicine. The medicine must be adjusted to the disease; both must be united to form a harmonious whole, just as in the case of man and woman. If the physician finds such a remedy, he is complete.[52]

The seeds of the man and the woman, "each according to its nature," form the child in the womb. The child as homunculus, embodying the attributes of both parents, develops all aspects of the complete human being endowed by God's grace "with spirit, reason, understanding, and all attributes of the soul." However, even while in the womb, it is "burdened with the potentialities of every disease" because "all [physical and spiritual] diseases are inherent in its nature"; but it "could not be born alive and healthy if an inner physician were not hidden in it."[53] Although one may say that the female body is more prone to disease than the male body, such

---

[51] Paracelsus, *Selected Writings*, p. 18. Whereas the animal body is linked to the mysteries of earthly life, the sidereal body is linked to the mysteries of the Great World. The first matrix is water on which the spirit of God was borne; it is the maternal womb in which heaven and earth were created. The second matrix is heaven and earth in which the first human being was formed by the hand of God. Woman was created by that same Hand out of man; she became the maternal womb of all human beings. Although man and woman are different, "both suffer as creatures beloved by God" (pp. 23–5).

[52] Paracelsus, *Selected Writings*, pp. 23, 33, and 73–4. Paradoxically, Paracelsus identifies woman with the earth and the elements, but she is also the "tree of life," which is superior to man by virtue of its fruits (p. 25). "He who contemplates woman should see in her the maternal womb of man [humanity]. How can one be an enemy of woman—whatever she may be? This world is peopled with her fruits, and that is why God lets her live so long, however loathsome she may be" (p. 26). "A good tree produces good fruit, but those fruits may produce bad seeds infected by the devil or good seeds sent by God" (p. 29).

[53] Paracelsus, *Selected Writings*, pp. 27, 30, and 76.

sexual differentiation is ultimately irrelevant to any concept of perfectibility in which the human being aspires to an integral whole. Life cannot exist without both the male and female as progenitors, and neither masculine nor feminine qualities of being human can be eliminated in this quest for wholeness. The astral magician-physician cannot give preferment to the male or the female without losing that essential quality of wholeness of all binary attributes of human identity including the transcendent *animus* with the *anima* in the unity of the Self.[54]

Similarly, he cannot eliminate disease; he can only unite it with its remedy as "wife and husband" to create a greater physical and spiritual harmony. Paracelsus argues that most of nature's secrets are beyond the scope of empirical reason and natural philosophy. The realization of that sublime harmony, albeit in the domain of the divine, is a transcendent state to which the astral magician-physician aspires by using his imagination to make those invisible properties and potentialities into a more visible effect. To defend one's self against death, literally as the desire to live a healthy life and figuratively as a desire for human perfectibility, one must control both the physical and spiritual efficacy of the curative medicine. Thus the astral magician-physician must aspire to a "psycho-somatic" perfectibility of one's physical and spiritual health as a manifestation of his divine work to restore the essential wholeness to human nature through the symbolic forms of celestial powers interpreted by the imagination.[55]

Paracelsus argues that the astral magician is justified to pursue those aspirations. Astral magic is a creative process designed to open the mind to its outermost limits and interpret the divine significance of those ineffable powers that animated nature's mutable forms. This interaction between natural and occult philosophy also inspired Henry Cornelius Agrippa to argue that the modalities of human perfectibility could be revealed through the interpretive powers attributed to astral magic. Agrippa's "dignified *magus*" expresses a higher degree of perfectibility

---

[54] In modern psychological theories, the archetypal human is not differentiated by gender; the authentic Self is a unified whole of the female *anima* and male *animus*. This point is frequently repeated by Carl G. Jung and Gerhard Adler, in *The Archetypes and the Collective Unconscious*, vol. 9 of *The Complete Works of C.G. Jung*, trans. R.F.C. Hull, Bollingen Foundation (Princeton: Princeton University Press, 1981); *Psychology and Alchemy*, vol. 12 of *The Complete Works* (1980); *The Structure and Dynamics of the Psyche*, vol. 8 in *The Complete Works* (1970); and *Symbols of Transformation*, vol. 5 of *The Complete Works* (1977).

[55] "It is not God's will that His secrets should be visible; it is His will that they become manifest and knowable through the works of man who has been created in order to make them visible" (*Selected Writings*, p. 109). Paracelsus seems to anticipate the idea in twentieth-century "alternative medicine" that the conscious mind can "conjure" through "guided fantasies" its own unconscious psychic powers acting through its "auto-immune system" to cure the biological and corresponding mental illnesses of the body when conventional medical sciences fail. See: O. Carl Simonton, Stephanie Matthews-Simonton, and James L. Creighton, *Getting Well Again* (New York: Bantam Books, 1978/1980); and Joseph Murphy, *The Power of Your Subconscious Mind* (New York: Prentice-Hall, Inc., 1987).

through a continual process of seemingly miraculous spiritual transformations in artistic approximations that had been considered inexpressible in purely rational terms. However, neither the moral perfection of the *magus* nor the technological perfection of astral magic is possible in absolute terms. Human perfectibility is a never-ending process of imaginative interpretations, not a finite state-of-being.[56] Although all natural beings possess the potentiality for their perfectibility they are also subject to time and their own dissolution. Astral influences may be the projected cause for an improvement in human nature, but they are inferior to the Christian conception of salvation through God's grace.[57]

As Paracelsus progressed from his interpretations of the natural world into the spiritual domain of the sacred, he was less certain that his interpretations of astral

---

[56] Francis Bacon (1561–1626) and later René Descartes (1596–1650) argued that empirical methodology and mathematics could objectify the subjective formulations of the alchemical- magician, but they too could only approximate the teleological perfection of the natural world. Bacon admitted that his grand investigation could never reach an ultimate closure because new knowledge and inventions continually reopened those axioms for further development. "For I could not be true and constant to the argument I handle, if I were not willing to go beyond others; but yet not more willing than to have others go beyond me again." Francis Bacon, *The Advancement of Learning*, XXV.25, ed. G.W. Kitchin (London: J.M. Dent & Sons Ltd., 1973; Totowa, NJ: Rowman and Littlefield, 1974), p. 221. In the *Discourse: On the Method* (1637), Descartes linked objective method with human moral perfectibility (part IV, 170–77). However, he admitted that although reason may persuade one about the truth of an idea (referring to Galileo's persecution by the Inquisition), other belief systems (such as religious doctrine) may distort that which reason discovers (part VI, 191). Furthermore, knowledge like desire cannot be ultimately satisfied (part VI, 193). "I am quite willing it should be known that the little I have hitherto learned is almost nothing in comparison with that of which I am ignorant, and to that knowledge of which I do not despair of being able to attain" (part VI, 195). Although he had faith in his ability to discover truth in objective science (part VI, 196), he admitted that the subjective imagination of one man may not be equal to the task of realizing that truth (part VI, 199) and that his future readers will distort his accomplishments (part VI, 201). *Discourse: On the Method of Rightly Conducting Reason and Seeking Truth in the Sciences*, [*Discours de la Méthode pour bien conduire le raison et chercher la Verité dans les sciences*], 1637, trans. John Veitch, *The Method, Meditations, and Philosophy of Descartes* (New York: Tudor Publishing Co., 1901).

[57] Henry Cornelius Agrippa, *De Occulta Philosophia*, II.50 (Cologne, 1533), pp. 230–31. Agrippa was attacked as a "black magician" because his defense of astral magic did not adequately attempt to synthesize his magical attributes with Christian doctrine (II.4, pp. 215–7). Agrippa's "dignified magus" reveals the good life, or embodies the good life, followed the archetypal regenerated man of Orphic and Dionysian mystery cults (III.1–3, pp. 253–4). Ficino, in *Theologica Platonica*, and Pico in *Heptaplus*, were also attracted to the Dionysian and Pseudo-Dionysian conceptions of human regeneration rendered explicitly in occult magic. However, both Ficino and Pico denied that the regenerative process of redemption reached its apotheosis in occult transformations. Also see: M.H. Keefer, "Agrippa's Dilemma: Hermetic 'Rebirth' and the Ambivalence of *De Vanitate* and *De Occulta Philosophia*," *Renaissance Quarterly*, 41(1988): 614–53.

symbolism could lead to human perfectibility.[58] He was skeptical about the adequacy of his imaginative arts and sciences to provide the true signification of celestial influence, especially because both the subjective imagination and the conception of free will empowered by magical processes were closely identified with the human disposition to do evil. Thus he warns his would-be magician to first struggle with the contrary nature of his "rock-like heart" that ascended with goodness and descended with evil of its own free will before he could approximate the laws of nature in so-called transcendent and magical forms.[59] This moral *psychomachia* was a crucial impediment to his success as a magician.[60] In the words of Koheleth: "I gave my heart to know wisdom and to know madness and folly: I perceived that this also is a vexation of spirit. For in much wisdom is much grief: and he that increaseth knowledge increaseth sorrow" (Ecclesiastes 1:17–18). If the practice of astral magic could only approximate the enigmatic properties of metaphysical causality, which the imagination conceived as a transcendent form of knowledge, then those approximations involve a circling process of self-perpetuating reinterpretations to reach an indefinite center that appears forever elusive.

John Dee also based his theory of human perfectibility on a process of understanding nature through astral magic that aspired to extend the human being's intellectual excellence to its utmost.[61] He assumed that God's "dignities"

---

58 "How can a man say, 'I am certain,' when he is so far from certainty." Paracelsus, *Selected Writings*, p. 206. Also see: Henry Cornelius Agrippa, *Of vanitie and uncertaintie of Arts and Sciences*, trans. James Sanford (London: John Daye, 1589); and Charles G. Nauert Jr. (1965). This problem of lingual dysfunction is not caused by the reflected vision but by the intermediaries of an inferior intellect seeing and comprehending, which are imposed between essence and object. See: Plato, *Republic* 515b—518d, in *The Collected Dialogues of Plato*, pp. 747–51.

59 Because the human heart was divided by the contrary attractions of good and evil, the divine "magic" of Jesus' ministry, revelation, and passion were necessary to effect the supernatural perfection of nature and the redemption of the human being. Paracelsus, *Selected Writings*, pp. 159–65, 191, 193. In the Greek myth of the flood, "innocent and worshipful" Deucalion and Pyrrha are commanded to repopulate the world by throwing "your mother's bones behind you." Deucalion interprets this impious order as casting stones, the "bones of mother earth" behind them. "The stones the man had thrown turned into men,/ The stones the woman threw turned into women,/Such being the will of God. Hence we derive/The hardness that we have, and our endurance/Gives proof of what we have come from." Ovid, *Metamorphoses* I: 318–418, trans. Rolfe Humphries (Bloomington: Indiana University Press, 1963), pp. 12–15.

60 "Know therefore that the rock upon which the sheepfold is built cannot have been established by man, and that no man has ever undertaken to create a rock. But whether they were good or bad, they always placed the burden on the rock which God had given them … and here they have always let the matter rest, entrusting themselves to the rock and believing in Him whom God sent." Paracelsus, *Selected Writings*, p. 189.

61 In *Acts and Monuments* (London, 1563), John Foxe branded Dee as a "great conjurer" for his seeming confusion of astral magic and science. Drawing on the works of Ficino, Pico, Agrippa, Paracelsus, and Ramon Lull, Dee insisted that his esoteric practice

(goodness, wisdom, power, and immortality) were modes of divine creativity through a hierarchy of celestial and earthly spirits. By interpreting the occult sympathies of those spirits as a form of "telepathic communication," his astral magician could ascend above matter through the celestial spheres to his apotheosis in God.[62] In the *Mathematicall Preface* (1570), Dee argues that human beings participate with spirits and angels in the quest for perfectibility because "they were all created in the image of God."[63] Although the "original image" was lost in the Fall, Dee's experiments in astral magic aspire to rediscover the "star demon" within his nature in order to become "like God" again.[64] The *magus* could access this "secret wisdom" through alchemical experimentation and astrological observations without trespassing on the sacred domain of the Divine Will, without asserting the Protestant heresy of self-inclusion in divine election, and without claiming the miraculous powers of a Catholic saint. By studying the sympathies and antipathies of all natural objects, the magician could perform through his own artificial methods "miraculous" discoveries of the unifying principles

---

of kabbalistic magic dealt with angelic hierarchies and not with conjuring demonic spirits. Queen Elizabeth considered Dee to be a pious physician and astrologer-magician and defended his reputation. For a study of Dee's stature in Elizabeth's court and in later periods, see: Peter French, *John Dee: The World of an Elizabethan Magus* (New York: Dorset Press, 1972/1989), pp. 7–10, 13–5, 22. For a discussion of Ramon Lull's influence on Dee, see pp. 47–8. Also see: Wallace Notestein, *A History of Witchcraft in England: From 1558–1718* (New York: Thomas Y. Crowell Co., 1968), pp. 52–3; and Keith Thomas, *Religion and the Decline of Magic* (Hammondsworth: Penguin Books, 1971/1973), pp. 265–9.

[62] Dee's theory of astral magic was influenced by Ficino's *Corpus Hermeticum*, and in the first part of the *Corpus Hermeticum*, *Pimander*, Pimander instructs Hermes in the transcendent powers that are invested in the *magus*. "Thus unless you make yourself equal to god, you cannot understand god; like is understood by like. Make yourself grow to immeasurable immensity, outleap all body, outstrip all time, become eternity and you will understand god. Having conceived that nothing is impossible to you, consider yourself immortal and able to understand everything, all art, all learning, the temper of every living thing. Go higher than every height and lower than every depth. Collect in yourself all the sensations of what has been made, of fire and water, dry and wet; be everywhere at once, on land, in the sea, in heaven; be not born, be in the womb, be young, old, dead, beyond death. And when you have understood all these at once—times, places, things, qualities, quantities—then you can understand God." *Corpus Hermeticum*, "Tract XI.20," in *Hermetica*, p. 41.

[63] Dee also assumes that the Hermaphrodite Adam and the gender-differentiated Adam and Eve were created in the image of God and possessed an essential unity (oneness) in the nature of their humanity.

[64] John Dee, "'Mathematicall Preface' to the *Elements of Geometrie of the most auncient Philosopher Euclide of Megara*," tr. Sir Henry Billingsley, ed. John Dee, (London, 1570) sig. C.iii and C.iiii. In *De occulta philosophia*, Agrippa argues that the key to operating in the angelic realm is the "dignifying of men to this so sublime vertue and power" (III, 350–51). Their ability to participate in astral magic symbolizes their potentiality to be possessed by a perfected morality and form (III, 357–8).

within all being in the universe. He could reconcile the contrary qualities of all material objects through their inherent affinities and reveal their potentialities for purification. He argues that his magical operations are "not mythical" (meaning fantastical), but mystical and based on "the *logos* of the creative word (God's word) [that] works by rules so that [human beings], godly-minded and born of God may learn by straight-forward work and by theological and mystical language [reasoned speech]."[65] Mathematical formulae, like the Kabbalist's interpretation of letters and words, possess a transcendent signification that can be used to interpret the mutable forms of nature.

Dee's complex magical formulations in *Monas Hieroglyphia* (1564) are intended to elevate the human consciousness of the divine in the natural world. He believed that his natural magic did not violate the so-called "laws of nature," but could transcend nature by illuminating the relationship between celestial and earthly bodies. He asserts that the creative power of the divine word is encoded in the symbolic "hieroglyph," which similar to kabbalistic *gematria*, could be used to interpret the "divine Oneness" of the super-celestial world.[66] In his complex mathematical interpretations of the hieroglyph, Dee uses his seemingly arbitrary mathematical designations of word/image and symbol as a form of sublime *gnosis* that is mystical and religious.[67] Nicolaus Cusanus (1401–1464), Pico, and Agrippa also assert that no interpretation of natural and celestial causality could be made without mathematics.[68] Through this so-called "mystical-mathematical

---

[65] John Dee, *Monas Hieroglyphia*, trans. C.H. Josten, *Journal of the Society for the Study of Alchemy and Early Chemistry* (1964): 199–200.

[66] *Monas Hieroglyphia*, 12, 135. The ideal of the human being's spiritual regeneration through his ability to commune with the divine "Oneness" of the universe, based on the works of Plato, Iamblichus, Orpheus, and works attributed to Hermes Trismegistus in the *Corpus Hermeticum*, was the central issue in Dee's *Monas Hieroglyphia*. It was also a main issue in his study of Paracelsus' synthesis of alchemy and kabbalah, and attempt to implement Agrippa's *De occulta philosophia* (II.iii). Also see: Peter French (1972/1989), pp. 78, 80.

[67] *Monas Hieroglyphia*, 135. Also see: Frances A. Yates, *Giordano Bruno and the Hermetic Tradition* (London: Routledge and Kegan Paul, 1964), pp. 44–61.

[68] Dee identified himself with Agrippa, who in *De occulta philosophia* had synthesized the study of the physical-elemental world with the mathematical celestial-middle world and the Pythagorean super-celestial world. Agrippa argues that: "The Doctrines of Mathematicks are so necessary to, and have such an affinity with Magick, that they [who] do profess it without them, are quite out of the way, and labor in vain, and shall in no wise obtain their desired effect." *De Occulta Philosophia*, , *Three Books of Occult Philosophy*, Vol. II, p. 167. Citing Boethius' thesis that knowledge of divine things is impossible without mathematics, Nicolaus Cusanus, in his *De mathematica perfectione*, argues that: "*Nihil certi habemus in nostra scientia nisi nostram mathematicam*" [Nothing can be know for certain by the human mind where mathematics fails]. Cusanus argues that mathematics enhances the study of philosophy with a true knowledge and perfected precision (formulation) of the universe. *Opera* (Paris, 1514; rpt. Frankfurt, 1962), p. 259. Also see: Ernst Cassirer (1927/2000), pp. 7–45.

language" Dee believes that he could discover the potentiality of all being to realize its perfectibility, first in thought, then in word, and finally in a suitable mathematical form.

In the *Mathematicall Preface*, Dee argues that mathematical reasoning disciplines the imagination to create a "perfect demonstration of truths" and provides a sublime knowledge of the operation of nature.

> God through Numbrying produced orderly and distinctly all thinges. For his Numbryng then, was his creatyng of all thinges. And his Continuall Numbryng of all thinges, is the Conservation of them in being…The mathematicall minde, [can] deale Speculatively in his own Arte: and by good meanes, Mount aboue the cloudes and sterres: And thirdly, he can, by Order, Descend, to frame Naturall thinges, to wonderfull uses: and when he list, retire home into his own centre: and there, prepare more Meanes, to Ascend and Descend by: and, all to the glory of God, and our honest delectation in earth.[69]

Through mathematical notations the harmonic order and occult sympathies between elemental matter and its animating spirit could be revealed. The mathematician could experience "the spirit within nature" as a magical form of telepathy between the inherent excellence of the natural object and the intuitive spirit of the mathematically enlightened imagination.

Although Francis Bacon (1561–1627) criticized Dee's "mystical-mathematical language" as a superstitious and speculative philosophy unverifiable by sensual measurement, both Bacon and Dee shared a profound belief that natural philosophy could have major influence on the perfectibility of human beings.[70] In the *New Atlantis* (1624), the practitioners of Bacon's "scientific method" aspire to reveal the "secret wisdom" of nature "for the love of God and men." The Elder of the House of Salomon declares that "The End of our Foundation is the knowledge of Causes, and the secret motion of things; and the enlarging of the bounds of Human Empire, to the effecting of all things possible."[71] Many of the experiments conducted by Bacon's scientists concern health (576), medicine (578), and heat, light, and optics (579), and involve the imagined interaction of physical matter and celestial influences. For Bacon, the perfection of the "arts of science" in his systematic method of observations and experimentation could lead to the creation

---

[69] John Dee, "Mathematicall Preface," sig.C.iii–v.

[70] In *The Advancement of Learning* (1605), Bacon criticizes astral magic for "being fraught with much fabulous matter, a great part not only untried, but notoriously untrue, to the great derogation of the credit of natural philosophy with the grave and sober kind of wit" (IV.10). Bacon's criticism focuses on astrological signs, dreams, omens, and retributive judgments, which he characterizes as false, sophistic, and superstitious. Francis Bacon, *The Advancement of Learning*, IV.10–12, , pp. 29–30. Also see: Francis Bacon, *Novum Organum*, I.xlvi, in *Selected Writings of Francis Bacon*, introduction by Hugh G. Dick, (New York: Modern Library, 1955), p. 472.

[71] Francis Bacon, *New Atlantis*, in *Selected Writings of Francis Bacon*, p. 574.

of verifiable axioms of true natural processes. For Dee, however, those who believed that empiricism was sufficient to understand the true nature of all being deceive themselves.

In *Propaedeumata Aphoristica* (1558), Dee argues that the imagination is the primary mental faculty through which the spiritual illuminations of celestial powers coalesced, as in a mirror, to reveal their wonders.[72] The imagination functioned like the "seal of Hermes" in the *Monas Hieroglyphia* as the ultimate creative power uniting the subjective symbol with objective matter thereby creating its transformations.[73] However, Dee's theory of the magical powers of the imagination raises serious questions. Could the imagination actually transform natural objects into their perfected form in the world or did it operate only within the "enlightened consciousness" of the astral magician as a subjective assertion of the objects' potential perfectibility? Furthermore, if the imagination was capable of manipulating "celestial spirits" to perfect nature, could it also manipulate "chthonic spirits" that would destroy the natural order and condemn the astral magician to perdition? Dee believed that chthonic spirits were inferior to celestial spirits, and although chthonic spirits could influence human behavior in the world, they had no real ability to transform human nature. In other words, astral magic had no potency if used for impious intentions, which would render the idea of human perfectibility and the purification of matter through their agency meaningless. Although his mathematical, alchemical, and astral magical experiments were considered helpful human inventions, particularly in the field of medicine, his concern for the moral and spiritual transformations of human beings to live a better and more informed life did not achieve the practical results he sought. Dee's description of Archimedes' "mathematical magic" might well be used to describe his idealization of astral magic as an eternal process of approximations: "In great matters it is enough to have had the intention."[74] Although his experiments in alchemy, transforming impure matter into its perfected form, and interpreting astrological influences of superior beings upon inferior beings were indeterminate, Dee maintained his theory that human perfectibility could be affected by astral influences working through the magician's imagination. Dee may be considered a good mathematician and an inadequate scientist; but above all, he was considered a wise man.

---

[72] See: *John Dee on Astronomy: Propaedeumata Aphoristica (1558–1568) Latin and English*, sigs. I.ii.r–v, ed. and tr. Wayne Shumaker (Berkeley: University of California Press, 1978). "*tum lumen tum sine lumine: non ad visum solum, sed ad alios interdum sensus, & praecepue in Spiritu nostro imaginali, tanquam Speculo quodam coalescunt, seseque; nobis ostendunt, & in nos mirabilia agunt.*" Dee's 120th aphorism present a detailed explanation of his theories about how the physical universe functions according to magical principles. Also see: S.J. Tester (1987), 227.

[73] For Ficino and Dee, the imagination is the mental faculty through which the magician merged symbol and reality. For example, Ficino believed that the talisman possessed a power to attract celestial influences, and Dee believed that the Hermetic seal could emanate celestial influences. Both the talisman and the seal took on the reality of that which they symbolized. See: Peter French (1972/1989), *John Dee*, pp. 93–100.

[74] Cited in Peter French (1972/1989), *John Dee*, p. 125.

In their works on astral magic, Pico, Paracelsus, and Dee interpret human nature subjectively as the divinely created "image of God" aspiring to recover the "creative spirit of God" through the imagination as the truly magical measure of human perfectibility. Albeit in different modes of perceptions and inventions, astral magic denotes how ineffable divine mysteries are expressed in actual forms. One thing that does emerge from their speculations on human perfectibility is the absolute necessity to break down all forms of binary oppositions, be they celestial and earthly, angelic and bestial, or masculine and feminine in the refashioning of the authentic self in nature. Such dualism inhibits both the physical being and the imagination from actualizing their true potential for creativity. For Pico, Paracelsus, and Dee, astral magic is not limited to speculative prognostications and alchemical transformations degraded as an inferior "mechanical science." They believed that it effects a higher level of human understanding in the domain of the *phantastic*, which based on potentiality and possibility reveals qualities in the natural world that are truly better than actual existence. As an art, astral magic is based on the Neoplatonic philosophical ascent of the soul, the mystic's ecstatic subjective vision, and kabbalistic valorization of language and mathematics, as well as occult hieroglyphics. All of these systems depend on the enlightened imagination to navigate between ideas and forms to conceive of realities beyond the scope of reason and empirical experience, and to identify the potentialities within all being to realize its higher order of excellence.

In renaissance theories of human perfectibility, the principal goal is to affect a union with the divine based on the interaction of faith and grace, and refashion moral behavior to improve the ethical social order as an integral whole. The essential imperfections of the world are attributed to the human being's fragmentation in terms of oppositions between the soul and the body, social oppositions between masculine and feminine identities and qualities, and political and religious oppositions within the social order. Astral magic aspires to reconnect the "dots," so to speak, and put the fragments of the divine and the human, the male and the female, the soul and the body, and the imperfect qualities of animate and inanimate nature back together in their perfected analogical relationships. For Pico, Paracelsus, and Dee the true astral magicians could assume the role of "a greater human being" whose intellectual, intuitive, and imaginative powers reveal how the animating "spirit of divine presence" within all being elevates earthly existence to a celestial level of presumed excellence. It is easy to see that such a vision of human perfectibility appears magical for only by invoking superior celestial powers could one aspire through one's own volition to a union with God and achieve an essential wholeness within the self where in all binary oppositions are eliminated. Astral magic aspires to this condition of universal wholeness in which God, humanity, the earth and stars, souls and bodies, masculine and feminine qualities, and all matter find their proper affinities through the agency of the imagination.

Chapter 2
Guillaume Postel, the Shechinah, and the Feminine Principle

Alain Ekorong

Born near Barenton at the beginning of the sixteenth century, Guillaume Postel was not only an original thinker, but also a very public figure. After he studied oriental languages, he was commissioned by King François 1 to buy manuscripts in the Near East. Notably, Postel mastered Arabic, Hebrew, Syriac, and many other Semitic languages. In 1536, seeking an alliance with the Ottoman Turks, King Francis I named him official interpreter to Suleiman the Magnificent in Constantinople. This enabled him to publish in 1538 *De originibus seu de hebraicae linguae et gentis antiquitate*, the first of several publications in French, Latin, and Hebrew on the affairs of the Middle East. In the early 1540s, he formulated his theory, drawn from his knowledge of the Turks, that peace will be achieved through a universal religion. In this universal religion, Jews, Muslims, and heathens could be converted to Christianity, through careful reasoning and logic and not war, by demonstrating to all common foundations in all religions, and that Christianity best represented these similarities. This will be developed in his major work *De orbis terrae Concordia* (1543–4). After briefly contemplating becoming a Jesuit, he travelled around the Middle East, Italy, and Eastern Europe. He was interrogated by the Inquisition in 1555 for his religious views then judged to be insane and sent to prison for 4 years in Rome. Postel was also prolific in his translation of several Greek, Hebrew, and Arabic texts. Most notably among them, works on astronomy by al-Tusi and other Arabic astronomers, and his Latin translations of the *Zohar*, the *Sefer Yetzirah*, and the *Sefer Bahir*, the three most fundamental texts of the Jewish Kabbalah. From this moment on, Postel will become a staunch advocate of the integration of magic and Kabbalah in the quest for world peace and harmony.

As one of the most influential Christian kabbalists of his time, Guillaume Postel has been largely ignored by scholars who often discard his work as too obscure to be seriously analyzed. It was only at the start of the twentieth century that comprehensive research on his work was launched, notably under the efforts of French scholar François Secret.[1] Recently, works by William Bouwsma,

---

[1] François Secret has published an important body of work on Postel that includes titles such as, "Le Zôhar chez les kabbalistes chrétiens de la renaissance," in *Mémoires de la société des études juives*, III (Paris: Librairie Durlacher, 1958); *Les kabbalistes chrétiens de la Renaissance* (Paris: Dunod, 1964); *Guillaume Postel (1510–1581) et son interprétation du candélabre de Moyse* (Nieuwkoop: B. De Graaf, 1966); *Le thrésor des prophéties de*

Marion Kuntz, and Yvonne Petry,[2] among others, have shed more light on his vast enterprise. A prolific author, he published more than 60 books, a renowned publicist, Guillaume Postel represents what one could call the "other" French Renaissance, a renaissance whose humanism draws some of its foundational principles heavily from medieval thought. As Bouwsma puts it, "he was a sort of mystic truly entrenched in the problems of his time."[3] It is this mystical understanding of these issues that often pushed him to the margins of sanity and put him at odds with both political and religious authorities. Jean Dupebe, in his study of Postel's troubles with both political and religious authorities "*Poursuites contre Postel en 1553*," successfully demonstrates the unique nature and context of his work. He writes:

> Le vendredi matin 7 avril 1553 apres Pâques, l'avocat du Roi, Me Denis Riant apporte a la Grand-Chambre du Parlement "letters dudict seigneur (…) par lesquelles le Roy aiant entendu que ung nomme Postel auoyt fait et compose ung liure plain dheresies et blasphemes contre lhonneur de Dieu et de la Religion crestienne et iceluy faict imprimer en ceste ville de Paris contre les inhibitions et defenses cideuant faictes par ledict seigneur (…) mande a ladicte court faire prendre ledict Postel prisonnier et en faire punition exemplaire a tous aultres et aussi limprimeur qui a imprime ledict liure."[4]
>
> (On Friday morning the 7th of April 1553 after Easter, the King's lawyer, Denis Riant, brings to attention of the Chamber of the Parliament "letters of the aforementioned lord (…) Having heard that a certain Postel, ignoring his inhibitions and prohibitions, had written and published in this city of Paris a book full of heresy and blasphemy against the honor of God and the Christian Religion, the King summoned the court to send its author to prison and to punish the others, including the publisher of this book…")

As Dupebe shows, the two books that land Postel in troubled waters are *Les très merveilleuses victoires des femmes du nouveau monde* and *La doctrine du siecle doré*.[5] The apparent scandal stems from Postel's original understanding of the role of women: in his quest for *Harmonia mundi* or World Peace, Postel's

l'univers, a manuscript published with his introduction and notes (Archives Internationales d'Histoire des Idées. No. 27. La Haye: Martinus Nijhoff, 1969); *Bibliographie des manuscrits de Guillaume Postel* (Genève: Droz, 1970).

[2] See important works by William J. Bouwsma, *Concordia Mundi: The career and thought of Guillaume Postel (1510–1581)* (Cambridge, MA: Harvard University Press, 1957); Marion L. Kuntz, *Guillaume Postel: Prophet of the Restitution of all Things, His Life and Thought* (London: Martinus Nijhoff, 1981); and Yvonne Petry, *Gender, Kabbalah and the Reformation: The Mystical Theology of Guillaume Postel (1510–1581)* (Leiden: Koninklijke Brill, 2004).

[3] Bouwsma, p. 57.

[4] Jean Dupebe, "Poursuites contre Postel en 1553," *Guillaume Postel, 1581–1981: actes du colloque international d'Avranches, 5–9 septembre 1981* (Paris: Editions de la Maisnie, 1985), pp. 29–39 (30). All translations of French quotes in this essay are my own.

[5] Dupebe, 31. See also Guillaume Postel, *Les très merveilleuses victoires des femmes du nouveau monde* (Geneva: Slatkine Reprints, 1970).

most controversial view lies in his theory of the Feminine Principle. Borrowing primarily from kabbalistic theories and alchemy, Postel believed that World Peace could only be reached through the Shechinah or the *Indwelling Presence* of God. It is this gendered quest toward universal harmony that this essay intends to explore. I will investigate Postel's understanding of the concept of the Shechinah, its function, and its use in the construction of this harmonious world. In this essay, I contend that beyond Postel's "folie" or eccentricity,[6] his desire to elevate the Feminine Principle in a genuine attempt to find World Peace or *Harmonia Mundi* is unique within the French Renaissance. I wish to depart from Yvonne Petry's understanding of gender roles[7] within his work by focusing my analysis on a number of foundational principles of the Kabbalah. But what is Kabbalah? And why was it so important to Postel?

Meaning literally "receiving," the Kabbalah is generally understood as a body of esoteric principles purportedly handed down from generation to generation, and designed to rationally bridge the gap, through teaching and studying, between the Unknowable Infinite Creator (the *Ein Sof*) and the Finite Universe. It is an attempt to comprehend the paradox between these two worlds, and to understand the nature of the relationship between God and humans. What attracted Postel is precisely the possibility of attaining harmony by understanding this paradox. For this same reason, the concept of the Shechinah was fundamental in this quest. Generally defined as a nest for the "Indwelling Presence" of God within the universe, the Shechinah fascinated Postel precisely because of this Infinite possibility she carried within her.

In her book *Gender, Kabbalah and the Reformation*, Yvonne Petry suggests that Postel "retained the Neoplatonic world-view with regard to male/female relationships [...] however, he transformed it into an entirely unique and personal theology."[8] If it is true that Postel, in his quest for world harmony and unity, borrows some of its foundation from Neoplatonism, it is important to underline the kabbalistic nature of his discourse on women in *Les très merveilleuses victoires des femmes du Nouveau Monde*. Marion Kuntz, William Bouwsma, and Yvonne Petry demonstrate, in their work, the inherent contradictions of Postel's views on women, which occur when attempting to reconcile his religious views with his political ideologies:

> By unraveling his thought processes and comparing his religious and political opinions, we can gain some insight into the problems he encountered and his attempts to resolve them. Points to consider are how Postel applied male/female symbolism to the political realm, how this related to his idea of power in the world, and finally, what his actual relationships were with rulers of his day.[9]

---

[6] See here an excellent article by Peter A. Redpath "The nature of woman and her role in religion according to Guillaume Postel," published in a special volume of *Actes du Colloque International d'Avranches (Guillaume Postel, 1581–1981)*, 137–49.

[7] See Yvonne Petry in her book *Gender, Kabbalah and the Reformation*.

[8] Petry, p. 53.

[9] Petry, p. 51.

In my view, because Postel's views on women evolved with time, it is counterproductive, at least from a philosophical standpoint, to attempt to understand his positions as a male/female dichotomy. Such a reading would do some disservice to the author's struggles to translate some important, inherent, and fundamental contradictions into a powerful discourse on equality and peace. This is what Peter Redpath attempts to demonstrate: "Eccentric elements in the thinking of Postel are easy to discover since they seem to appear on almost every page he writes. What is difficult to discover about Postel, however, is what he is actually saying behind all his symbolism and enigmatic language."[10] For Redpath, because "the victories [of women] are primarily spiritual ones [in *Les très merveilleuses victoires des femmes du nouveau monde*]," it makes more sense to analyze Postel's thought within a "meditative and metaphysical" framework.[11] However, Redpath's analysis of Postel's views of women never goes beyond a traditional understanding of male/female dichotomy. This traditional view tends to create a clear separation between man and woman based on either male or female gender even though Postel, as we will show later, clearly transcends this apparent division. This misunderstanding is evident when the Redpath discusses Postel's discourse on the Animus and the Anima. Although he is able to capture Postel's subsequent subdivisions of the Animus and the Anima,[12] he fails to bring the kabbalistic dimension of this discourse evident in the figure of Mother Johanna, the influential Venetian woman Postel met while in Italy. Moreover, his conclusion on the "nature and role" of women is rather disappointing:

> Granted, Postel may have mental problems, still, I think the metaphysical and spiritual background of Postel accounts for much of his peculiar way of expressing himself. On the metaphysical side, it is not uncommon for neo-Platonic and Augustinian thinkers to attempt to drive their readers into an aporia. Rather it seems a pedagogical necessity. If Postel does not make sense, one reason for this is that Postel does not want to make sense.[13]

But I would argue that Postel could make sense and if he does not *succeed* in making sense, it is precisely because his contemporaries *and* modern researchers generally do not integrate kabbalistic doctrines into this discourse. Similarly, when scholars do take into consideration the Kabbalah as Petry does, it is pushed into the background.[14] In an attempt to fully integrate Postel's own kabbalistic theories in his discourse, my essay will mostly focus on *Les très merveilleuses victoires des femmes* because this text constitutes one of the rare instances where

---

[10] Redpath, p. 137.

[11] Redpath, p. 138.

[12] Redpath, pp. 140–41.

[13] Redpath, p. 149.

[14] Petry's book is quite interesting in this regard. Although she refers to the kabbalistic context quite successfully, an analysis of important kabbalistic concepts (such as the *Shechinah)* valued by Postel is nonexistent.

the "eccentric" author clearly purports to use these ancient Jewish philosophies to demonstrate rationally the centrality of the Feminine Principle in the Restitution of all things. This inner movement clearly borrows from Lurianic Kabbalah[15] its threefold evolution of the universe: Tzimtzum (or Contraction of God that formed a metaphysical void), The Shevirat-ha-Kelim (or the Breaking of the Vessels that created a separation of the opposites, in particular, a split between the masculine and the feminine aspects of both God and the Primordial Man), and the Tikkun-ha-Olam (or the Restoration of the World overcoming chaos and evil, giving meaning to that which is senseless, and concretizing abstract values, thus assuring the completion of *Ein-sof* or the Infinite God).[16] The idea of Restitution, then, should be fully comprehended through these kabbalistic lenses.

From the outset of the book, Postel sets the framework of his discourse on women. A quick look at the chapter titles reflects this predisposition. Titles such as "Des admirables excellences & faictz du sexe féminin & comment il faut qu'il domine le monde," "Satisfaction de la commune querelle dont l'on charge à tort le sexe feminin," "Des souverains biens qui son venus au monde par les femmes," "Des femmes d'esprit & entendement singulier & la cause pourquoi," "Particulieres histoires des sages femmes," "Histoires des prudentes & savantes femmes," are perfect examples of Postel's attempt to delve into the debate on women from an original angle, at least within this historical context. His intention is to transform the so-called inferiority of women into a powerful case for their centrality or even their superiority. In Postel's view, positioning women in higher dimensions or realms is important in the *Restitution* of all things. As Yvonne Petry suggests,

> There is a rather paradoxical attitude at work in Postel… This paradox lay at the core of his theology. He combined the concept of women's inferiority with recognition of the paradoxical message in the New Testament. He argued that the virtues extolled by Jesus were more often found in women than in men. In this way he defended women, arguing that since they were more humble they were ultimately more spiritual. He was still using the Aristotelian paradigm, but reversed its meaning through reference to the New Testament theology. Postel used women's inferiority as a rhetorical device.[17]

Postel' stance on women is complex and his discourse goes far beyond mere rhetoric. The foundation of his positions lies with the enigmatic figure of Madre

---

15 Isaac Luria (1534–1572), also known as the "Ari Zaal" or "Divine Rabbi Isaac" developed a complex doctrine called the Shevirat-ha-Kelim or the Breaking of the Vessels in which the main idea revolves around a three-phased evolution of the world: 1) contraction, 2) shattering (similar to twentieth century Big Bang theory), and 3) repair. This doctrine has greatly influenced subsequent kabbalistic theories.

16 See here Gershom Gerhard Scholem, *On the Kabbalah and Its Symbolism* (New York: Schocken Books, 1996).

17 Petry, p. 145.

Zuana [Joanna].[18] As Yvonne Petry notes, "Postel's discussion of knowledgeable women turns out to be an introduction to the person of Joanna."[19] For Marion Kuntz, "As Postel worked on his translation of the Zohar, he became ever more convinced that the restitution of all things as interpreted by his Mother Johanna was confirmed not only in the 'most divine and rare books of the Zohar', but also in the books of the ancient [Jewish] interpreters."[20] It is here that any investigation of Postel's theory of women must be launched. Bouwsma shows how Postel developed an extraordinary story concerning the Venetian woman known as Madre Zuana (Joanna).[21] According to Bouwsma, Postel thought Madre Zuana was responsible for the divine grace believed to have descended upon Venice, a city in which she was working for the poor. For Postel, thanks to Mother Joanna's mysticism, Venice had been chosen by God to be the New Jerusalem. He went so far as to call Mother Joanna the Virgin of Venice. In fact, throughout his work, Postel constantly glorifies the city as a sanctuary for this new Virgin upon which the Spirit of God has descended, and in which the living Christ is supposed to have found his palace. This process, often called immutation, is believed to have occurred in Venice in 1540 in a small hospital named by Postel *Xenodochius* because it was used by the Venetian Virgin (Mother Joanna) to "receive foreigners."[22] He refers to her as, "the moon that reflects rays of the sun."[23] For Postel, "[…] il faut qu'a tous Jesus soit Pere mental et Jehanne mere spirituelle, Adam nouveau et Eve nouvelle, deux en une spirituelle chair" ("It is important that Jesus be the spiritual father and Johanna the spiritual mother, the new Adam and the New Eve, two in one spiritual flesh").[24] This description of the Venetian Virgin, in order to be rationally linked to the Christ and to the figure of Eve, uses the kabbalistic theory of the Shechinah to ground Postel's argumentation. This technique is borrowed from Giovanni Pico della Mirandola and subsequent Christian Kabbalists who believed that Christian dogmas could be better and rationally explained through magic and kabbalah. Pico is credited with having initiated this strand of Christian Cabala[25] in Renaissance Florence. His intentions were to harmonize Christian beliefs with magic and

18 According to Postel, while in Venice, he received guidance from an illiterate woman called Madre Zuana, or Mother Joanna, the "Venetian Virgin." He frequently refers to her as the mother of the world, the Shechinah, and the second Messiah.

19 Petry, p. 142.

20 Kuntz, p. 84.

21 See Bouwsma, *Concordia Mundi.*

22 Guillaume Postel, *De Orbis terrae Concordia: libri quatuor…*(Basel: Oporinus, 1544), p. 432.

23 *De Orbis*, p. 433.

24 *De Orbis*, p. 8.

25 When referring to the Christian recuperation of the Jewish Kabbalah, critics usually write Cabala. We use this form here only.

kabbalah, which he saw as the most primal form of Jewish theosophy started since Moses and foreshadowing, in his opinion, the teachings of Jesus.[26]

This connection is clearly made by Postel himself in chapter 14 of *Les très merveilleuses victoires des femmes*. At the end of this chapter, Postel explains in great detail the original position held by women in his theory of restitution of all things.

> Vray est que dedans les livres des auditeurs de Moyse en lieux innumerables est de *ladicte Mere du monde*[27] *parlé. Mais tres-clairement se voit tel mystere caché par le Sainct Esprit dedans Jeremie, 23:33 où il repète les mesmes sentences du Messie soubz masculin genre*, & en apres *soubz le feminin*, disant : Voicy les jours viennent, dict le Seigneur Dieu, & je susciteray pour David le Germe Le Juste & le Germe La Juste, & regèra Roy, & fera estre sage, & fera jugement & justice en la terre... Par cecy se voit que la Nature feminine au 33e chapitre, & la Nature masculine au 24e doit regner. *Mais il y ha infiniment plus d'excellence de regne dedans & avec le regne feminin que avec le masculin*; car Dieu par moindre force se monstre, & se veult, pour accroistre sa gloire, manifester plus excellent que par la plus grande. Et par ainsi adjoint la *mesme difference masculine & feminine* disant : & c'est icy le Nom qu'ils appeleront LUY (au 23e c.) & qu'ils appeleront ELLE (au 24e c.), Jehovah ou le Seigneur *Tetragrammaton* est nostre Justice... *L'arbre des Noms divins*, le *Zohar* et le *Racanati*, avec *les commentaires de Ruth* et le livre *Bahir* enseigneront le reste.[28]
>
> (It is true that in the books compiled by the interpreters of Moses, *the name of the Mother of the World* is mentioned in several places. One can clearly see such a mystery hidden by the Holy Spirit in Jeremiah 23:33, in which the same sentences are repeated using the masculine and feminine gender in this manner: Here comes the days, said the Lord, I will instill in David *the Germ of the Masculine Just and the Germ of the Feminine Just*, will create a wise being, will provide judgment and justice on earth... Through this, one observes that in chapter 33 the Feminine and in chapter 24 the Masculine must reign. But *there is infinitely more excellence within the Feminine reign than there is in the Masculine reign*, because God, in order to increase his glory, more easily manifests his excellence in the bigger reign. Thus, he attributes the same masculine and feminine difference by saying: here is the Name they will call HIM (c. 23) and the one they will call HER (ch. 24), Jehovah or the *Tetragrammaton* Lord is our Justice... The *tree of The Divines Names*, the *Zohar* and the *Recanati*, with *commentaries of Ruth and the Book of the Bahir* will teach the rest.)

---

[26] Pico will develop, in his *900 Theses*, a comprehensive use of magic and the kabbalah with the goal of rationally proving the divine and messianic essence of Jesus. For more on Pico's theses, as well as an excellent English translation, see Stephen Alan Farmer, *Syncretism in the West: Pico's 900 Theses (1486): The Evolution of Traditional, Religious, and Philosophical Systems, with Text, Translation, and Commentary* (Tempe, AZ: Medieval and Renaissance Texts and Studies, 1998).

[27] My emphasis.

[28] Postel, *Les très merveilleuses victoires des femmes*, pp. 70–71.

Three main elements can be drawn from this excerpt. First, the Feminine is essentially equal to the Masculine. Therefore, it is possible to repeat, as was the case in Jeremiah 23, the "same sentences" under both the masculine and the feminine. At this point, one must recognize Postel's belief that both the Masculine and the Feminine carry the "same difference." Here, the concept of "same difference" can be understood as a hyphen (*trait d'union*) between radical alterity and sameness, a hyphen in which difference would be located within the Potential and not in the distance and the trace. The importance of the hyphen lies in its dual and somewhat paradoxical function: it both differentiates and connects at the same time, thus carrying with its essence the notion of potentiality. As a connector, the hyphen (here the "same difference") establishes a potential union whereas as a separator, it creates a difference in which something is waiting to *happen*, a potential or a possibility or reunion. In French, it's much easier to visualize this dichotomy in the phrase *trait d'union* (the "trait" as in the expression "tirer un trait," to "draw a line" constitutes separation; and "union" reunites). Postel's "same difference" is therefore not simply a repeating of difference but rather a sort of derridean *differance*, a difference void of concept precisely because God's infinite nature transcends human narration. Put differently, and borrowing from John Caputo's analysis in *The Prayers and Tears of Jacques Derrida*, it seems that what Postel argues for here is the recognition of the Potential not as a "transcendental ulteriority" because it is "deferred," but really a "quasi transcendental anteriority"[29] since the divine presence has already filled the feminine. Second, since the divine presence dwells in the feminine (the Shechinah), the Potential can be understood as the immanent force or energy capable of recreating the divine union. This Potential is similar to the sap that flows through the sephirotic tree of life.[30] Postel also states that the Feminine Potential is filled with much more excellence than the Masculine one. In other words, the potential difference of the Feminine allows far more effectively the Divine Reign. Third, in reading this excerpt, one senses that Postel prepares the reader what he will argue later: both the Feminine and the Masculine are essential principles that can be found in both the Male and the Female because, as the Lord promises, "je susciteray pour David le Germe Le Juste & le Germe La Juste."[31] Here, Postel is subtly asserting the notion that Feminine and Masculine qualities transcend gender dichotomies. In other words, the separation of the masculine and the feminine does not necessarily translate into a male/female dichotomy.

At this point, a reading of the *Zohar* or Book of Splendor, "widely revered as a sacred text of unquestionable value"[32] and its affirmation of this transcendence is useful:

---

[29] John Caputo, *The Prayers and Tears of Jacques Derrida* (Bloomington: Indiana University Press, 1997), p. 3.

[30] The sephirotic tree of life is presented later in this essay.

[31] Postel, *Les très merveilleuses victoires des femmes*, p. 70.

[32] Scholem, *On the Kabbalah and Its Symbolism*, p. 1.

> And you may ask if the sojourner is not both *male and female*[33], *will the Shechinah then leave him?* [34]
>
> *Come and behold: He who goes on a journey should pray to the Holy One, blessed be He, BEFORE HE LEAVES, so as to draw upon himself his Master's Shechinah, when still at home and still both male and female. And when he prayed and praised, and the Shechinah rests upon him, then he can go on his way. Now that the Shechinah is with him, he can be male and female* in the city, THAT IS, AT HOME and in the field, ON HIS JOURNEY. BECAUSE THE SHECHINAH IS JOINED TO HIM, it is written: "Righteousness shall go before him," with RIGHTEOUSNESS REPRESENTING THE SHECHINAH, "and then he shall place his footsteps on the way."[35]

The *Zohar* seems to refer to the metamorphical stature of the Shechinah, her ability to embody and transform the living spirit into a potentially dual gender. It is this capacity of the Shechinah to infuse both genders with the sap of the Holy One that attracts Postel. In this regard, even though his political posture seemed at times hypocritical, his philosophical discourse on women, especially in *Les très merveilleuses victoires des femmes*, purports to adopt a vertical movement that follows the mystical path of the Shechinah described in the *Zohar*. This sort of analysis is justified by Postel himself, who, in the excerpt previously quoted, seeks the authority to validate such a discourse. He invokes four foundational kabbalistic texts: *The Tree of the Divine Names*, the *Zohar*, and the *Recanati*, with commentaries of Ruth, and the *Book of the Bahir*. Once again, Pico della Mirandola had a great influence on Postel here. As Gershom Scholem asserts in his book *Kabbalah*, "Pico began his kabbalistic studies in 1486, and when he displayed his 900 famous theses for public debate in Rome he included among them 47 propositions taken directly from kabbalistic sources, the majority from the Recanati's commentary on the Torah, and 72 more propositions that represented his own conclusions from his kabbalistic research."[36] Thus, even though the framework of this essay is not vast enough to accommodate the type of investigation Postel proposes, it is vital to, at the very least, understand the substance and the nature of the relationships that link the Divine Names in the tree of life.

According to kabbalistic theories, the *sephirots* (or "enumerations," Sephiroth, Sefiroth, singular: Sephirah, in Hebrew), are the ten attributes that God (who is referred to as *Ein Sof*, "Limitless Light, Light Without End") created and through which he can manifest himself not only in the physical but also in the metaphysical universe. The tree is divided in Upper Sephirots (1. Keter, "Supreme crown," 2. Hokhmah, "Wisdom," 3. Binah, "Intelligence"), Middle Sephirots

33 All italicized excerpts in quotes are my emphasis.

34 *Zohar* 3, Beresheet B:51. All citations from the *Zohar* are drawn from: http://www.kabbalah.com/k/index.php/p=zohar

35 *Zohar* 3, Tehilim 85: 14.

36 Gershom Scholem, *Kabbalah* (New York: New York Times Book Co., 1974), p. 197.

(4. Gedullah or Hesed, "Greatness," 5. Gevurah or Din, "Power," 6. Tiferet or Rahamim, "Beauty"), and Lower Sephirots (7. Nezah, "Lasting Endurance," 8. Hod, "Majesty," 9. Yesod, "Foundation of the World," and 10. Malkhut, "Kingdom").[37] Keter, or Supreme Crown, is the highest sephirot and the closest to the Ein Sof. Hokhmah, or Wisdom, as the first created sephirah, is the medium through which God's Will flows up to Malkhut. According to the *Zohar*, she is the "sap of all creation" and the "potentiality of that is" (I:2a). Thus the importance of the word "potentiality," which is directly connected to the concept of the Potential mentioned above. Binah or Intelligence is conceived as a "palace" erected around Hokhmah to receive and distribute the "sap" to the lower levels of the tree. From a cognitive standpoint, Binah is an expansion or the realization of Hidden Thought (also believed to be the "sap") in Hokhmah. She is also viewed as the reasoning process itself, a dialectical movement in which intellectual attributes of God are put in motion in order to recreate a "perfect world." Equally fundamental is the belief that Binah, when in relationship with the last Lower sephirot Malkhut (or Shechinah), is actually the Celestial Mother. In other words, Binah seems to transmit to the Shechinah a combination of feminine and masculine virtues because the Celestial mother, albeit carrying with her maternal qualities, generally embodies the most fundamental divine metaphors.

By analyzing Postel's thought within kabbalistic discourses, it is possible to assert that the dichotomy superior/masculine versus inferior/feminine does not translate into an affirmation of women's inferiority. As various relations within the tree show, there are two Mothers: a Celestial (Superior) Mother, Binah, and a Terrestrial (Inferior) Mother, Malkhut, also called Shechinah. The structure of the Sephirotic tree clearly shows that there is in fact, in each human being, the Archetypal Mother, which is none other than the divine presence, the sap circulating within the body. This apparent, but necessary, contradiction stems from the complexity of the Shechinah (the tenth and last sephirah) herself. According to Scholem, "the Shechinah – literally in-dwelling, namely of God in world – is taken to mean simply God himself in His omnipresence and activity in the world and especially in Israel."[38] Therefore, she has a dual movement within herself. Arthur Green in *A Guide to the Zohar*, suggests that "as Malkhut ("kingdom"), it represents the realms over which the King (Tif'eret) has dominion, sustaining and protecting her as the true king takes responsibility for his kingdom. At the same time, it is this sephirah that is charged with the lower worlds."[39] In this sense, "the tenth sephirah is a passive-receptive female with regard to the sefirot above Her, receiving their energies and being fulfilled by their presence within Her. But She is ruler, source of life, and font of all blessing for the worlds below, including

[37] I am using as my model Gershom Scholem's structuration of the tree of life in his work *Kabbalah*. I also adopt his terminology throughout this essay in order to facilitate the argument.

[38] Scholem, *Kabbalah*, p. 105.

[39] Arthur Green, *A guide to the Zohar* (Stanford: Stanford University Press, 2004), p. 50.

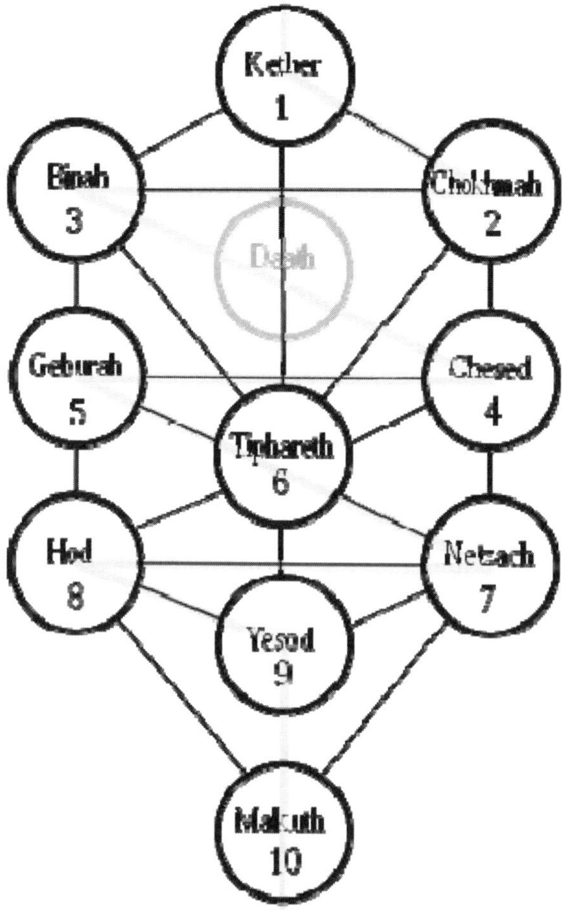

Fig. 2.1 The *sephirots*.

the human soul."[40] Therefore, one possible explanation of internal contradictions within Postel's discourse on women is this inward-outward essence of the Shechinah. In fact, one has to understand Postel's distinction between feminine and masculine as prehuman since the Shechinah is indeed the link between the higher and the lower worlds. This is the reason why, as Green notes, "the kabbalist

[40] Green, p. 52.

sees himself as a devotee of the Shechinah, a spiritual knight of the Matronita."[41] This devotion might well explain the fact that Postel actually claimed that Mother Joanna descended upon him and took possession of his body. To kabbalists this possession of the body by the Mother symbolizes the normal outcome of the mystic voyage of the sap.

These Divine Names sought by Guillaume Postel are none other than the quest for the *Harmonia Mundi* or World Peace. The imperious presence of the Shechinah (or the Feminine) in the World, is a vital part of this quest, as Postel emphasizes in chapter 13:

> Au surplus, j'ay au precedent chapitre monstré comme mesme intelligence, esprit, ange ou vertu qui presidoit en Saiinct …combien qu'il y ha six cens ans que à tres-grand regret *ladicte Sechinah, ou esprit feminin ne trouve sur qui aller* …mais principalement depuis l'election … le Pape Paule, *passant par la mere du monde … est venue en Elie Pandochien* …Car *le pere Jesus conduit Jehan Cain, & la mere Johanna conduit Jehan Abel.* [42]

> (Moreover, I have shown in the previous chapter how even intelligence, spirit, angel and virtue presided over the life of Saint John, the first annunciator of the Lord. Thus, it is with great regret that for six hundred years the Shechinah *or the feminine principle has been in exile.* However, since the election of Pope Paul *through the Mother of the world*, her spirit *descended* upon her son Elias Pandochian. From this moment Mother Johanna directs John Abel the way Father Jesus directs Cain.)

The italicized segments evidently show the centrality of the Shechinah in the process of Restitution of all Things. The idea is that, according to Postel, the Feminine Spirit descends (as an indwelling presence) upon the World in order to extend to humans the "sap" of the Good. As we suggested previously, in this excerpt Postel "receives" a prophetic mission and is filled with the same divine presence that lies with the Shechinah. For Postel, if Jesus instructs and directs Cain, similarly, Mother Johanna instructs and directs Abel. There is an obvious desire by Postel to transform a story of fratricide into a more harmonious relationship. But above all, he wants to emphasize the power of the Shechina, and her ability to "pass" her divine nature on to the world. This excerpt is almost a paraphrase of the Zohar, which constantly refers to the exile of the Shechinah and the imperious necessity for her to find a body. Postel's notion of immutation thus finds its justification within this sacred kabbalistic text.

The paradoxical position suggested by Petry is therefore a necessary one and pertains to the positionality of the Shechinah/Malkhut within the relational organization of the Divine Names of the Tree. One must remember that in the midrashic tradition, Malkhut, also called the Crown, the Face of Israël, or "Knesset Yisrael" (" the Community of Israël"),[43] has come to symbolize the mystery of

[41] Green, p. 52.

[42] Postel, *Les très merveilleuses victoires des femmes*, pp. 62–3.

[43] Scholem, *Kabbalah*, p. 111.

the union of the Sons and Daughters of Israël with God, and a tension towards harmony. In this context, the Shechinah also represents the Eternal God. She is not only an image of God, but his Love. If Postel sometimes represents the Shechinah as inferior, it is precisely because according to the *Zohar*, there are in fact two Shechinahs who are in exile with the children of Israel:

> HE FURTHER EXPLAINED: Come and behold. There is the Shechinah below and above THE CHEST OF ZEIR ANPIN. The Shechinah above abides in the twelve borders of the holy Chariots and the twelve supernal living creatures. The Shechinah below abides in the twelve holy tribes. The Shechinah includes of above and below and they all shine simultaneously. AND THEN, "THE WHOLE EARTH IS FULL OF HIS GLORY" (YESHAYAH 6:3), AND THE SHECHINAH IS REVEALED BELOW IN THIS WORLD. When the children of Yisrael were in exile, the Shechinah was not perfected below or above. This is because the Shechinah is in exile with them. [44]

The Servant-Shechinah corresponds to the last Sephira (feminine for Sephirot) called Malkhut or the Crown of Israel. She is both inferior (external) and immanent (internal). This dualism is highly important in Postel's understanding of the Feminine Principle. As the King's Daughter but also his Inner part, Malkhut, understood through the medium of the third Sephira Binah (Intelligence), represents the Transcendent Face (*Arich Anpin*) within the sephirotic hierarchy. In kabbalistic language, to see the Inner Shechinah is similar to seeing the *Panim*, or Faces, that are constantly hidden from the Lower Worlds or from Human Intelligence; and to see the Outer Shechinah is similar to seeing the *Ashorim* or Backsides that represent the ordinary human vision.[45] Thus, understanding Postel's discourse on women requires a complex association of elements, drawn from the *Zohar*, and centered around the Shechinah. If Postel is able to link Mother Joanna to Eve, it's precisely because the zoharic concept of the Shechinah also carries with it qualities generally attributed to the Virgin Mary: Femininity, Candor, Humility, and Charity. Like the Virgin Mary, the Shechinah is the perfect medium because she represents God's desire to communicate with Israel.

Postel, in his quest for "world unity," has visions of the Shechinah, visions similar to those Ezekiel has in his dreams. Therefore, one should not underestimate both the power and the importance of these visions. As the *Zohar* asserts:

> Come and behold: It is said of Isaiah, "and I saw Hashem" (Yeshayah 6:1), WHICH IS THE SHECHINAH, CALLED "ET (LIT. 'THE')." And of Ezekiel it is written: "And I saw visions of Elohim." Here "Et" IS THE SHECHINAH, and there "visions" IS THE SHECHINAH, for what one saw, so did the other, NAMELY ONLY THE SHECHINAH. Happy is the portion of Moses. There was no prophet as perfect as he, FOR HE SAW THE ILLUMINATING MIRROR, WHICH IS ZEIR ANPIN.[46]

---

[44] *Zohar* 9, Vayetze: 27.

[45] Scholem, *Kabbalah*, p. 76.

[46] *Zohar* 19, Yitro: 19.

In fact, here, the Shechinah has a messianic mission. She is charged with the task of bringing God's love to Israel and therefore saving them from their sins. It is for this reason that Postel seeks in Mother Joanna a form of redemption. For "la mere Johanna conduit Jehan Abel" ("Mother Joanna directs John Abel," cited above). Chapter 11 is, for this matter, an evident intertext of the *Zohar*:

> C'est donc le moyen par lequel *ladicte Dame & espouse de l'Aigneau* aura victoire de tout le *monde inférieure & corruptible*. C'est pourquoy Dieu ha voulu que les armes, lettres & imprimeries feussent en souveraine excellence préparées avant que les *deux enfantz* ressuscitassent, l'un pour l'authorité sacrée ou Papale, l'autre pour la temporelle & Royale, affin que par de telz moyens peussent contraindre tout le monde à l'obédience de l'eternelle loy & au vray usage de la raison ...[47]
>
> (Thus, it is the medium through which the aforementioned Lady and Spouse of the Lamb will conquer the inferior and corruptible world. This is why God wanted arms, letters, and printing houses to be perfectly prepared before the two children could be resuscitated, one for the sacred or Papal authority, the other for the temporal and Royal authority, so that through this medium, everyone could be forced to obey the eternal law and constrained to the true use of reason.)

In this excerpt, the association of "ladicte Dame" and "espouse de l'Aigneau" borrows from the Zohar the necessary union of the human world ("monde inférieure & corruptible") with the spirit of God indwelled into the Shechinah for a final victory. The Shechinah is the "illuminating mirror" referred to in the Zohar through which the human world will be again reunited with the divine world. The Shechinah is not only a prophet and a pope, she is the second Messiah. And, since Postel also sees Mother Joanna as the Shechinah, he himself becomes a prophet because, in his mind, she has descended upon him in a process we have called immutation. For Kuntz, "Joanna's prophecy confirmed his own previously formulated beliefs about world peace; later, after his spiritual immutation in 1551, he became a prophet with a clearly defined [goal that] had Joanna at its centre."[48] In Postel's view' "Ladicte Dame & espouse de l'Aigneau," is in fact Joanna and thus a figure of the Shechinah, and her messianic mission is clearly revealed. She is indeed charged with the task of saving the "monde inférieure & corruptible" (the lower and corruptible world). The two "enfants" ('infants') are of course Abel and Cain, who represent, beyond the myth of Good and Evil, Postel's attempt to reach a peaceful end to a tragic relationship.

Thus, for Postel, "contraindre tout le monde à l'obédience de l'eternelle loy" ("to force everyone to respect the eternal law") is to assert that the Shechinah is linked to a messianic vision in a special way because she is the path to redemption and salvation. As one reads in the Zohar:

---

47 Postel, *Les très merveilleuses victoires des femmes*, p. 49.

48 See, Kuntz, p. 100.

> We have learned that Yisrael are detained in exile for three things: For treating the Shechinah with contempt in exile; for turning away their face from the Shechinah, AS IT IS WRITTEN, "FOR THEY HAVE TURNED THEIR BACK TO ME, AND NOT THEIR FACE" (YIRMEYAH 2:27). Finally, for defiling themselves before the Shechinah, WITHOUT CONSIDERING THAT THE SHECHINAH IS WITH THEM IN EXILE. We explained them all in our Mishnah.[49]

The moment "Yisrael" sinned, it also confined the Shechinah to exile by separating Her from God. Thus, the era of reunion of the Shechinah and the Holy One is a messianic period because,

> The Holy One, blessed be He then exiled the King's children, NAMELY YISRAEL, together with the Queen, WHO IS THE SHECHINAH, and swore He shall not return to His place until the Queen return to Hers. THUS a man who is charitable with the Shechinah and repents, and in all Her Torah and precepts MEDITATES only on redeeming the Shechinah FROM EXILE, acts with piety towards his Maker and it is as if he redeemed Him and His Shechinah and His children FROM EXILE.[50]

Postel is evidently struggling to incorporate this powerful concept of the Shechinah into his (perhaps nationalistic and imperialistic) attempt to achieve world peace. I believe that one can find fault in this nationalistic endeavor because after all, as Petry and others have rightly asserted, Postel's vision is fundamentally based on his belief that the French held a certain supremacy over the rest of the world: "Postel argued for French supremacy on the basis of inheritance and primogeniture."[51] However, one should not ignore why some of his views were so controversial. One foundation of this controversy lies with the power invested in the Shechinah, notably her apparent dualism that allows her to transcend gender dichotomies. For Postel then, in *Les très merveilleuses victoires des femmes*, this tension between male and female is essentially transitory because it lays down the foundation for unity. Thus, when inferiority is invoked, it is not, I believe, a hierarchical difference but rather, a necessary internal arrangement within the tree of life.

Once this fundamental and essential position of the Shechinah is established, Postel can then justify his argument by invoking feats accomplished by important women in the history of Europe. Postel makes his position clear:

> C'est une commune querelle qu'on ha contre le dit sexe, de dire & ecrire que les Femmes ont perdu & gasté le monde, ce que n'ayant esté faict en nulle sorte, qu'il n'y aye eu plus d'hommes, ou pour le moins autant de consentantz à la malice comme de Femmes, il fault accuser les plus & non les moins coulpables. Cela est pour certain que là où elles sont le plus accusées, est en ce qu'elles ont seduict

---

49 *Zohar* 32, Acharei Mot: 56.

50 Zohar 49, Ki Tetze: 22.

51 Petry, p. 53.

> les hommes, & par eulx ainsi seduicts, faict ou faict faire de grandes ruines & alterations au dict monde. Mais, on debvroit à mon tres-certain jugement en beaucoup plus accuser les hommes qui ont esté si lourdautz et malusantz de la plus grande excellence que Dieu leur ha baillée [...][52]
>
> (It is a common accusation people have against the aforementioned gender, to say and write that Women have caused the Fall and perverted the world... but since there are as many consenting guilty men to this supposed malice, we must blame the latter more and not less. It is certain that because they seduced men and consequently caused through them great ruins and alterations of the world, one must, in my opinion blame men more because of their laziness and misuse of the greatest excellence given to them by God.)

Here, Postel wants to shift to men the blame constantly attributed to women. For him, if women are to blame for the Fall, men should bear a greater responsibility. In the context of the Reformation, this position departs from that of his contemporaries. If it is true, as Petry suggests, that seeds of such a position can be found in the medieval period, it is equally important to realize that when interpreted within the kabbalistic context, his discourse is quite original. One could argue that if Postel confers to men a greater responsibility, it is precisely because they are supposedly superior.

However, there is an evident *aporia* in Postel's position: it is a dialectical attempt to transcend a contradiction in order to reach his *harmonia mundi.* In other words, Postel seems to suggest that one must transcend the dichotomy that occurred during the Fall in order to restore unity. For men must first recognize their essential flaw by regaining the Shechinah's inner faith. Put differently, this "excellence" that was granted by the Holy One was none other than the Shechinah, the Face of God. Once again, Postel insists on the fact that this Feminine Principle can be found in both male and female and that it transcends gender:

> Il est pour certain que l'homme ou masle est comme le monde superieur & inferieur : le tout reduict en un souverain abregé ; toutefoys l'abregé du monde inferieur y est moins puissant que le superieur, & au contraire est la Femme en laquelle domine le monde inferieur. Cela est aussi tout certain que l'un & l'autre, tant *l'homme comme la Femme*, ha formelle partie divisée en deux parties : l'une la raisonnable ou supérieure, l'autre la sensuelle ou inferieure.[53]
>
> (It is certain that the man or male is composed of both the higher and the lower worlds: the whole reduced to an abridged omnipotent: yet the abridged version of the lower world is not as powerful as the higher world; contrary to the Woman in which the lower world dominates. It is also true that in both *the Man and the Woman*, the formal aspect of their being is divided in two parts: one reasonable or higher, the other sensual or lower.)

---

52 Postel, *Les très merveilleuses victoires des femmes*, p. 8.

53 Postel, *Les très merveilleuses victoires des femmes*, p. 15.

Thus, both man and woman carry within them both the higher and the lower worlds. As we have demonstrated, this is clearly borrowed from the *Zohar*. Postel's idea of salvation through the Feminine Principle has some of its roots in "medieval notions of sexuality,"[54] since he clearly glorifies virginity. However, Postel, at least in the context of *Les très merveilleuses victoires des femmes*, also departs from what Petry calls a desire to elevate "virginity as the highest female virtue."[55] He clearly refutes this by insisting on women's intellectual and mystical attributes. While discussing Mother Joanna's unique abilities, Postel writes:

> Et quant à parler du *sçavoir feminin*, si *tres-grand et eminent* estoit en elle. Quant aux choses divines, avec toutes les doctrines secretes & depuis plus de trois mille ans cachées & propres des *72 auditeurs de Moyse* `a tous les Latins …, icelle qui n'apprint oncques latin, ne Grec, n'Hebreu, ne autre langue ou lecture, me scavoit tellement ouvrir & declarer quand je tournoys le *Zohar*, livre tres-difficile et contenant l'ancienne Doctrine Evangelique en latin […] elle ne m'eust *clairement exposé*.[56]

> (Regarding *feminine knowledge*, it was *great and eminent* in her [Mother Joanna]. As for divine matters, all the doctrines specific to the *72 auditors of Moses* and hidden for more than three thousand years kept secret from the Romans… a woman who had never studied Latin, Greek, Hebrew or any other language was not only able to open and read in Latin the *Zohar* to me, a very hermetic book containing the ancient Evangelic Doctrine, but also *clearly expound upon it*.)

There are two highly important elements in this excerpt. First, Postel views "feminine knowledge" as "great" and "eminent." Furthermore, this high knowledge is actually part of her essence (note the imperfect "estoit," which suggests an ontological presence). Second, he mentions Mother Joanna's ability to explain the most difficult of all books: the *Zohar*. This is not innocent. According to kabbalists, an understanding of the *Zohar* places its reader in the highest spheres of knowledge. The view that women also possess Reason/Intelligence is clearly stated at the beginning of the book when Postel attempts to demonstrate that both men and women are infused with this "superior intellect": "La Mente donc ha deux degrez, l'un pour l'homme, l'autre pour la Femme& l'Esprit semblablement" ("The Mind has two levels, one for the man, and the other for the woman and the spirit similarly").[57] A bit further in the book, he links this "superior intellect" to the debate on Anima and Animus.

> L'Ame (anima) despend du corps & est constituée dedans le sang ; l'Anime (Animus) est immortel divinement crée & *uni en une nature avec l'Ame*, comme

[54] Petry, p. 104.

[55] Petry, p. 107.

[56] Postel, *Les très merveilleuses victoires des femmes*, p. 89.

[57] Postel, *Les très merveilleuses victoires des femmes*, p. 17.

> l'element de la terre avec l'eau ; la Mente ou Vertu Supérieure, ou l'Intellect Agent respond au feu & se conjoinct avec l'Anime ; l'Esprit respondant à l'air se conjoinct à l'Ame comme avec la terre.[58]

> (The Soul (anima) depends on the body and is formed in the blood; the Spirit (Animus) is immortal and divinely created and *united in one nature with the Soul*, the same way earth is united with water; Mind or Superior Virtue, or Intellect Agent is associated with fire and unites itself with the Soul; the Spirit, associated with air, unites itself with the Soul the same way earth unites with water.)

Even though Postel was not always consistent in his entire work with his use of the Anima and the Animus,[59] one must recognize the originality of the introduction of "Menthe ou Vertu Supérieure" in his discussion. I would like to suggest that this concept is directly linked to his understanding of the *Zohar*, especially, to the idea that the "essence" or "sap" of God is believed to circulate through the tree of life. I contend that this "menthe" is none other than the Shechinah, the necessary and missing ingredient in his quest for unity and peace, at least as he envisions it. Far from separating the Animus from the Anima, Postel insists on their unity ("uni en une nature avec l'Ame"). He also borrows from alchemy its lexicon in order to attain this essential unity: air, water, earth, and fire are all part of the alchemist's quest for the Great Work. One could argue that the "menthe," analyzed within this quest, constitutes the fifth and vital element required to find the Philosophical Stone. However, this would not be in contradiction with the *zoharic* nature of his work. In fact, Postel always claimed, after his "immutation" with Mother Joanna, to be a *magus*. This was the purpose of naming himself Rorispergius (or "Sovereign Astrologue"). As such, he would perform the magic of calling all humans to find the Truth (or God's Image). This explains why he saw the *Zohar* as "alchemical manuscript."[60] In his view, his work was similar to that of an alchemist in his lab. As Kuntz puts it "in Postel's terminology the magician is he who discover the pure gold of nature, the laboratory which God has provided for man."[61] We now know that the development of what is usually referred to as Christian Kabbalah was also influenced by various hermetic traditions, including alchemy and neoplatonism. Christian kabbalists "believed that they had discovered in the Kabbalah an original divine revelation to mankind that had been lost and would now be restored, and with the aid of which it was possible not only to understand the teachings of Pythagoras, Plato, and the Orphics […] but also the secret of the Catholic faith."[62] It is evident that he is greatly influenced by the concept of the two Shechinah put forth by the *Zohar*. There is, in *Les très merveilleuses victoires*, a conscious effort to constantly explore and represent these two levels:

---

58 Postel, *Les très merveilleuses victoires des femmes*, p. 37.

59 Petry, p. 57.

60 Kuntz, p. 168.

61 Kuntz. P. 170.

62 Scholem, *Kabbalah*, p. 197.

> Donc il faut y aye deux *degrés de raisonnabileté & deux de sensualite*. Pour parler correct & bien distinctement j'appelle la superieure partie Animus ou l'Anime, & l'inferieure Anima ou l'Ame, comme feirent les anciens Italiens. *Donc il y ha en l'un [l'homme] & l'autre [la femme] trois parties*. L'anime, l'ame & le corps, lequel corps est aussi divisé en deux parties : l'une insensible comme les humeurs, les os, la moelle, la semence, les cheveux & poilz avec substance du cerveau & l'autre sensible, comme les nerfs, veines, arteres, muscles, peau & toute espece de chair...[63]
>
> (It follows that there must be two levels of reasonability and two levels of sensuality. In truth and to speak clearly, I call the higher degree Animus or Spirit, and the lower degree Anima or Soul, the same way ancient Italians did. Therefore, there are one (the man) and the other (the woman) three parties. The spirit, the soul and the body, which in turn is divided in two parts: one insensitive part composed of things such as humors, bones, the marrow, the seed, hair and bristle with the substance of the brain; the other sensitive part composed of things such as nerves, veins, arteries, muscles, skin and any kind of flesh...)

For Postel, there are in both man and woman three parts: the Animus, the Anima, and the Body. The latter is in turn divided in two parts: insensitive and sensitive. Although one could dispute this arbitrary separation, what is constant is his desire to represent a similarity between both genders. In truth, Postel's quest for world harmony is deeply entrenched in a sort of alchemical quest for the Androgynous Man (or Rebis). His allusion to the Four Elements, his bridging of opposites through the concept of the Potential coupled with the quintessential reunion with the Divine presence in the Shechinah all point to the alchemical nature of his entire work.

For Postel, women's attributes transcend maternal qualities and he intends to demonstrate their divine nature by recounting their feats:

> J'ay mis [...] le Chapitre précédent [...] pour les sages Femmes, c'est à sçavoir qui ses sont adonnées au sçavoir d'immortalité, pour les distinguer de celles qui non-seulement aux divines lettres, mais aussi aux humaines, ont été très-excellentes, ou encore de présent sont.[64]
>
> (I dedicated the previous chapter to intelligent Women, those who devoted themselves to the knowledge of immortality so as to distinguish them from those who have excelled or continue to excel not only in divine letters but also in human ones as well.)

Women, according to him, have excelled in many areas and he wants to celebrate them. A quick look at the list of women he mentions confirms this desire to celebrate women's intellectual attributes. First, he tells the story of Luigia Sigea:

63 Postel, *Les très merveilleuses victoires des femmes*, p. 15.

64 Postel, *Les très merveilleuses victoires des femmes*, p. 21.

> Laquelle l'an 22 de son aage, l'an 1548, par expérience monstra, escripvant au Pape Paule (de respondre en Arabic & en Chalde, à laquelle fus par ledict Pape prier) en Latin, en Grec, en Hebreu, en Chalde & en Arabic par tout doctissimement, combien il y ha en elle de sçavoir. Car oultre la congnoisance des dites langues, elle a veu tous les cours des disciplines & sacrées & humaines, chose qui montre que à la Femme n'est rien impossible.[65]

> (Which from the age of 22, in the year 1548, showed by experience and by writing to Pope Paul in Latin, Greek, Hebrew, Chaldean and Arabic with such learning, what knowledge she had. For other than the knowledge of the aforementioned languages, she was exposed to all sorts of subjects, both sacred and profane, proof that to Woman nothing is impossible.)

Here, Postel refers to Luisa Sigea, a renowned Spanish poetess who spent most of her life serving Maria de Portugal (1521–1577). She was known for her precocious and libertine intelligence. As a humanist, she is believed to have represented a case of an exceptionally learned woman of the Spanish Renaissance seeking to perform in a nonreligious milieu. For example, Sigea's vernacular poems, such as "Un fin, una esperanza, un como, un cuando" and "Pasados tengo hasta ahora", can be viewed as an attempt to revisit and to challenge the traditional poetic female subject often used in Petrarchan poetry. Here, as Mar Martinez Gongora states, "she revises the traditional trajectory of the Petrarchan poetic subject in order to replace the elusive woman, viewed as a passive object of the male gaze and ultimately responsible for his spiritual perfection, into a female subject able to articulate her own poetic voice, a voice impregnated by melancholy and sorrow."[66] Sigea refutes the Aristotelian concept of melancholy as an exclusive male artistic genius, by constructing a female subject that would embody special characteristics she viewed as powerful and unique. According to Góngora, "his use of melancholy coincides with her personal frustration with the lack of professional opportunities open to a female humanist in the Spanish courts of the Renaissance."[67] One notes the insistence on the knowledge ("congnoisance") of many languages, a clear sign of intellectual ability. Most striking though, is the firm assertion that "à la Femme n'est rien impossible," to a woman nothing is impossible.

This limitless and infinite possibility is obviously borrowed from the Zohar, since, as we have shown, the Shechinah is said to have inherited from the Ein Sof his infinite nature. One could even argue that here, one senses that Postel wants to posit himself as an advocate for women, for the recognition of their ability. This is perhaps the reason he invokes the next woman: "signora Isabella Rosera, gentilfemme Espagnole." It is said that Isabella Rosera devoted herself to the conversion of the Jews, dazzled multitudes with her eloquence in the cathedral

---

[65] Postel, *Les très merveilleuses victoires des femmes*, p. 24.

[66] Mar Martinez Góngora, "Poesía, Melancolía y Subjetividad Femenina: La Humanista Luisa Sigea," *Neophilologus*, 90/3 (2006): 423–43 (423).

[67] Góngora, p. 423.

in Barcelona, and expounded the subtleties of Duns Scotus before prelates and cardinals at Rome.[68] Postel then concludes with a powerful woman, Marguerite of France: "Mais qui congnoistra Madame Marguerite de France, la pourra vrayement estimer le Parangon des lettres & heritiere de l'excellent siecle ..."[69] ("Yet, anyone who meets Mme. Marguerite of France will no doubt consider her as the Model of letters and the heiress of this great century..."). It is fundamental to underline the word "parangon" of letters. Postel sees her not only as a literary model, but also as a gem or a precious stone representing the intellectual elite. Such an elevation cannot be ignored in a century where women were still struggling for social recognition and deference. This is perhaps the reason why *Les très merveilleuses victoires des femmes* created a scandal. It is certainly one of the reasons he was cast as heretic and fell from grace. Jean Dupebe, quoting Antoine Couillard in his attempt to justify Postel's fall from grace in the political sphere, writes: "Par audacieuse presumption il auait non seulement publicquement presché, mais aussi escript & faict imprimer un oeuvre, qui a bon droict fut incontinent censuré, comme le plus depraué & scandaleux, qu'oncque ait esté veu en toutes le(s) Gaulles" ("...because of his audacious presumption, he had not only publicly preached, but also written and had published a work, which was rightly censured, as the most depraved and scandalous that had ever been seen in all of Gaul").[70] The book, addressed to Marguerite of France, certainly annoyed political authorities as its censure clearly suggests. But more importantly, this book was negatively received in religious circles since it was evident that Postel was attempting to connect the virtues and intelligence of Marguerite of France to Mother Joanna's mystical knowledge of the divine.

In a final analysis, one can see that in *Les très merveilleuses victoires des femmes*, Guillaume Postel, far from viewing women as inferior, intends to laud their intellectual qualities. There is no doubt that his views on women changed with time and context but what stands out in Postel's discourse on women is how his quest in women seems to be the foundation for world harmony. In this regard, his use of both alchemy and kabbalah is original in that the feminine principle is the single important element in achieving peace among human beings. His discourse is unique in that it touches at least three very important areas of human society: religion, politics, and science. The reason Postel was considered a heretic was mainly because of the place he gave to women in the restitution of all things. In a time when women were mainly portrayed as evil, one must admire Postel's courage. Politically speaking, his whole body of work, and particularly *Les très merveilleuses victoires des femmes*, created outrage, as we have shown, in political circles. Because he devoted the great part of life to establishing a universal

68 See René Maulde-La-Clavière and George Herbert Ely, *The Women of the Renaissance: A Study of Feminism* (London: Swan Sonnenschein & Co., Ltd., 1900), p. 409.

69 Postel, *Les très merveilleuses victoires des femmes*, p. 22.

70 "Poursuites contre Postel en 1553," p. 38.

monarchy,[71] it is safe to assume that political authorities also feared the centrality of women in such a structure. Postel, with his diplomatic duties and his knowledge of Turkish culture, was among the firsts to raise the concept of a European Union. In his *Republique des Turcs*, Postel makes a very modern argument on the type of relationship that could be possible with the Turks.[72] With regards to science, Postel's quest for knowledge was remarkable because it was driven by this view of the importance of the feminine. His attraction to oriental languages and philosophies was certainly based on his desire to demonstrate the importance of the restitution of all things: most notably Hebrew as a divine language and the feminine principle. It is no surprise that Postel has now been acknowledged as "the first Orientalist and the first comparative linguist."[73] Considering the context of the Renaissance, Postel can quite easily be called a "feminist" because of the way he inverts, subverts, or even transcends gender roles. In my view, the kabbalistic (and also alchemical) nature of his understanding of the universe, and his attraction to the concept of the Shechinah set this book apart. I would argue that perhaps his idea of Restitutio, borrowed from lurianic kabbalah and its concept of the Tikkun (Restoration), constitute the sort of triumphant esotericism that makes Postel both controversial and appealing.

---

[71] Kuntz, p. 171.

[72] Guillaume Postel, *De la Republique des Turcs, et là ou l'occasion s'offrira, des meurs et loy de tous Muhamedistes…Histoire et considération de l'origine, loy et coustume des Tartares, Persiens, Arabes, Turcs…*(Poitiers: Chez E. de Marnef, 1560).

[73] Kuntz, p. 172.

Chapter 3
Odd Bodies: Reviewing Corporeal Difference in Early Modern Alchemy

Kathleen P. Long

Art, anatomy, and archeology come together in the sixteenth century to create a conception of the human body that is radically different from that presented in medieval medical works. This conception of the human body is idealizing, based as it is on classical sculptural representations of the gods, and it will come to dominate early modern, and arguably modern, medical notions of the normal, healthy body. Thus, well before the modern era, the stage is set for a narrowly normalizing view of how the human body should look. This normalizing view also focuses primarily on an idealized masculine body, with the feminine version presented as an afterthought. For example, in Andreas Vesalius's *De humani corporis fabrica libri septem* (Basel, 1543), the female body is only represented in a discussion of reproductive organs, with only a torso view of that body. Relative to all other parts of the body, the masculine form is the norm. This way of conceptualizing medicine has in fact predominated to the present day; it is only recently that medical studies have focused on women's bodies other than the reproductive organs. In the early modern period, illustrated alchemical treatises offered an alternative to the masculine, strongly idealizing, norm presented in medical manuals. Feminine and feminized masculine bodies are frequently represented, and even forms deemed monstrous, such as the hermaphroditic double-headed rebis, are presented as central to the alchemical process. Those crippled by injury or illness, for example a diseased king, are often also presented as images of the alchemical process. Whereas the diseased or radically different body had only a limited place in medical illustrations of the sixteenth century, these bodies are omnipresent in alchemical works. In this study, Michael Maier's alchemical emblem book, the *Atalanta fugiens*, because of the striking nature of its visual images and their relation to the work of Vesalius, will serve as an example of the alchemical corpus. This corpus offers an alternative to the predominantly normalizing and masculinizing images of the human body found in the most widely disseminated treatises on anatomy.

Lawrence M. Principe and William R. Newman opened a debate in their article "Some Problems with the Historiography of Alchemy" (2001)[1] concerning the

[1] Lawrence M. Principe and William R. Newman, "Some Problems with the Historiography of Alchemy," in *Secrets of Nature: Astrology and Alchemy in Early Modern*

validity of reading alchemical symbolism as anything other than a straightforward code for the materials and the processes of alchemical practice. This insistence on the "chemical" meaning of alchemical imagery and language was a corrective to anachronistic psychoanalytic readings of alchemical treatises, but in some sense Principe and Newman may have overcorrected. Hereward Tilton takes on their arguments in his book on Michael Maier, contending that the larger cultural context in which these works were created should also enter into consideration. I would agree with Tilton that alchemical symbolism can be read in a number of ways and as having a number of meanings,[2] some inherently a part of various aspects of the alchemical process, and some "accidental" (that is to say, clearly not referring to the alchemical process itself). I will be reading the *Atalanta* in a wider context, partly because alchemical symbolism was echoed in the wider context of court poetry and political polemic[3] and partly because this symbolism was itself drawn from that wider context. While it is hard to know whether alchemical imagery deliberately provided a critique of other cultural productions (such as anatomical treatises) or whether the reuse of these productions was merely fortuitous, the truth is that alchemy provides a repository of images and ideas that often serve as alternatives to those arising from more officially sanctioned milieus (the University, in the case of anatomical treatises, as well as religious and political notions of acceptable gender roles).

In this reading of the *Atalanta*, I diverge from some previous readings of the work, most particularly that of Sally G. Allen and Joanna Hubbs, who read Maier's images and commentary, and by extension all alchemical works, as relentlessly masculinist:

> Alchemical symbolism, rich in both mythological and biological allusion, presents the image of the opus as the wresting of an embryo from the womb of the earth, embodied in women, a birth from a man-made alembic. This recurrent symbolism in alchemical works suggests an obsession with reversing, or perhaps even arresting, the feminine hegemony over the process of biological creation.[4]

I have also pointed out the frequent effacement of the feminine in some alchemical works, particularly those of Paracelsus.[5] But I would also strongly agree with Didier Kahn, who presents alchemy as a complex web of practices that change

---

Europe, William R. Newman and Anthony Grafton, eds. (Cambridge, MA: MIT Press, 2001), pp. 385–431.

2 Hereward Tilton, *The Quest for the Phoenix: Spiritual Alchemy and Rosicrucianism in the Work of Count Michael Maier (1569–1622)*. Christoph Markschies and Gerhard Mueller, eds. Arbeiten zur Kirchesgeschichte 88 (Berlin: Walter de Gruyter, 2003), p. 14.

3 Kathleen P. Long, "Lyric Hermaphrodites," in *Hermaphrodites in Renaissance Europe* (Aldershot, UK: Ashgate Publishing, 2006), p. 163.

4 Sally G. Allen and Joanna Hubbs, "Outrunning Atalanta: Feminine Destiny in Alchemical Transmutation," *Signs* 6/2 (1980): 213.

5 Long, *Hermaphrodites*, pp. 119–23.

over time and according to the varied contexts in which they arise.[6] The central role given to the figure of the *rebis*, or alchemical hermaphrodite, at least following the publication of the *Rosarium philosophorum* (1550)[7] on (if not from much earlier), can only render the notion of an all-encompassing masculinist ideology in alchemy problematic at best. Particularly significant is the fact that the hermaphrodite, which represents the stage of conjunction (of Sol and Luna, mercury and sulphur) of the masculine and feminine principles or elements, retains two distinct gender identities in one body.

I would further argue that, while the various images of feminized masculinity, of the union of the sexes, and the exhortations to the (supposedly male) alchemist to do "women's work" can be read as appropriations of women's role in procreation, they are also queer in the sense of constantly shifting gender roles and effacing gender boundaries. A pregnant man is not a simple masculinist effacement of the feminine. And, in fact, the repressed feminine returns constantly in the *Atalanta*, not only as the Earth nursing the Philosopher's Stone or as a woman working, but as the sister of the conjunction, as Luna who fights the dragon alongside Sol, as Aphrodite joining with Hermes to create the rebis. In emblem 42, the alchemical philosopher follows Nature (represented as a woman) rather than mastering her.

The fact is that alchemy was such a vast range of practices, both in geographical and what we would call today "disciplinary" scope, that its images and commentaries were often inflected to suit particular contexts. So, while the penultimate image of the *Rosarium philosophorum* is the Father, Son, and Holy Mother (presumably the Virgin Mary),[8] in keeping with the emphasis on the conjunction of masculine and feminine that pervades the treatise, the insistently masculine *De Lapide Philosophico Libellus* ends with the Father, Son, and the male Guide (presented as a sort of angel or Holy Spirit).[9] There is no feminine figure in Lambsprinck's work, while the feminine is a constant presence in the *Rosarium*; this contrast is merely a sample of the vast range of alchemical imagery.

Furthermore, consideration of alchemical works in the context of other scientific images and discourses reveals some pronounced differences in emphasis. A quick survey of some of the best-known medical treatises of the period reveals that the female body is represented only when the reproductive organs are in question; for

---

6 Didier Kahn, *Alchimie et paracelsisme en France (1567–1625)* (Geneva: Droz, 2007), p. 7: "Définir l'alchimie n'est pas chose aisée. Cette discipline mouvante a toujours su s'adapter à tous les contextes, se fondre dans le milieu ambiant, se mêler aux doctrines ou aux sciences les plus proches. Il est en fin de compte plus facile de dire ce qu'elle n'est pas." ("It is not an easy thing to define alchemy. This mutable discipline has always known how to adapt itself to every context, to melt into the surrounding environment, to mix with the doctrines and forms of knowledge closest to it. It is, finally, easier to say what it is not.")

7 Joachim Telle, ed., *Rosarium Philosophorum: Ein Alchemisches Florilegium des Spätmittelalters, Faksimile des illustrierten Erstausgabe Frankfurt 1550* (Weinheim: VCH Verlagsgesellschaft, 1992).

8 Z3v (p. 182 in the facsimile edition of the Rosarium).

9 Lambsprinck, *De Lapide Philosophico Libellis* (Frankfurt: Luca Jennis, 1625), emblem 15.

the rest of the body, the male serves as the example for both sexes.[10] It is intriguing that, while images of the male body come to dominate anatomical works in the second half of the sixteenth century, and the first half of the seventeenth, images of the female body and the feminized male body invade the alchemical realm. These bodies are presented alongside others that are strikingly different from the Vesalian male norm: the hydropic man, the figure of Saturn as an amputee from Maier's *Symbola Aureae Mensae*,[11] the double-headed hermaphroditic rebis. The alchemical corpus becomes a significant repository for images of various bodily differences, and a means of contemplating the various potential significances of those differences.

By means of scrutiny of some of these images, I hope to nuance some current arguments concerning the advent of an idealizing form of normalcy, for which I discern roots in early modern medical manuals. By the late eighteenth and early nineteenth centuries, the new science of statistics is put to use defining the normal human body, and eventually enforcing an idealizing norm. At the same time, alchemy falls by the wayside, considered an outdated mode of scientific inquiry. In recent criticism, the critique of enforcement of idealizing norms relative to the human body has been focused primarily on modern practices. As Lennard Davis points out in his essay on "Constructing Normalcy," the modern notion of the "average man" – a notion that both fueled and was fueled by the mania for statistics – evolved into an idealizing notion of normalcy. The eugenicist Sir Francis Galton (1822–1911) transformed the interpretation of statistics from perceiving the average as normal to promoting above-average traits as normal:

> In an "error curve" the extremes of the curve are the most mistaken in accuracy. But if one is looking at human traits, then the extremes, particularly what Galton saw as positive extremes – tallness, high intelligence, ambitiousness, strength, fertility – would have to be seen as errors. Rather than "errors," Galton wanted to think of the extremes as distributions of a trait.

Davis describes revisions Galton made to his system in order to privilege these traits (height, intelligence, ambitiousness, strength, fertility), which he deemed superior. He goes on to discuss the implications of these revisions:

> What these revisions by Galton signify is an attempt to redefine the concept of the "ideal" in relation to the general population. First, the application of the idea of a norm to the human body creates the idea of deviance or a "deviant" body.

[10] This is true for Jacopo Berengario da Carpi's *Isagogae breves, perlucidae ac uberrimae in anatomiam humani corporis* (Bologna: Benedictus Hector, 1523); for Charles Estienne's *De dissection partium corporis humani libri tres* (Paris: Simon Colinaeus, 1545); for Juan Valverde de Amusco's *Anatomia de corpo humano* (Rome: Ant. Salamanca and Antonio Lafrery, 1560); and for Andreas Vesalius's own *De humani corporis fabrica libri septem* (Basel: Joannes Oporinus, 1543). The images from all of these treatises are easily available for scrutiny at the National Library of Medicine website, *Historical Anatomies Online*: http://www.nlm.nih.gov/exhibition/historicalanatomies/browse.html

[11] *Symbola Aureae Mensae Duodecim Nationum* (Frankfurt: Luca Jennis, 1617).

> Second, the idea of a norm pushes the normal variation of the body through a stricter template guiding the way the body "should" be. Third, the revision of the "normal curve of distribution" into quartiles, ranked in order, and so on, creates a new kind of "ideal." This statistical ideal is unlike the classical ideal which contains no imperative to be the ideal. The new ideal of ranked order is powered by the imperative of the norm, and then is supplemented by the notion of progress, human perfectibility, and the elimination of deviance, to create a dominating, hegemonic vision of what the human body should be.[12]

This vision is put into action first by the eugenicists, who wish first to eliminate those who deviate from the norm, both the "feeble bodied" and the "feeble minded," by means of sterilization, incarceration, and even by means of what they call euthanasia, practiced massively by the Nazis in the 1930's against the first victims of the Holocaust, the disabled.

While Davis is correct in observing particular modern means of marginalizing physical difference, his idealization of the past does not hold up under scrutiny of that past. Early modern anatomical treatises can be considered possible precursors for our own understanding of the norm, and some alchemical works can be seen as alternatives to normalizing depictions of the human body. As Davis suggests, there are political and social implications to our Enlightenment ancestors' choice of statistic-driven ways of representing the body over other possibilities. In this regard, the argument in this essay differs from that of William R. Newman, in his book, *Promethean Ambitions*.[13] While alchemical belief in the perfectibility of nature and of human nature may have played a role in the rise of idealizations of the norm, how that perfectibility manifests itself in alchemical treatises is radically different from the notion of perfection represented in medical manuals.

In Western Europe, the practice of annual dissections of a human cadaver began sometime in the course of the fourteenth century.[14] Some of these exercises were deemed illicit, and students prosecuted for sacrilege; others were permitted by university statutes, for example those of Montpellier in 1340. By the end of the fifteenth century, the annual dissection was a regular practice in medical faculties, and there is some evidence that it became quite widespread. Leonardo da Vinci began performing a number of dissections and making anatomical drawings based on them around 1487. His representations, while often mechanistic, are relatively realistic. But these images were not widely available.[15]

---

12 Lennard Davis, "Constructing Normalcy: The Bell Curve, the Novel, and the Invention of the Disabled Body in the Nineteenth Century," *The Disability Studies Reader* (New York: Routledge, 2006), p. 8.

13 William R. Newman, *Promethean Ambitions: Alchemy and the Quest to Perfect Nature* (Chicago: The University of Chicago Press, 2004).

14 Nancy G. Siraisi, *Medieval and Early Renaissance Medicine: An Introduction to Knowledge and Practice* (Chicago: The University of Chicago Press, 1990), p. 86.

15 Siraisi, p. 97.

Before the advent of what we would consider to be relatively accurate anatomical representations, medieval medicine was dominated by schematic drawings of the internal workings of the body, known as the "Five-Figure" series (because they consisted of five figures, representing the muscles, the skeletal system, the veins, the arteries, and the nervous system). These figures were often joined by a sixth, an image of a pregnant woman. These seem to have arrived in Europe via Persian manuscripts, but resemble images from Chinese and Indian medical treatises. These images are based on other images, rather than on direct observation of the human body. They are quite schematic, and not useful for surgeons in particular who might need a more accurate understanding of the human body.[16]

One might think that once dissection of the human body had become a fairly regular feature of medical training, representations of the body would have more closely resembled actual, even ordinary, human bodies.[17] What happens is more complex, and related to the discovery of classical sculptures representing gods from the Greek and Roman pantheon. The most widely disseminated anatomical images in early modern Europe were those from Vesalius's treatise, *De humani corporis fabrica*. These images dominated early modern medical treatises for at least a century, republished and imitated in other works such as Caspar Bauhin's treatise on human anatomy, cleverly titled *De corporis humani fabrica*, thus avoiding accusations of overt plagiarism while capitalizing on the popularity of Vesalius's work.[18] Bauhin's version was published in 1590 in much smaller format and on cheaper paper, and thus was suitable for use by medical students. Vesalius's original edition was a prohibitively expensive book, more intended for rich patrons than for medical students, and thus not as widely available as the works of his imitators. Bauhin's work itself was anthologized with treatises by other authors, and so was disseminated throughout Europe;[19] and his work is only one example of the many medical treatises appropriating the images in Vesalius's work. As we shall see, these images were also disseminated and imitated in a far wider range of texts than merely medical treatises.[20]

---

[16] Siraisi, pp. 92–3.

[17] Siraisi, p. 94.

[18] Caspar Bauhin, *De corporis humani fabrica*...(Basel: Sebastianum Henricpetri, 1590). This and later versions of Bauhin's anatomical treatise were illustrated with imitations of Vesalius's work, done by Theodor de Bry.

[19] For example, in the *Mikrokosmographia: a description of the body of man: together with the controversies and figures thereto belonging / collected and translated out of all the best authors of anatomy, especially out of Gaspar Bauhinus and Andréas Laurentius*, Helkiah Crooke, ed. (London: printed by R.C. and are to be sold by Iohn Clarke .., 1651).

[20] For a brief overview of anatomical treatises in the sixteenth century, see Andrew Wear, "Early Modern Europe, 1500–1700," in *The Western Medical Tradition, 800 BC to AD 1800* (Cambridge: Cambridge University Press, 1995), pp. 280–81. For another take on Renaissance anatomy, see Jonathan Sawday, "The Renaissance Body," in *The Body Emblazoned: Dissection and the Human Body in Renaissance Culture* (London: Routledge, 1995), pp. 16–38. See also Katharine Park, *Secrets of Women: Gender, Generation, and the Origins of Human Dissection* (New York: Zone Books, 2006).

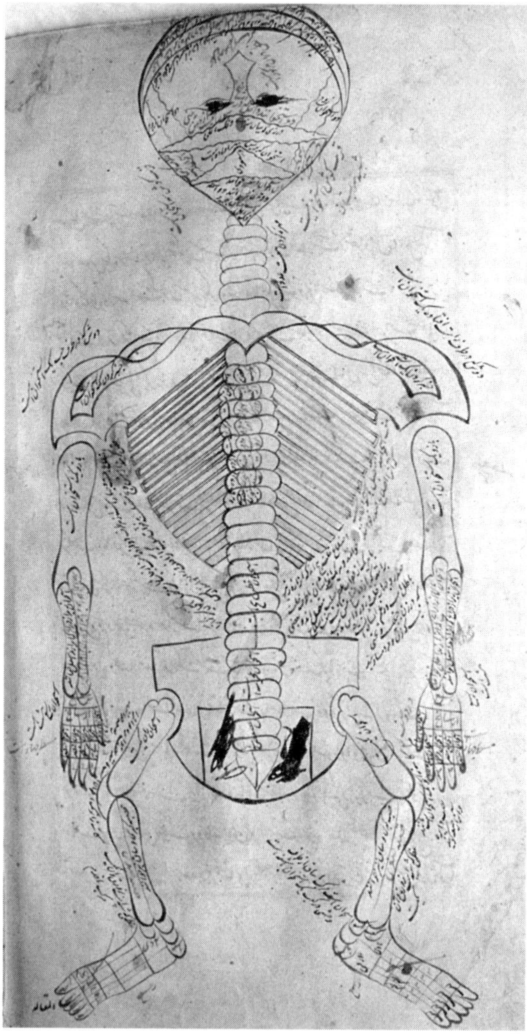

Fig. 3.1 The Skeletal System: An Image from a Five-Figure Series, from Mansur ibn Ilyas, *Tasrih-I badan-I insan* (*Anatomy of the Human Body*). Courtesy of the National Library of Medicine.

But where did these images come from? In an attempt to market his work, Vesalius hired artists to create the images, among them Johannes Stephanus of Calcar, a student of Titian's.[21] Stephanus imitated classical sculpture, such as the Belvedere Torso, in his depiction of the human body. The Apollo Belvedere, a Hellenistic or Roman copy of a fourth century B.C.E. bronze sculpture, rediscovered in the late fifteenth century,[22] was also a popular model for anatomical illustrations, as the "Flayed Man" from Juan Valverde de Amusco's *Anatomia del corpo humano*,[23] itself imitated in other treatises, demonstrates. The Apollo Belvedere's posture and musculature are also echoed in the famous Vesalius/Stephanus image of the "Muscle Man." Valverde de Amusco's work also appropriated this and other Vesalian images.

The Vesalian "Muscle Man" is in fact echoed fairly widely in the late sixteenth and early seventeenth centuries. Theodor de Bry used it extensively in his *America* series, an illustrated edition of every single account he could gather of the discovery, exploration, and conquest of the Western Hemisphere by Western Europeans. His idealizing portrait of a Virginian (that is, Native American) king echoes the proportions and the posture of the "Muscle Man," while adding some more mannerist-style musculature (see figure 6 in Sean Teuton's essay). This image is from the first part of the series, published in 1590, also known as the *Admiranda narratio*, and based on Thomas Hariot's accounts of the English encounters with the natives of Virginia.[24] The fact that de Bry intended to present the more welcoming Virginians as ideal in body as well as behavior, particularly compared to their cannibalistic Brazilian counterparts, who are portrayed as having shorter limbs and longer torsos, as well as rounder heads, indicates that this classicizing representation of the body was seen as an ideal (see Teuton, figure 7).[25] In some other, similar, images, the Virginians are even overtly compared to predecessors of

---

[21] A recent article by Patricia Simons and Monique Kornell, "Annibal Caro's After-Dinner Speech (1536) and the Question of Titian as Vesalius's Illustrator," *Renaissance Quarterly,* 61/4 (2008): 1069–97, summarizes much of the scholarship on the subject, as well as putting to rest the question of Titian's involvement in the project. The fact that Titian's name has even been invoked relative to the *De humani corporis…* underscores the symbiotic nature of art and anatomy in this period.

[22] Roberto Weiss, *The Renaissance Discovery of Classical Antiquity* (Oxford: Oxford University Press, 1969), p. 103.

[23] Juan Valverde de Amusco, *Historia de la composicion del cuerpo humano…* (Rome: Salamanca and Lafrery, 1556). Republished as *Anatomia del corpo humano* (Rome: Salamanca and Lafrery, 1560). Images from this text are available on the website run by the National Library of Medicine: http://www.nlm.nih.gov/exhibition/historicalanatomies/valverde_bio.html

[24] Theodor de Bry, ed. and illus., *Admiranda narration, fida tamen, de commodis et incolarum ritibus Virginiae…Anglico scripta sermone à Thoma Hariot…*(Frankfurt: J. Wechel, 1590).

[25] Theodor de Bry, ed. and illus., *America tertia pars memorabilem provinciae Brasiliae historiam continens…*(Frankfurt: M. Becker, 1605).

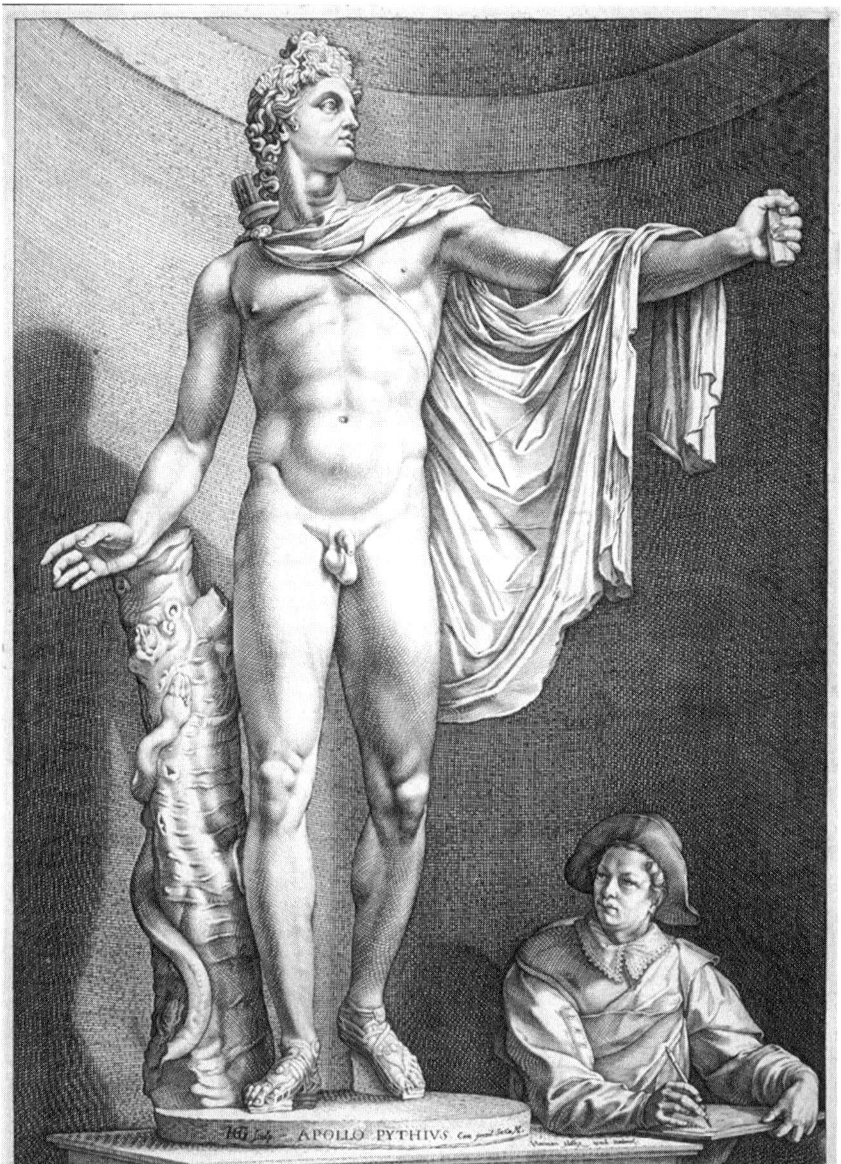

Fig. 3.2 *Apollo Belvedere*, Hendrik Goltzius, copy by Herman Adolfz, from *Antique Statues in Rome*, ca. 1592, dated 1617. Courtesy of the Bryn Mawr College Collections.

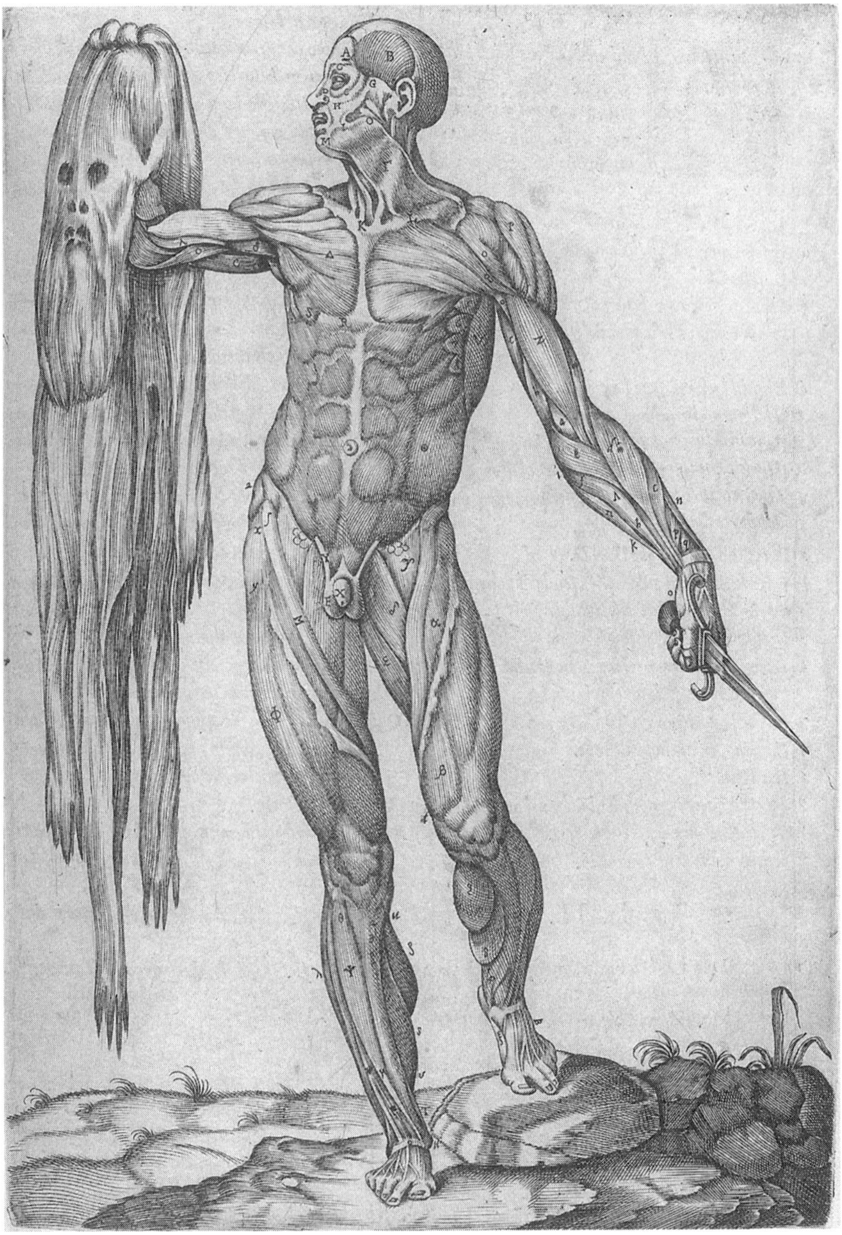

Fig. 3.3 The Flayed Man, from Juan Valverde de Amusco, *Anatomia del corpo humano* (Rome: Salamanca and Lafrery, 1560), plate 1, vol. 2. Courtesy of the National Library of Medicine.

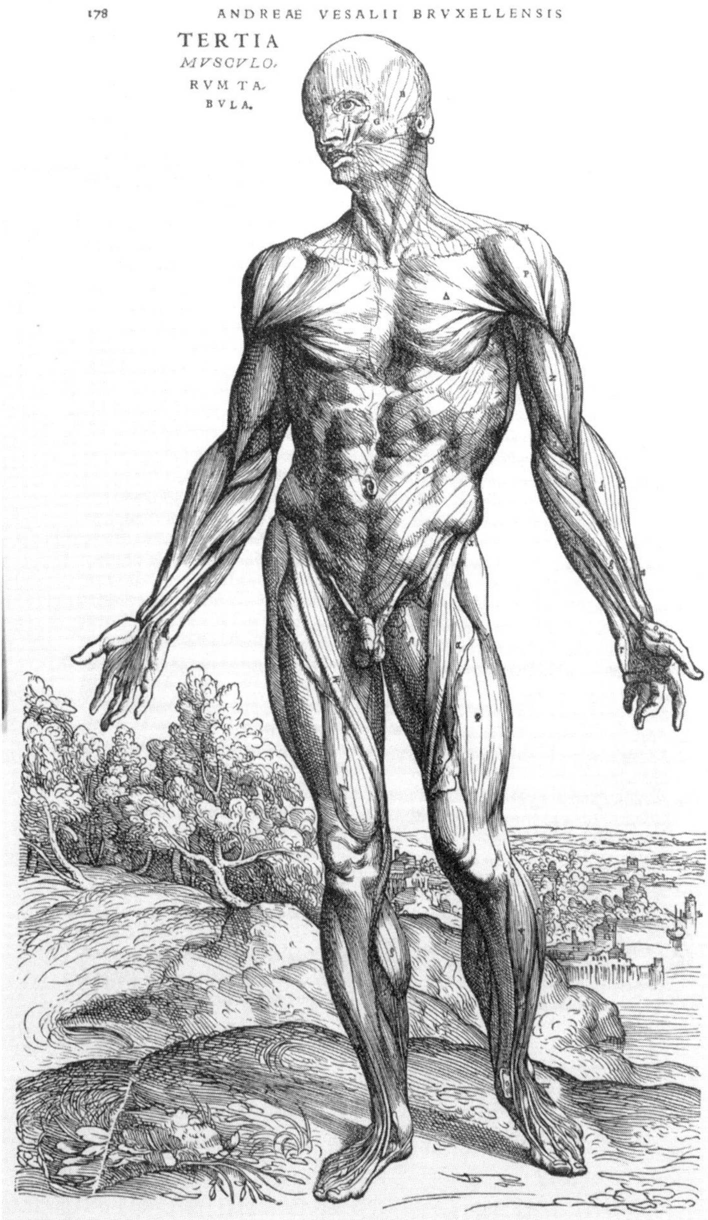

Fig. 3.4 "The Muscle Man" ("Tertia musculorum tabula") from Andreas Vesalius, *De corporis humani fabrica* (Basel: I Oporini, 1543). Courtesy of the Division of Rare and Manuscript Collections, Cornell University Library.

the early modern Europeans, particularly the Picts, who tattooed themselves much as some Native Americans did.

Not surprisingly, given that the de Bry family imitated Vesalius both in their medical illustrations for Bauhin's anatomical treatises and in their *America* project, they also imitated the *De humani corporis fabrica* in alchemical illustrations. Probably the best-known example of an illustrated alchemical treatise is Michael Maier's *Atalanta fugiens* (*Fleeing Atalanta*), first published at Oppenheim in 1617 by the de Bry family and illustrated by engravings done by a de Bry son-in-law, Matthäus Merian. Maier himself, born in 1568, was no marginal figure, but was the court physician to the Holy Roman Emperor Rudolph II, a noted patron of alchemy and of the arts.[26] The fact that Maier was court physician recalls that alchemy was more than the search for ways to turn lead into gold. It was also known as "chemical medicine," and this branch of the art consisted of seeking out medicines, made out of chemical compounds, herbs, and other ingredients, to restore the body's equilibrium and thus its health. For Maier, alchemy also had a spiritual significance, based on the belief that contemplation of certain ideas or images would improve the individual's understanding of the universe and of his or her place in it. This alchemical regime, playing as it does with gender and other corporeal norms, often seems to present an alternative to the predominant regimes organized by Church and State, most particularly the theological as well as legal privileging of the masculine over the feminine. These three branches of alchemy, the search to create higher forms of materials from lower ones, to find medicines to cure the body of illness, and to improve one's understanding through contemplation of complex ideas and images, were intertwined in many alchemical works of the late sixteenth and early seventeenth centuries., although the *Atalanta fugiens* seems to privilege the philosophical.

The *Atalanta* is an odd work for modern readers unfamiliar with alchemical emblem-books, consisting of a series of 50 emblems representing stages of the alchemical process as symbolic figures, with a motto, an epigram, and a long explanatory discussion, all in Latin but also translated into German. The further complication of this work is that all 50 epigrams are set to music (fugues, to be precise, in keeping with the title of the work). The reader was apparently expected to sing the epigram while contemplating the emblem; this means that the viewing of the emblem was supposed to be more than a casual glance. This methodology resembles some early modern meditative practices more than it does modern scientific methods of experimentation, thus suggesting the possibility not only of transformation of materials external to the practitioner, but also the inducing of a state of mind within the practitioner. That being said, I would not want to follow a Jungian approach to the texts; rather, I would hope to reinstate these works in their original context, that is to say, a period when meditation was becoming a

[26] For more background on Maier, see Hereward Tilton, cited above, and Bruce T. Moran, *The alchemical world of the German court: occult philosophy and chemical medicine in the circle of Moritz of Hessen (1572–1632)* (Stuttgart: F. Steiner, 1991).

significant part of religious practice (one need only think of the *Spiritual Exercises* of Saint Ignatius of Loyola). As strange as all this is, this work was popular enough to be published in 1617 and again in 1618, and yet again in 1687 and 1708.[27] In this reading of Maier, I depart from Allen and Hubbs by placing Maier in the context of the scientific and theological discourses of his time. By means of his repeated invocation of the four elements, which are omnipresent in the *Atalanta*, as well as the precise way in which this invocation is presented, Maier demonstrates a connection to Hippocratic, as well as Aristotelian traditions, in which fire, air, water, earth correspond to hot, dry, wet, and cold, as well as the humors of yellow bile, blood, phlegm, and black bile.[28] In this context, the balance of the four elements, with air and fire representing the masculine and earth and water the feminine, is crucial rather than the mastery and effacement of some elements by others. The constant rebalancing of the elements throughout the process explains the repetitive nature of the imagery in many alchemical treatises. For example, in the *Atalanta*, the stage of conjunction is evoked repeatedly in the images of the marriage of brother and sister (emblem IV), of Sol and Luna (emblem XXXIV), of Mercury and Venus (emblem XXXVIII), as well as in the image of the alchemical rebis (emblems XXXIII and XXXVIII). It should also be noted that the elements are often presented as ambiguous or mixed in nature; thus, the masculine Wind is presented as a pregnant Man, the feminine Water is presented as a hydropic man, rather than a woman, and the rebis, associated with Fire, is hermaphroditic.

The bodies themselves also call for some contemplation, disrupting as they do, and did in the sixteenth century, our expectations of bodily normalcy as evoked by the images in Vesalius's treatise. In this, we can see the idealized body, represented in much of what Renaissance artists knew of classical sculpture, becoming the norm that Lennard Davis discerns in modern culture. But alchemy represents bodies that are somehow strange, and it could be argued that alchemical illustrations normalize strangeness by offering it for contemplation, as part of the alchemical process. So, Vesalius's Muscle Man becomes the Wind, the first emblem in the *Atalanta*. His hair and his hands designate him as the airy element, even as he seems to dissolve into that element, and the child in his belly indicates his centrality to the generative process. The positioning of his feet, the aspect of this figure that most resembles the Apollo Belvedere, suggests the possibility of flight or lightness, as the heels of both feet are lifted slightly off of the ground. The arms, also echoing the placement of the arms in the Apollo Belvedere, end in gusts of wind, represented by spiraling clouds. The classical sculpture, with its emphasis on lightness and movement,

---

27 See H.M.E. de Jong, *Michael Maier's Atalanta fugiens: Sources of an Alchemical Book of Emblems* (York Beach, ME: Nicolas-Hays, Inc., 2002; reprinted from the Leiden edition, Brill, 1969), p. 5.

28 Vivian Nutton, "Medicine in the Greek World, 800–50 BC," in Lawrence I. Conrad, et. al. *The Western Medical Tradition: 800 B.C. to A.D. 1800* (Cambridge: Cambridge University Press, 1995), pp. 23–5.

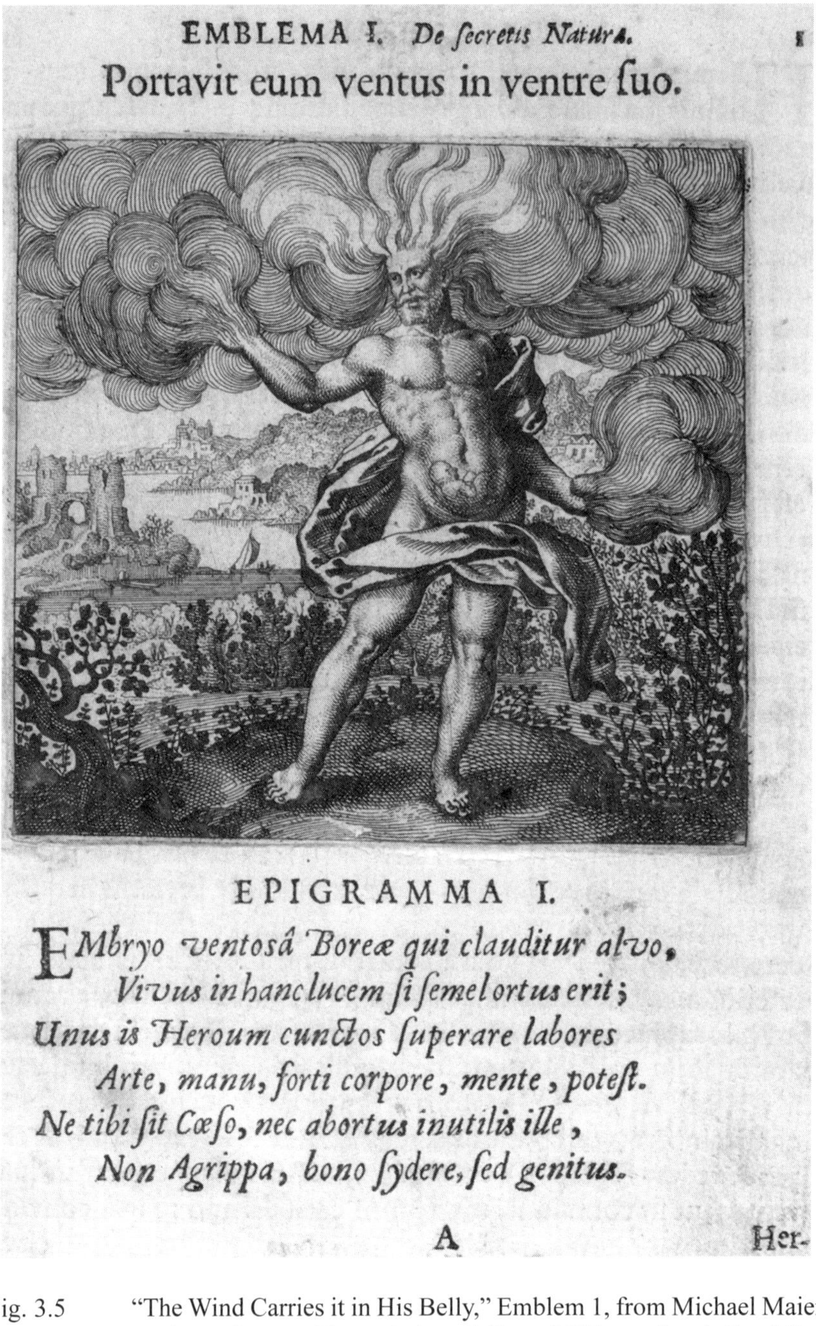

EMBLEMA I. *De ſecretis Naturæ.* I

Portavit eum ventus in ventre ſuo.

EPIGRAMMA I.

EMbryo ventoſâ Boreæ qui clauditur alvo,
Vivus in hanc lucem ſi ſemel ortus erit;
Unus is Heroum cunctos ſuperare labores
Arte, manu, forti corpore, mente, poteſt.
Ne tibi ſit Cæſo, nec abortus inutilis ille,
Non Agrippa, bono ſydere, ſed genitus.

A Her-

Fig. 3.5 “The Wind Carries it in His Belly,” Emblem 1, from Michael Maier, *Atalanta fugiens* (Oppenheim: Gallery, 1617; reprinted, Frankfurt, 1687). Courtesy of the Division of Rare and Manuscript Collections, Cornell University Library.

serves as the perfect model for an image of the Wind as a semi-divine, elemental force in the production of the Philosopher's Stone.

The motto that accompanies the emblem, "The wind carried it in its belly," is a line from the earliest extant alchemical treatise, the *Emerald Table* (or *Tabula Smaragdina*), probably dating from around the fourth century AD. This work describes the Philosopher's Stone, the goal of every alchemical process, as the child of the Sun and the Moon, borne by the Wind and nourished by the Earth.[29] All aspects of nature are necessary to the production of the stone, just as an understanding of the various mathematical disciplines – arithmetic, music (considered a mathematical discipline in early modern Europe), geometry, and astronomy – perfects the philosopher's understanding of the world. At any rate, this is the lesson Maier offers in his commentary on the image.

In his depiction of the Wind, Matthäus Merian has only departed slightly from the classical ideal, but the pregnant man, a popular concept in early modern culture,[30] twists the Vesalian model in a new direction. The Wind leads logically to the nurturing Earth, as the *Atalanta* evokes the Aristotelian elemental foundations of the alchemical process: earth, air, water, and fire. This Earth is not at all classical in form; the contrast with the Wind is striking. Her form oscillates between emphasis on the human body as a world, and the world as a human body: note that one arm is human, and seemingly independent from the globe of the body; the other arm arises from the globe itself. Her feet are more solidly on the ground, and the composition in the foreground of the engraving emphasizes downward movement or grounding. Nonetheless, traces of the depiction of the Wind remain in the background, in the form of clouds and upwardly sweeping mountains. The third emblem introduces the elements of water and fire, with the fire and smoke sweeping upwards, and echoing the Wind in the first emblem with its billowing clouds, while the water pours downwards, thus echoing the movement in the second emblem. While, by the time of the Renaissance, earth and water came to be associated with the feminine and fire with the masculine, all of these elements needed to be in balance, according to Hippocratic medicine, newly revived in the sixteenth century.[31] It is significant that all of the elements, including Earth, are crucial to the alchemical process, which does not consist of a shedding of the lower elements, earth and water, themselves linked to the feminine in most other philosophical discussions of the time. These emblems also suggest that the Philosopher's work should reflect the functioning of nature, not dominate or eliminate it.

---

[29] De Jong, p. 55.

[30] See, for example, Sherry Velasco, *Male Delivery: Reproduction, Effeminacy, and Pregnant Men in Early Modern Spain* (Nashville, TN: Vanderbilt University Press, 2006).

[31] The revival of Hippocrates is linked to representations of gender by Lorraine Daston and Katharine Park in their article, "The Hermaphrodite and the Orders of Nature: Sexual Ambiguity in Early Modern France," *Gay and Lesbian Quarterly* 1 (1995): 419–38.

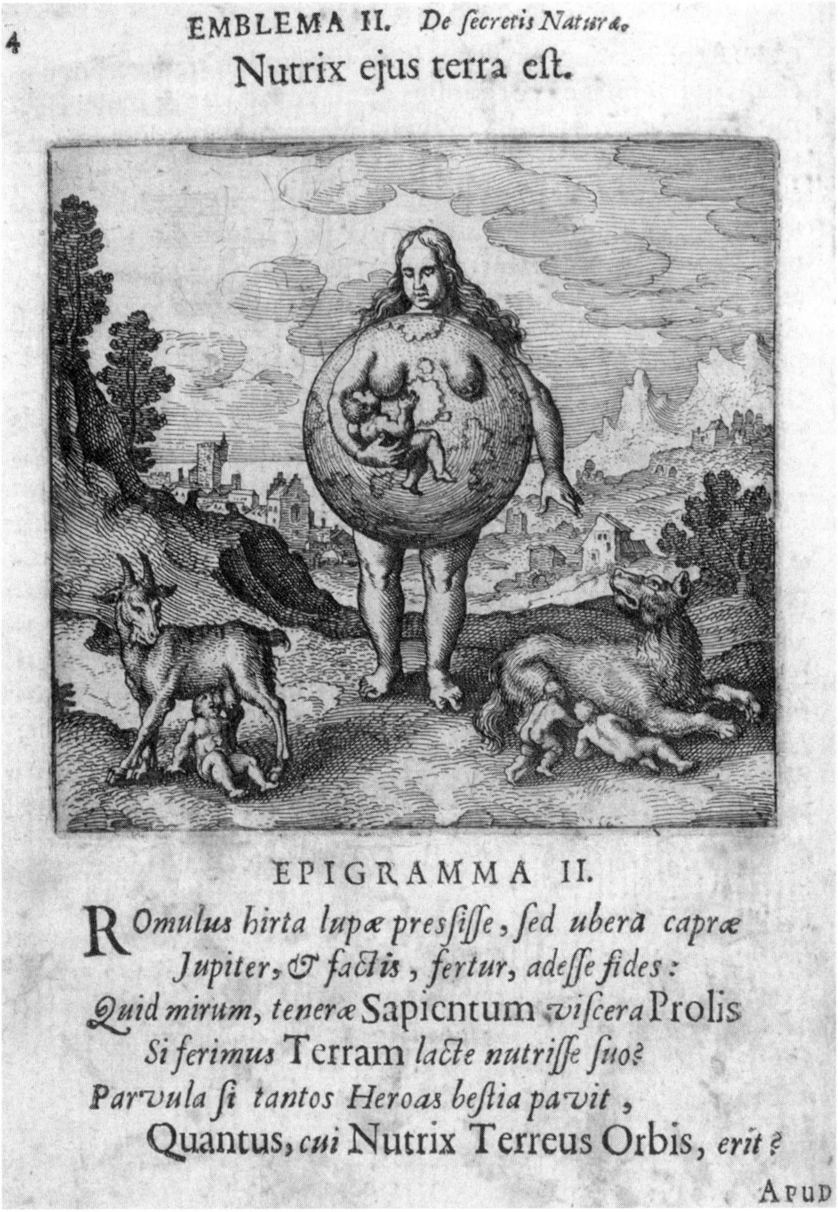

4

EMBLEMA II. *De secretis Naturæ.*

Nutrix ejus terra est.

EPIGRAMMA II.

R*omulus hirta lupæ pressisse, sed ubera capræ*
Jupiter, & factis, fertur, adesse fides:
Quid mirum, teneræ Sapientum *viscera* Prolis
Si ferimus Terram *lacte nutrisse suo?*
Parvula si tantos Heroas bestia pavit,
Quantus, *cui* Nutrix Terreus Orbis, *erit?*

APUD

Fig. 3.6 "The Earth is its Nurse," Emblem 2, from Michael Maier, *Atalanta fugiens*. Courtesy of the Division of Rare and Manuscript Collections, Cornell University Library.

The emblems of the *Atalanta* also reflect a play with categories or boundaries, particularly those involving the human body. While the first emblem underscores the dissolution of the human body into its surroundings (or, conversely, the coalescence of the wind into a human form), the boundaries dissolved in the second emblem are between the human and the animal, as wolves and goats nurture human babies (or divine, as in the tales of Romulus and Remus, and of Zeus/Jupiter, himself nurtured by a goat), and between the human microcosm and the natural macrocosm. The effacement and reestablishment of boundaries is a common theme in alchemical treatises, and so these works offer images of incest (brother/sister in the *Atalanta*, to symbolize Sol and Luna, Apollo and Diana, gold and silver; and mother/son in the *Rosarium philosophorum*), and of effeminacy, as in the case of the hydropic man (emblem XIII; see Teuton, figure 2), whose bloated body resembles that of a pregnant woman. This emblem also adds the element of water to the air/earth mix, as the hydropic man is both washed – that is bathed in water or dissolved in it, just as a chemical substance would be – and purged of his own disease, represented by excess fluid. This sort of paradox of adding and removal of elements is not uncommon in the alchemical process. The elements, earth, water, air, and fire, all dominate the emblems and are represented as the very bases of existence as well as the catalysts necessary for the alchemical process. The elements themselves are still gendered, with the earth represented as female (emblem II), water represented by an effeminate man (emblem XIII), air as masculine (emblem I), and fire most closely associated with the hermaphroditic rebis (emblem XXXIII). Thus, representations of the effacement and redrawing of boundaries in this treatise often involve an interplay between the masculine and the feminine.

Most striking among these representations of the human body is the rebis, a central figure in the alchemical process, representing the stage of conjunction of sulphur (Venus) and mercury, considered opposing elements but also the bases of existence in alchemical treatises of the early modern period. This conjunction of opposites leads to the production of the Philosopher's Stone, which symbolizes physical and spiritual perfection. The rebis is always represented with two heads, one male (generally with short hair) and one female (generally with long hair). Merian is careful to represent his rebis as hermaphroditic, that is, as having two sets of genitalia, one male and one female. This representation, in keeping with commentaries on the stage of conjunction in a number of alchemical treatises, suggests that while the elements are fused, they also retain their individual properties. This contrasts with the Ovidian myth of the hermaphrodite, in which the female Salmacis is subsumed into the male Hermaphroditus, who is weakened by her presence but retains his essential, and essentially masculine, identity.[32]

[32] Ovid (Publius Ovidius Naso), *Metamorphoses*, ed. William S. Anderson (Leipzig: Teubner, 1985) bk. 4, l.383.

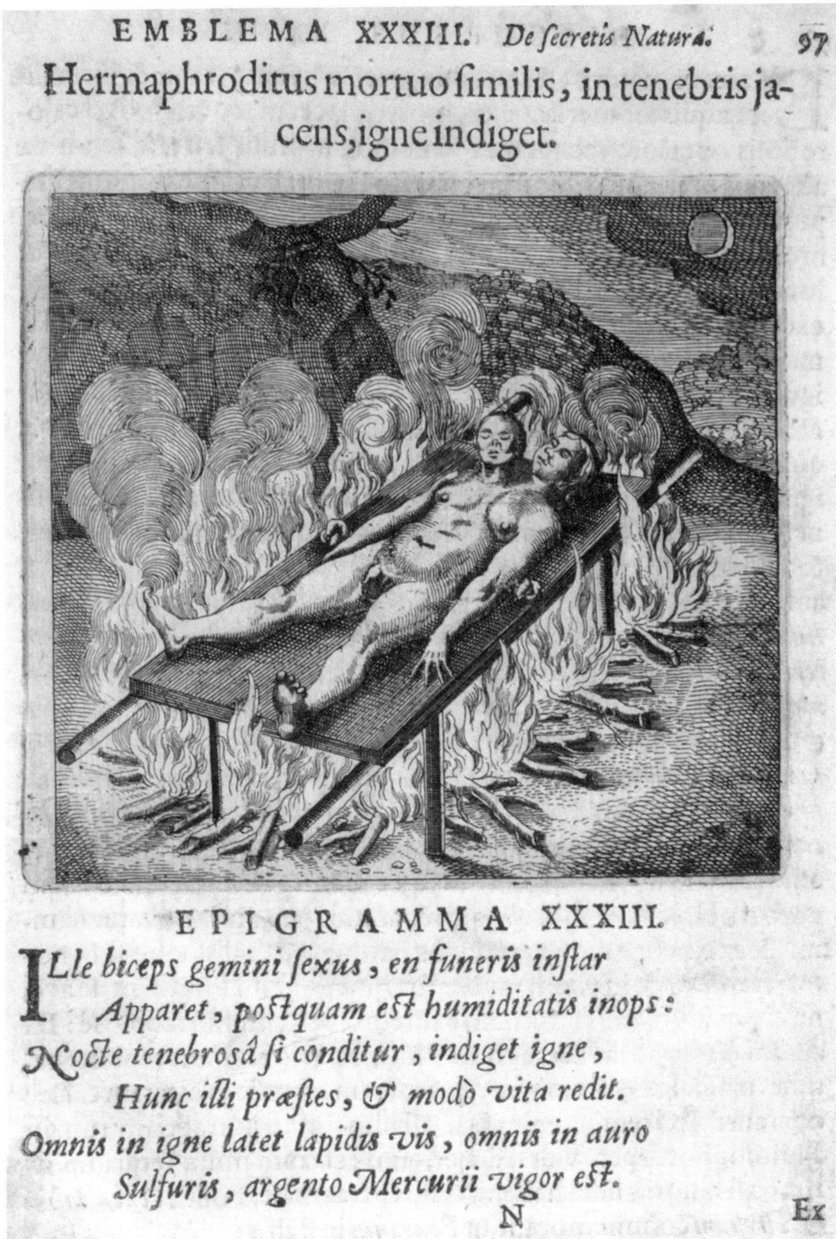

EMBLEMA XXXIII. *De ſecretis Naturæ.* 97

Hermaphroditus mortuo ſimilis, in tenebris jacens, igne indiget.

EPIGRAMMA XXXIII.

ILle biceps gemini ſexus, en funeris inſtar
Apparet, poſtquam eſt humiditatis inops:
Nocte tenebroſâ ſi conditur, indiget igne,
Hunc illi præſtes, & modò vita redit.
Omnis in igne latet lapidis vis, omnis in auro
Sulfuris, argento Mercurii vigor eſt.

N Ex

Fig. 3.7 The Hermaphrodite in the Stage of Putrefaction or Dissolution, Emblem 33 of the *Atalanta fugiens*, Michael Maier. Courtesy of the Division of Rare and Manuscript Collections, Cornell University Library.

Ovid's version is in line with the Aristotelian notions of gender, which present the female as a defective or lacking male.[33]

The alchemical rebis defies this vision of gender, by offering two distinct forms in one body. If the feminine aspect were merely a defective or lacking version of the masculine aspect, it would disappear into the masculine form, as Salmacis does into Hermaphroditus. The fact that the feminine aspect remains evident in the rebis, underscored both by the presence of female genitalia and one female breast, as well as by long hair, suggests that this figure is the union of two truly distinct forms, which retain that distinction even when joined. In this interplay between distinction and effacement of difference, most frequently resulting in a union of opposites that nonetheless allows those opposites to retain their distinct identities, Maier extends the representation of gender roles to a broader array of questions suggested by the imagery of the *Atalanta*, such as codependence of species (emblem II) and the problematic power and vulnerability of the king (emblems XXIV, XXVIII, XXXI, and XLVIII). The symbolic significance of the hermaphroditic rebis becomes quite capacious, as the ambiguity of the figure requires interpretation. In alchemical tradition, this hermaphroditic body is the ideal form. The Philosopher's Stone is often described as a hermaphrodite, as is the original God that created the universe.

I would like to argue that this anomalous body offers a potent political message, one echoed by Montaigne in a somewhat different context, his brief essay "On a Monstrous Child," the thirtieth essay in the second volume. After describing how this child, with a parasitic twin complete except for its head joined to him at the abdomen, is shown by relatives to anyone who will pay, he gives an interpretation: "This double body and its different parts, joined with one single head, could well provide a favorable prognostication to the King, that he might maintain under the union created by his laws these diverse parts and pieces of our state."[34] Montaigne is not overly optimistic about this possibility, but his vision of the union of disparate parts is not so distant from the alchemical notion of conjunction, where difference is joined together, but not assimilated into a uniform whole. He also argues, echoing St. Augustine's discussion of monsters in *The City of God*: "That which we call monsters are not such to God, who sees in the immensity of his creation the infinity of forms that he has included."[35] While Montaigne's "Monstrous Child" is

---

[33] Aristotle, *Generation of Animals*, in *The Complete Works of Aristotle*, Jonathan Barnes, ed. (Princeton, NJ: Princeton University Press, Bollingen Series, 1984) vol. 1, p. 1113 (716b 5).

[34] Michel de Montaigne, *Essais*, Pierre Villey, ed. (Paris: Presses Universitaires de France, 1978) vol. 1, p. 713: "Ce double corps et ces membres divers, se rapportans à une seule teste, pourroient bien fournir de favorable prognostique au Roy de maintenir sous l'union de ses loix ces pars et pieces diverses de nostre estat."

[35] "Ce que nous appellons monstres, ne le sont pas à Dieu, qui voit en l'immensité de son ouvrage l'infinité des formes qu'il y a comprinses."

the physical reverse of the alchemical rebis, being two bodies with one head, the lessons evoked by the two bear some resemblance.

What Montaigne's text makes clear is that, well before Hobbes, the body as metaphor for the body politic is not only current,[36] but already being turned in different directions by the use of unusual, disabled, or diseased bodies as metaphors for dysfunctional states. This problematic view of the body is evoked by Théodore Agrippa d'Aubigné in his epic on the Wars of Religion in France, *Les Tragiques*. He compares a France torn by civil war to a giant body afflicted by humoral imbalances and hydropsy.[37] While d'Aubigné more conventionally compares the dysfunctional state to a diseased body, Montaigne suggests that the unusual body of the "monstrous child" sends a different message: that of the potential harmony of the disparate factions in France at the end of the sixteenth century. In this context, the hermaphroditic rebis suggests a larger political arena for alchemical modes of thinking.

The lessons of Montaigne's monstrous child and of the alchemical rebis also bear some resemblance to those offered by Alice Dreger relative to conjoined twins. Western belief in the overriding importance of individuality may seem to drive the urge to surgically separate conjoined twins, as Dreger argues, but this urge also arises from the social importance of conforming to idealizing norms of corporeality, from a drive to efface individuals who are too different, too individual, as Davis has suggested in his essay on "Constructing Normalcy," cited above. This drive to create an individual who conforms to our view of bodily norms causes surgeons to impose often dangerous procedures on their conjoined twin patients, as well as on other individuals with "extraordinary bodies." Today, as in the early modern period, we still have difficulty accepting certain forms of difference. Yet conjoined twins often seem quite happy as they are. They almost always have two distinct personalities, with very different interests and impulses. This was true, for example, of Chang and Eng, the famous "Siamese twins" from the nineteenth century. Still, they learn from birth to compromise and to function as one, in order to survive, but ideally they do so without sacrificing their individuality, as present-day conjoined activists Abigail and Brittany Hensel do: "How do conjoined twins cope with their attachments? Like the rest of us who live in commitment with others, they work out explicit and tacit agreements about day-to-day living."[38] Yet, Dreger adds, "conjoinment does not automatically negate individual development and expression, any more than other forms of profound human relations do. Indeed, differing personalities and tastes are the rule among conjoined twins with

[36] For a critique of Hobbes's corporeal metaphors, see Moira Gatens, *Imaginary Bodies: Ethics, Power, and Corporeality* (London: Routledge, 1996), pp. 21–8.

[37] "Ce vieil corps tout infect, plein de sa discrasie,/ Hydropique…" ("This old body, completely infected and full of humoral imbalances, hydropic…"), ll. 146–7, from "Misères," in *Les Tragiques*, from the *Oeuvres*, H. Weber, ed. (Paris: Gallimard, 1969), p. 24.

[38] Alice Dreger, *One of Us: Conjoined Twins and the Future of Normal* (Cambridge, MA: Harvard University Press, 2005), pp. 38–41.

two conscious heads." The implications of this dual identity in one body, first suggested by Montaigne, are significant: in the relations we form and that are necessary to our existence, physical, familial, social, or political, it is possible to function as a unit without sacrificing difference. But this can only happen in a social and political context that embraces difference, rather than attempting to eliminate it, whether by means of eugenics or other means of limiting the lives or reshaping the bodies or minds of those who do not match up to our expectations. Pronounced bodily differences are a test of our capacity to accept difference; we are still in the process of working out how to include individuals with these differences in our societies. As Montaigne suggests, our capacity to embrace and comprehend physical difference has implications for a larger social arena, as a reader aware of Inquisition modes of torturing heretics would recognize when gazing on Maier's emblem of a rebis being calcinated by means of "mort à petit feu," or death by slow fire, a form of torture used both on heretics and recalcitrant natives of the Western hemisphere in the sixteenth and seventeenth centuries.

Alchemy, now rehabilitated as a proto-chemistry, a discipline without which chemistry might never have existed, by scholars such as Allen Debus,[39] William Newman, and Lawrence Principe, was mocked and discredited by Enlightenment and post-Enlightenment thinkers, particularly academics, and particularly those in the discipline of medicine. One need only read the opening pages of Mary Shelley's *Frankenstein* to see how far it had fallen out of grace even in the realm of popular culture by the early nineteenth century. Victor Frankenstein learns from his professors that his study of Cornelius Agrippa, Albertus Magnus, and Paracelsus, the greatest of alchemists, has been an utter waste of time: "Every minute … every instant that you have wasted on those books is utterly and entirely lost."[40] Alchemy was regarded as a monstrous practice. Yet it had been one of the few pursuits open to women, who were excluded from university studies and thus from the academic practices of science, as well as from the medical profession, and, increasingly,

---

[39] Allen Debus, *The Chemical Philosophy: Paracelsian Science and Medicine in the Sixteenth and Seventeenth Centuries* (New York: Science History Publications). This book was enormously influential in its redirection of modern understanding of the place of alchemy in the history of science. See also *Chemistry, alchemy and the new philosophy, 1550–1700: studies in the history of science and medicine* (New York: Variorum Reprints, 1987). For Lawrence Principe, see *The Aspiring Adept: Robert Boyle and his Alchemical Quest* (Princeton, NJ: Princeton University Press, 1998). William Newman's *Promethean Ambitions: Alchemy and the Quest to Perfect Nature* is a superb study of the relationship between early modern alchemy and modern scientific endeavors. A readable and cogent introduction to alchemy and early modern science is Bruce Moran's *Distilling Knowledge: Alchemy, Chemistry, and the Scientific Revolution* (Cambridge, MA: Harvard University Press, 2005). In terms of the larger social importance of alchemy, Tara Nummedal's recent study, *Alchemy and Authority in the Holy Roman Empire* (Chicago: University of Chicago Press, 2007) is the most comprehensive study to date.

[40] Mary Shelley, *Frankenstein* (New York: W.W. Norton, 1995), p. 26.

from midwifery. From the scholarship of Jayne Archer and Penny Bayer,[41] as well as many others, we know that quite a few women practiced alchemy both as a science, performing early versions of chemistry experiments, and as a philosophy, discussing what it meant for their place in the world. Thus, alchemy became a space for difference in a number of ways. Relative to women practitioners, it grants them a field in which to pursue scientific and philosophical inquiries, at a time when they remain shut out of official academic and scholarly circles, and as they are being excluded from domains of inquiry and practice formerly permitted to them, such as management of childbirth and other reproductive issues.

As has been mentioned above, alchemy had been for many centuries considered both a science and a philosophy of life, a process of perfecting nature and the self. While some alchemical treatises give precise "recipes" to follow for various chemical experiments, many, Michael Maier's *Atalanta fugiens* among them, were more like meditative exercises linked to the alchemical symbolism used in more practical manuals. What then, were individuals meditating on? One of the fundamental principles of alchemy is that both masculine and feminine elements are necessary for the perfection of any aspect of nature or man; another, that perfection arises out of imperfection and irreducible difference, not out of elimination of that imperfection or that difference. The constant representation of odd bodies in alchemical treatises – and Michael Maier's other treatises, as well as the works of other alchemists, foreground corporeal difference repeatedly – goes against the grain of idealizing and masculinizing representations of the body in medical works. It should be recognized that this privileging of radical bodily difference, including monstrosity (in the sense of cross-species hybrids), disability (in the sense of bodies that depart from an idealizing norm), and transgenderism all associate the feminine with the "monstrous" in alchemical lore. The difference from mainstream medical treatises is that the feminine and the monstrous are not judged to be inferior or defective, but valued as part of an ongoing process of perfection. Nonetheless, when alchemy is rejected as an outmoded and fantastical enterprise, not to be considered a science, the association of the monstrous and the feminine becomes grounds for denigration of the latter, rather than for reconsideration of what monstrosity might mean.

As Lennard Davis points out, the rationalizing impulses of the Enlightenment provided the context for the development of the science of statistics, and the perfection of means for measuring and categorizing human bodies. How differently

---

41 See the essays in this volume, as well as Penny Bayer's essays, "Jeanne du Port, alchemist daughter of Joseph du Chesne," *Rosenholmeren: Notiitser og Meddelelser fra Renaessancestudier ved Aarhus Universitet*, 6/7, (October 1999): 1–4, "Lady Margaret Clifford's Alchemical Receipt Book and the John Dee Circle," *Ambix* (November 2005): 271–84, and "From Kitchen Hearth to Learned Paracelsianism: Women's Alchemical Activities in the Renaissance,", in *"Mystical Metal of Gold": Essays on Alchemy and Renaissance Culture*, Stanton J. Linden, ed. (Brooklyn, NY: AMS Press, 2007), among other pieces. See also Jayne Archer, "Women and Alchemy in Early Modern England," unpublished PhD dissertation, University of Cambridge, 2000.

things might have turned out if alchemy, more imaginative, visual, and creative than many of the scientific disciplines devised by the Enlightenment, more inclusive of women as practitioners, and more open to diverse bodily forms, had not been discredited by the moderns. The eighteenth century saw the first clear elaborations of the concept of human rights in Europe, but the evolution of this concept in the West has often led to the exclusion from these rights of groups who don't fit into an idealized norm: women, openly gay, lesbian, bisexual or transgendered individuals, minorities, and the disabled. A number of modern medical practices, such as eugenics, forced sterilization, institutionalization, selective abortion, and aesthetic surgery, seem to have favored uniformity and elimination of differences; they go hand in hand with political and social systems that have privileged relatively narrow subgroups of people who fit a particular aesthetic ideal – one inspired at least in part by classical statuary such as the Apollo Belvedere. Alchemy offered the possibility of an exercise in familiarizing the strange, of embracing, rather than eliminating, difference. Let us embrace this aspect of alchemical thought as we face new challenges and an increasingly global culture.

Chapter 4
"Put Out of Her Course"[1]: Images of the Monstrous in de Bry's Illustrations of *Atalanta fugiens* and the *America*

Sean Teuton

In his introduction to the *America*,[2] Johann Theodor de Bry closes with the caveat:

> I ask most earnestly that if anyone else should be found attempting to pirate this book of mine (for nowadays there are many dishonest people who try to get the benefit of another's work), that no credit should be given to the counterfeit copy, for I have put secret marks in my drawings which will certainly cause confusion if they are omitted.

As engraver and publisher of the monumental volume describing for the people of Europe the land called America, de Bry offers the above warning to protect not only his investment but also his reputation. Surely, his "secret marks" will alert him to pirates, but how are his readers to know they are in the presence of the real text? How are they to identify the secret marks? Of course, if the engraver revealed the marks to his audience, they would no longer be secret. Now consider this odd paradox of textual secrecy in the warning to the anonymously authored alchemical treatise, *Rosarium philosophorum*:[3]

> Neither shall any man justly use slanderous and blasphemous words against me, for seeing that the Ancient Philosophers have written so obscurely and

[1] Francis Bacon, in his treatise *De dignitate et Augmentis scientiarum*, grapples with the categorization of monsters, and determines that the monstrous is nature "put out of her course."

[2] Stefan Lorant, ed. *The New World: The First Pictures of America* (New York: Duell, Sloan and Pierce, 1965), p. 228. All subsequent references to this book will appear parenthetically in the text. The *America* was a project to publish illustrated Latin versions of all known accounts of the "discovery," exploration, and conquest of the Western Hemisphere. This project was first undertaken by Theodor de Bry (1528–1598), in collaboration with his son Johann Theodor de Bry (1561–1623). The text cited constitutes selections from this project.

[3] http://levity.com/alchemy/rosary1.html (22 May 2006).

> confusedly that they are not understood, nor seem not to agree together, because diverse men searching after this most precious Art have either been deceived or terrified from their purpose…

Though undoubtedly not authored by de Bry, the *Rosarium*, like the *America*, is predicated on a hermeneutics of secrecy that strategically underwrites authorship while locating error in the reader. Both discourses – New World travel accounts and alchemy – share a similar tone of secrecy: alchemy has always demanded reading as a ritualized decoding of images; did New World travelogues borrow this theory of reading? And both forms elicit an attendant privacy. With the recent advent of print in early modern Europe, literacy, if not "visual" literacy, allowed reading to be a private, individual, even unique, act. Working during this time, de Bry pursues a unique authorship by stroking his signature into each depiction, sequestering it somewhere in the intricate engravings. But the public sphere challenged the secrecy and privacy of these discourses, so that although it was often declared "heretical," alchemy was a familiar and ancient science, predating Christianity, and discussions of travel to the Americas filled the collective minds of citizens, especially when an explorer set sail for "the Crown." So, it is ironic that in the midst of their declaration of boundaries between secrecy and revelation, alchemy and exploration also announce the arbitrary nature of socially designated boundaries and categories, and even encourage their transcendence. In the following pages, I offer an analysis of the shared characteristics of these two systems of representation – New World travel writing and alchemical treatises – as organized and authorized by Theodor de Bry and his son Johann Theodor de Bry, in order to explain how early modern Europe maintained a corpus of knowledge in the face of radical difference.

In an age that was opening up to many new worlds, Europeans in the sixteenth and seventeenth centuries found themselves staggering before multiple problems of difference: in scientific classification, in religious beliefs, in human form and behavior. While they explored and celebrated the idea of difference in alchemy, they confronted real difference in the New World. Since antiquity, alchemy had provided a safe form in which to explore a "theory" of difference; now that theory would be challenged with the introduction of lands and life more radically Other than Europeans had ever known. Tzvetan Todorov agrees: "[T]he discovery of America, or of the Americans, is certainly the most astonishing encounter of our history."[4] As Europeans broadened their experience geographically (and hence culturally) through trade and conquest, they were constantly forced to redefine their world: previous definitions of humans, animals, women, or men, and their "normal" behaviors were being called into question, and so definitions had to be written, categories invented, new boundaries drawn. But the troubling disintegration of boundaries designed to clarify for Europe the idea of civilized

---

[4] Tzvetan Todorov, *The Conquest of America: The Question of the Other*, trans. Richard Howard (New York: Harper, 1994), p. 4.

human culture was not only threatening; it was also liberating. Stephen Greenblatt, in *Marvelous Possessions*, understands that Europeans responded to encounters with the New World with "wonder" – an ambiguous, bodily response to the unfamiliar that brings simultaneously fear and attraction.[5] Interestingly, although it had provided this experience of wonder long before voyagers "discovered" the Americas, alchemy invokes the same reaction.

Contact with the New World greatly intensified the epistemological divisions that Europeans had been negotiating at least since the dawn of the Reformation; they had to deal with newly encountered lands and objects, peoples and practices that challenged their shared collection of assumptions regarding the known world. They had to remake their world. Through profoundly theory-mediated processes such as the discourses of alchemy and discovery, Europeans were able to re-present the previously unacceptable in compellingly safe, mimetic terms. In this way, through the often-suppressed implementation of systems of representation, the threat of difference was assimilated into European culture, taking shape in "neutral" texts that allowed for epistemic struggles to be played out. Both alchemy and exploration consisted of such texts, functioning as "pure" sites of signification in which Europeans sought freedom from the restraints of a culture in a time bound by rigid definitions of the world. Readers drawn to liberating manipulation in alchemy would be able to confirm its principles in New World travel writing, which also invited the free play of signs.

Of course, when we speak of a uniform and historically located European culture, such as "early modern Europe," we risk simplifying a complex region and era with diverse cultural, religious, and economic differences that no doubt influenced alchemical thought as well as the accounts of the Americas. For example, religious differences often determined the alchemical process of purifying baser substances into the Philosopher's Stone. According to Carl Jung, the Catholic Mass clearly parallels this experiment; the priest redeems the bread and wine so that they may be taken in perfection. But Jung, a Protestant, after reading the Offertory, suddenly declares "[t]here is no sign of that unworthy sinful man whom Protestantism has so often slandered in the past …"[6] The different religious representations of alchemy are further complicated by the fact that the alchemical process predates Christianity; *Atalanta fugiens*,[7] the alchemical text which was probably illustrated by Matthäus Merian, a son-in-law of the elder de

---

5 Stephen Greenblatt, *Marvelous Possessions: The Wonder of the New World* (Chicago: Chicago University Press, 1991), p. 16–20.

6 C.G. Jung, *Psychology and Alchemy*, trans. R.F.C. Hull (Princeton: Princeton University Press, 1968), p. 312.

7 Michael Maier, *Atalanta fugiens*, trans. and ed. Joscelyn Godwin (Grand Rapids: Phanes, 1989). All subsequent references to this book will appear parenthetically in the text. The full text is available only in Latin, in a facsimile version published in 1964 (Kassel: Bärenreiter-Verlag). The most complete commentary on the work is still H.M.E. de Jong's *Michael Maier's Atalanta Fugiens: Sources of an Alchemical Book of Emblems* (Leiden: E, J. Brill, 1969).

Bry, is largely rooted in Graeco-Egyptian legends of alchemical knowledge, but is also buffered with medieval versions of the ancient art. Accounts of the New World Americans reveal the same troubling difference of European religious influence. According to Frank Lestringant, Catholic accounts of the voyages to Brazil were frustrated with the relationship of cannibalism to the taking of the Eucharist,[8] while Protestant accounts often demonized Catholics and Native people alike for at least sharing the idea of this practice. But by any sampling of accounts, the conquerors of America were equally confident and brutal in their enterprise.

However, if early modern European readership constitutes something like a mass audience, demanding texts that publishers provided, then perhaps the diverse groups of Europe shared much more than a continent. This audience reveals a shared system of representation and a view of knowledge and a collection of values that de Bry's *Atalanta fugiens* and the *America* both demonstrate. After all, the engraver was not the sole author of his publications; instead, capitalizing on the needs and sensibilities of a European readership, he was instrumental in compiling multiple accounts of individuals repeating a similar narrative. *Atalanta* was a famous book, first published in Latin in 1617, and reissued with corrections only a year later.[9] According to Gordon Sayre, the *America* series enjoyed a wide popular audience, and was translated into multiple European languages.[10] Both texts were especially known for their fantastic pictures that also guaranteed a broad audience by capturing the interest of Europe's less literate sector. Still, even with these considerations in mind, I have tried to recognize representational differences where they might appear.

The work of Theodor and Johann Theodor de Bry forms the nexus between images of American peoples and those in alchemical formulae. As the enigmatic Flemish goldsmith, bookseller, and engraver of mid-sixteenth-century Europe, a persecuted Huguenot who had to flee his homeland, the elder de Bry occupies an interesting position as illustrator of texts both illuminating and heretical. He and his son searched widely for material for the *America* volumes and took tremendous poetic license in their eclectic renditions of the land and people of the New World, a world they never visited.[11] As stated above, another member of the de Bry family, a member of their workshop as well, also most likely took part in the engraving of the famous alchemical treatise *Atalanta fugiens* by the

---

[8] Frank Lestringant, *Cannibals: The Discovery and Representation of the Cannibal from Columbus to Jules Verne*, trans. Rosemary Morris (Berkeley: California University Press, 1997), p. 9.

[9] Godwin, preface to the *Atalanta fugiens*, p. 10.

[10] Gordon M. Sayre, *Les Sauvages Americains: Representations of Native Americans in French and English Colonial Literature* (Chapel Hill: North Carolina University Press, 1997), pp. 55–6.

[11] Bernadette Bucher, *Icon and Conquest: A Structural Analysis of the Illustrations of de Bry's Great Voyages*, trans. Basia Miller Gulati (Chicago: University of Chicago Press, 1981), pp. 7–9.

erudite Michael Maier,[12] works that bear unmistakable resemblances to the images of the *America*.[13] This essay will explore the characteristics these two texts share, and what the significance of these resemblances might be. How does alchemical thinking influence the "discoveries" and depiction of Europe's *terra incognita*? And how does the European encounter with people of different cultures, with often radically alien worldviews, challenge alchemical thought?

In many ways, de Bry's *America* helped to inscribe the monstrous view of the cultural Other. Europeans, shaped by prevailing ideologies of the period, hoped to confirm in the Americas their suspicion of things and life outside their sphere of understanding. They were both compelled and repulsed by that which evaded familiar nomenclature. So, although some European thinkers in the skeptical tradition (like Montaigne)[14] questioned their rigid epistemology, such New World phenomena were often simply defined as "monstrous." Jeffrey Jerome Cohen, in his introduction to the collection of essays on *Monster Theory*, identifies the cultural origin of the monster, the construction of which he finds to be part of a recurring cultural epistemic practice, in the failure of binary thinking; the monster defies interpretation: "The monster always escapes because it refuses easy categorization."[15] And the representation of the monstrous is not always preconscious, a simple reflex response to the inscrutable, though it may begin as such. Cohen instead argues that cultural and racial alterity are often deliberately categorized as monstrous for reasons of power: "In the United States, American Indians were presented as unredeemable savages so that the powerful political machine of Manifest Destiny could push westward with disregard." (Cohen, p. 8) The sixteenth-century French cosmographer André Thevet, whose narratives de Bry illustrates, solves the problem of monsters by devising a curious taxonomy of "singularity," in which each anomaly is assigned a category of its own. Lestringant describes Thevet's manner of interpreting the monstrous behavior of the indigenous people of Brazil: "The most violent condemnations … to be found on every page are nearly always neutralized a line or two later by eulogies …"[16] In his shifting between European definitions of human and nonhuman behavior, Thevet struggles to understand the ways of the American Others, and, like his contemporaries, he often fails. The distorting lens of conquest, in its demand to legitimate the destruction of life, corrupted cultural accounts, reducing them to fabulation.

---

[12] See Godwin, p. 15.

[13] Bucher, p. 55.

[14] See Montaigne's famous essay, "Des Cannibales," for a challenge to Renaissance positivist thinking.

[15] Jeffrey Jerome Cohen, "Monster Culture (Seven Theses)," *Monster Theory*, ed. Jeffrey Jerome Cohen (Minneapolis: Minnesota University Press, 1996), p. 6.

[16] Frank Lestringant, *Mapping the Renaissance World: The Geographical Imagination in the Age of Discovery*, David Fausett, trans. (Berkeley: California University Press, 1994), p. 58.

Satisfying his audience, not always fully literate, de Bry often dazzled his European readers with the abominable, but having never traveled to America, the engraver obtained all of his information from second-hand, frequently dubious, sources;[17] so the images of the monstrous that abound in the *America* speak largely to a pervasive fear of and fascination with the liminal. Although alchemy served to contain concerns about the monstrous, the *America*'s announcement of life in the New World more than likely rekindled the anxiety of Otherness. One could say that the European's discovery of America took place at a "fortuitous" time in the European imagination; Europeans were still enduring the Inquisition and were in the midst of hateful sectarian rivalries. The New World became an opportunity to focus on what was represented as a greater evil without than within European borders. De Bry's collection of accounts of the discovery and conquest of this new land forced Europeans to confront and account for a world that evaded the careful classifications that defined normalcy, and so the unfamiliar was often reduced to the category of monster, a catch-all for whatever evaded already established definitions of race, gender, national origin, or species. Represented in the pages were Native cultures that appeared to erode these arbitrary boundaries. Only monsters transgressed such boundaries. But readers would be pacified by the knowledge that the monstrous nonhuman at times could also be saved by their conversion to Christianity and subordination within European colonial hierarchies, controlling them and thereby making them less monstrous, less threatening. Let me now offer an analysis of two de Bry illustrations, one from the *America*, the other alchemical, but both representative of the European preoccupation with the monstrous.

In his illustrations of the New World in the *America*, de Bry shows "Hermaphrodites as Laborers,"[18] with a caption most likely of his own composition, although taken from the source. In the engraving, muscular males with feminized faces and long, flowing hair carry the bodies of dead or injured warriors. Due in part to their extreme physical strength, they are chosen for this task. And although they are considered "odious" and are used as "beasts of burden," the "hermaphrodites" seem to fulfill a spiritual, healing function: they attend the dead; they "look after those who have contagious diseases; they take the sick on their shoulders to places selected for the purpose and feed and care for them until they are well again" (Lorant, p. 69). Judith Lorber, in her discussion of the Native American "berdache," a man who dresses and behaves like a woman and has a male partner, says that the berdache's "social status is defined by work and dress and sometimes a sacred calling."[19] Here, the marginal status of hermaphrodites, really berdaches or what we would now call transgendered males, instills in them a sacred power unknown to those of a single gender. The hermaphrodites/

---

[17] Stefan Lorant, "Notes on Le Moyne, Le Challeux, de Bry," *The New World*, pp. 30–31.

[18] Lorant, p. 69, originally from Theodor de Bry, *America, Brevis narratio eorum quae in Florida Americae provincial Gallis acciderunt…* (Frankfurt: de Bry, 1591), plate 17.

[19] Judith Lorber, *Paradoxes of Gender* (New Haven: Yale University Press, 1994), p. 91.

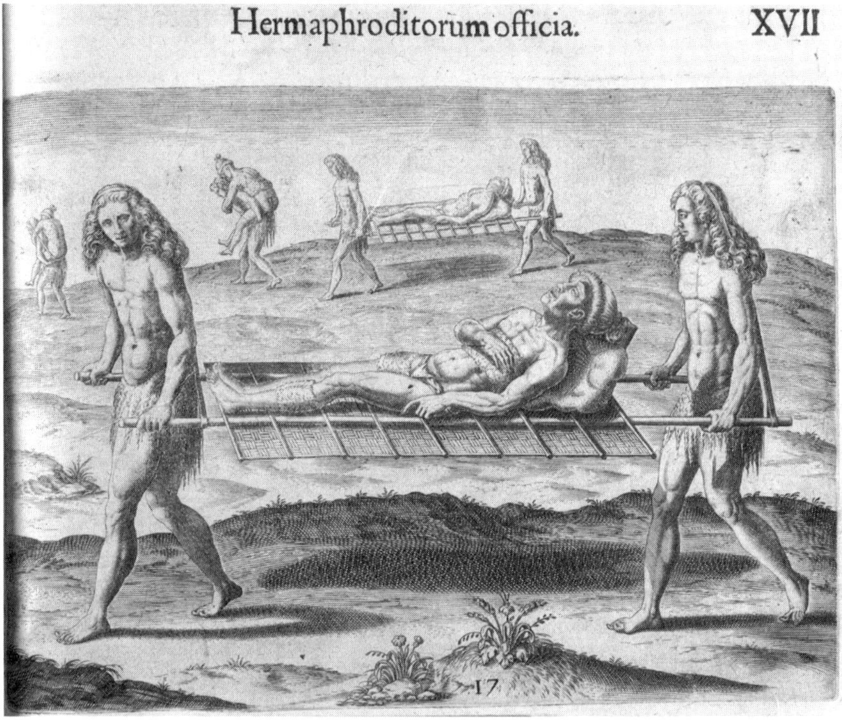

Fig. 4.1 The Tasks of Hermaphrodites, from Theodor de Bry, *America, Brevis narratio eorum quae in Florida Americae provincial Gallis acciderunt...* (Frankfurt: De Bry, 1591). Courtesy of the Division of Rare and Manuscript Collections, Cornell University Library.

berdaches painted themselves and often wore feathers: "How easy it must have been for Europeans, who conventionally associated such cosmetics with women, to think that all Indians were sodomites!"[20] Richard Trexler remarks. This display of apparently fluid gender boundaries receives the dual response of disgust and reverence, the kind of ambiguous reaction that Europeans often experienced in their contact with the Other.

Hermaphrodites, or beings of ambiguous gender, are represented in much the same way in alchemical treatises. See, for example, "Emblem 13. The Ore of the Philosophers is dropsical, and needs to be washed seven times in, just as the leper Naaman in the Jordan," which depicts a human of ambiguous sex, with a rounded, hairless, feminine body and the bearded head of a man.[21] S/he is the purifying agent

[20] Richard Trexler, *Sex and Conquest: Gendered Violence, Political Order, and the European Conquest of the Americas* (Ithaca, NY: Cornell University Press, 1995), p. 67.

[21] *Atalanta*, emblem 13, p. 131 in the Godwin edition.

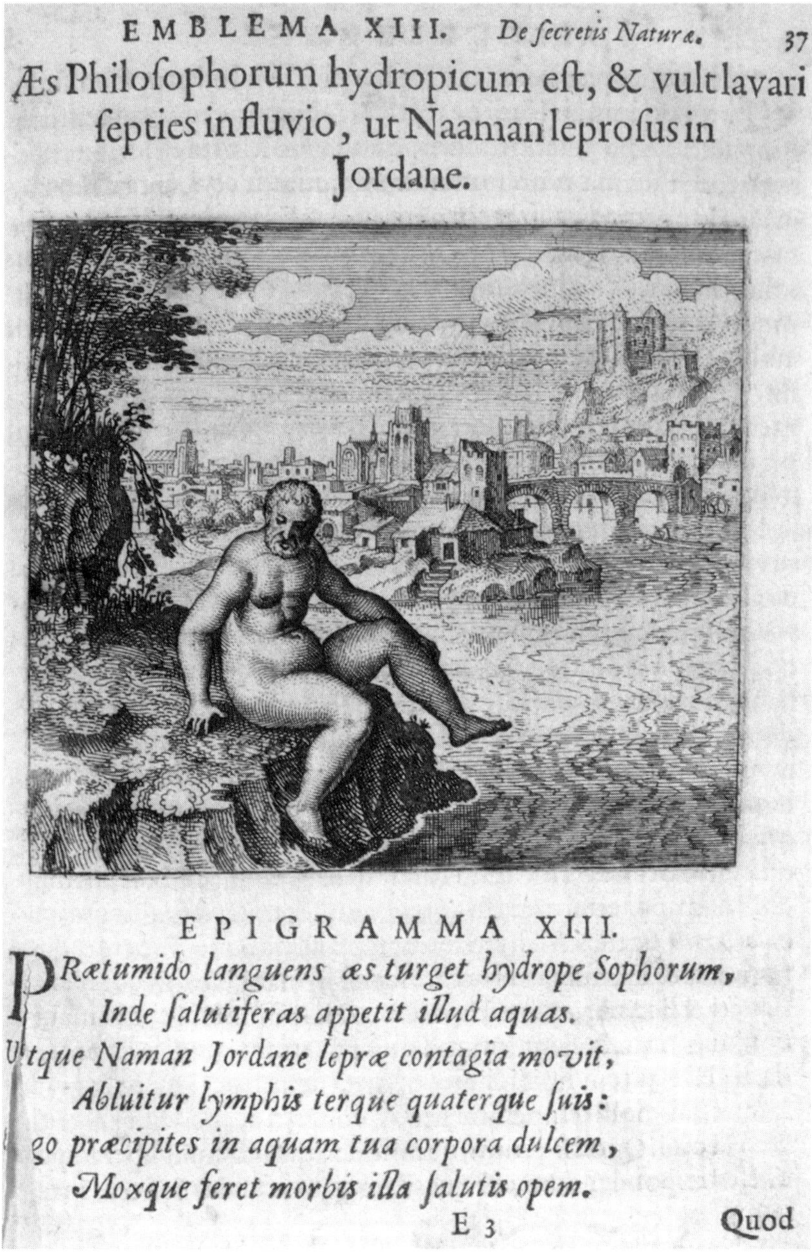
EMBLEMA XIII. *De ſecretis Naturæ.* 37

Æs Philoſophorum hydropicum eſt, & vult lavari ſepties in fluvio, ut Naaman leproſus in Jordane.

EPIGRAMMA XIII.

PRætumido languens æs turget hydrope Sophorum,
Inde ſalutiferas appetit illud aquas.
Utque Naman Jordane lepræ contagia movit,
Abluitur lymphis terque quaterque ſuis:
go præcipites in aquam tua corpora dulcem,
Moxque feret morbis illa ſalutis opem.

E 3 Quod

Fig. 4.2 The Hydropic Man, Emblem 13 of the *Atalanta fugiens*, Michael Maier (Frankfurt: De Bry, 1617; this illustration from a later edition (Frankfurt,1687)). Courtesy of the Division of Rare and Manuscript Collections, Cornell University Library.

of the "Ore of the Philosopher," the alchemist's gold. Having the liminal position of both male and female, occupying both symbolic roles, the hermaphrodite would seem to be the natural agent for the cleansing and purification of the Philosopher's Stone. Europeans used this alchemical view of gender to explain the unfamiliar gender formations among the autochthons of "Florida." In the eyes of European observers, the American hermaphrodite would be the natural agent to ease those who occupy a temporarily liminal state into a more comfortable place: from sickness to health or from life to death. Another striking engraving in *Atalanta* is that of a hermaphrodite in Emblem 33: "The Hermaphrodite, like a corpse, lying in the dark, needs fire" (see Long, Figure 3.7).[22] Merian seems to have taken his knowledge of the duties of "hermaphrodites" in the New World, and grafted it onto his alchemical image. Because the hermaphrodite cares for corpses, he is "like a corpse," occupying that same space between the living and the dead, mediating between the two realms. Vibrating between two symbolic realms, that of the sun and that of the moon, that of man and that of woman, he thrives in a perpetual death-rebirth cycle from dark to light, moon to sun. In the engraving, the hermaphrodite lies on a platform resembling the bench or cot used to aid in the treatment of the sick (plate 20 of the *Brevis narratio*) or a cooking platform much like that of the Native Americans cooking fish in de Bry's earlier engravings.[23] In fact, the platform echoes very closely a grilling platform depicted in one of de Bry's engravings of the cannibals of Brazil from part three of the *America*.[24] Thus, the boundaries between life and death, self and other veer into the eerie and grotesque.

How do we explain this link between the images? Alchemy offered early modern Europeans a suppressed epistemology designed to deal with difference. Since ancient times, alchemy has been relegated to the level of a superstition in a number of contexts: at worst a bogus system of medieval humbugs, at best a predecessor of modern science worthy of historical documentation.[25] But scientists and historians have until recently ignored the symbolic imagery and rhetoric that forms the basis for the process not just of turning baser metals into gold, but also of purifying nature by reuniting that which has been rent asunder, or reshaping nature by dissolving its substances and reassigning boundaries between them. The pursuit of alchemy involves an unending process of refinement enacted through the arcane and solitary contemplation of the alchemist. He must be of the proper mind; that is, his soul must be at peace while performing the process. Tied up in secrecy, alchemy's true formulae are shared only between those worthy of its secrets. All of this recalls the paradoxical warning in de Bry's introduction to the

[22] Godwin, p. 171.

[23] Plate 24 in the *Admiranda narratio, fida tamen, de commodis et incolarum ritibus Virginiae ... Anglico scripta sermone à Thomas Hariot* (Frankfurt: de Bry, 1590).

[24] *Americae tertia pars memorabilem provinciae Brasiliae historiam continens, Germanico primum sermone scriptam à Ioanne Stadio*...(Frankfurt: Matthias Becker, 1592, then 1605), no plate number.

[25] Kathleen Perry Long, "Salomon Trismosin and Clovis Hesteau de Nuysement: The Sexual Politics of Alchemy in Early Modern France," *L'Esprit Créateur* (Summer 1995): 9.

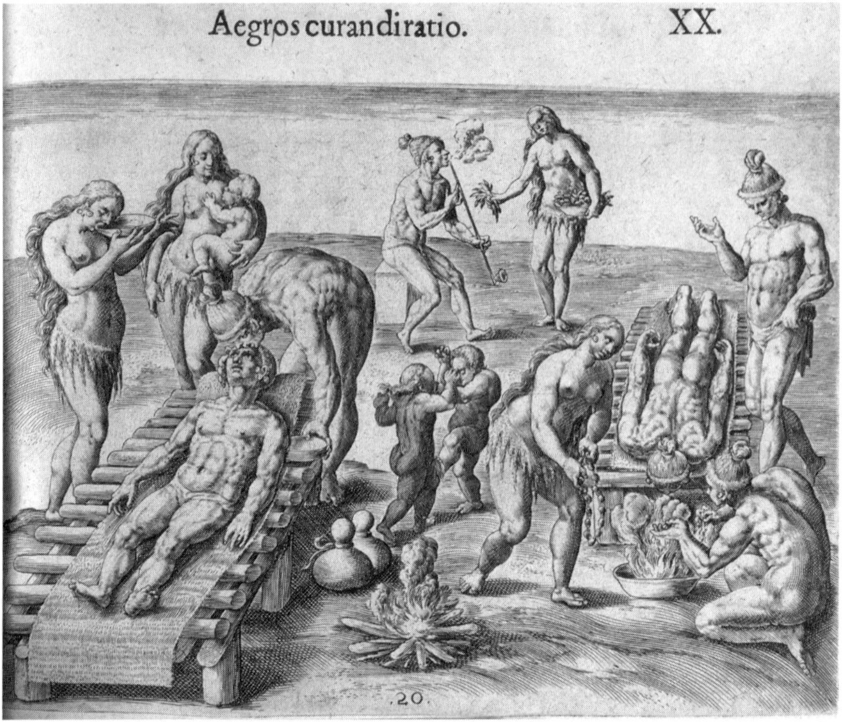

Fig. 4.3 Curing the Sick, from Theodor de Bry, *America, Brevis narratio eorum quae in Florida Americae provincial Gallis acciderunt…* (Frankfurt: De Bry, 1591). Courtesy of the Division of Rare and Manuscript Collections, Cornell University Library.

America: one only knows the secret if one knows the secret. Alchemy is replete with such seemingly absurd paradoxes. In his *Psychology and Alchemy*, Jung even declares alchemy to be "nonsense":

> Such is, superficially and in the roughest outline, the framework of alchemy as known to us all. From this point of view of our modern knowledge of chemistry it tells us little or nothing, and if we turn to the texts and the hundreds and hundreds of procedures and recipes left behind by the Middle Ages and antiquity, we shall find relatively few among them with any recognizable meaning for the chemist. He would probably find most of them nonsensical, and furthermore it is certain beyond all doubt that no real tincture or artificial gold was ever produced during the many centuries of earnest endeavor. What then, we may fairly ask, induced the old alchemists to go on laboring … if their whole undertaking was so portentously futile?[26]

[26] Jung, pp. 239, 241.

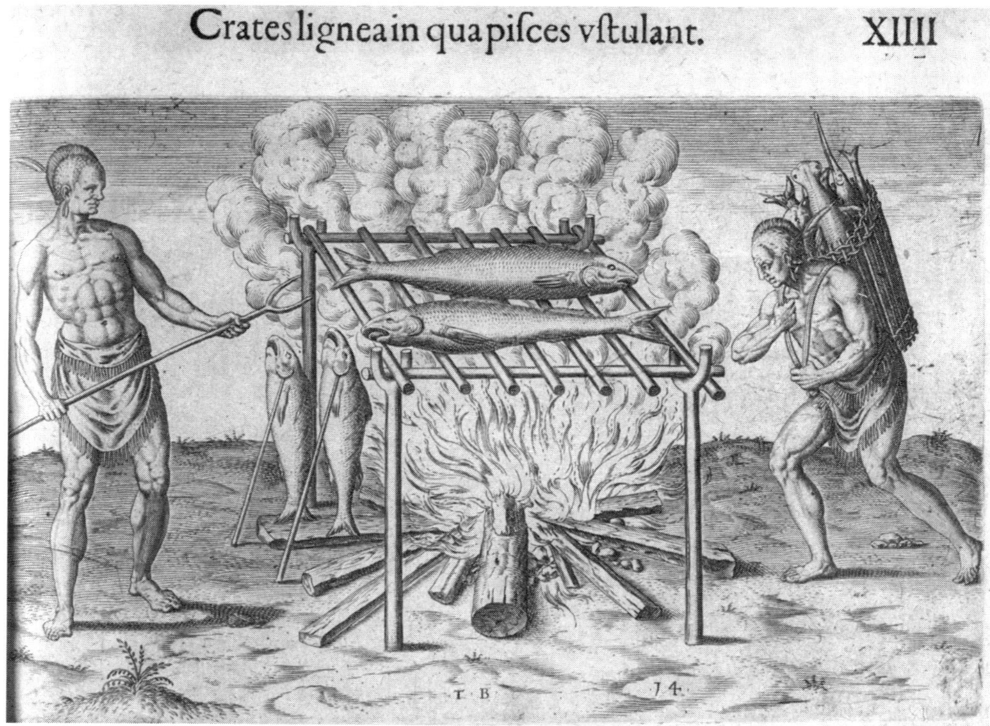

Fig. 4.4 Cooking Fish, from de Bry, *America, Brevis et fida narratio Virginiae* (Frankfurt: De Bry, 1591). Courtesy of the Division of Rare and Manuscript Collections, Cornell University Library.

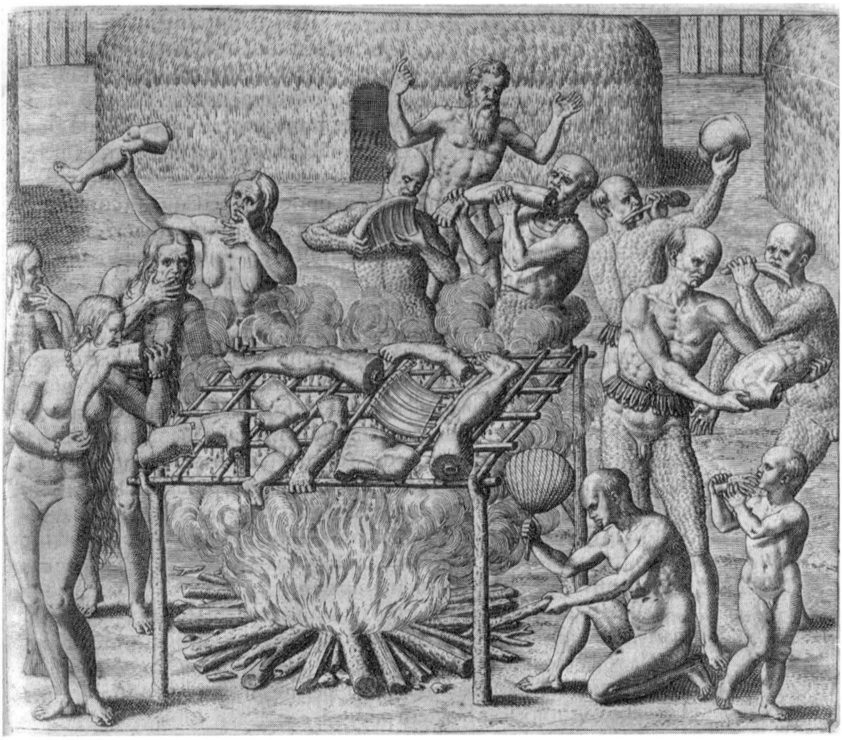

Fig. 4.5 Cannibals Cooking Humans, from de Bry, *America tertia pars, Historia navigationis in Brasiliam* (Frankfurt: de Bry, 1591). Courtesy of the Division of Rare and Manuscript Collections, Cornell University Library.

Jung answers himself: it was the "satisfaction born of the enterprise; the excitement of the adventure, of the *quaerere* (seeking) and the *invenire* (finding)."[27] In Jung's description of alchemy, one can perceive the project of seeking new worlds: alchemists and explorers alike persisting in the seemingly futile, proceeding for the sake of process, caught up in the "excitement of the adventure," in a (generally) vain hope of "finding." And nonsense was what both seekers often found. De Bry seems to proceed in his depiction of the New World with an alchemical authority and conviction, as if he is offering a gift of divine secrets known only to the chosen. We find other formal peculiarities of alchemy in de Bry's publications on the Americas.

Process, in the sense of one's deliberate and carefully sequenced actions, gives alchemy its performative form. To be successful, one must act out the formulaic sequence ritually, ceremonially. As much a part of things said are things seen. The

[27] Jung, p. 241.

visual aspect of alchemy is all-important, a fact that explains the explosive growth in publication of alchemical emblem-books throughout the sixteenth, seventeenth, and eighteenth centuries. For the *Atalanta*, aural dimensions play an equal part in the process. And so, alchemy calls for the absolute involvement of the subject in the role of the original alchemical philosopher, replicating the "experiment." Such ritualistic reenactment recalls the Catholic sacrament of the holy Eucharist, in which one ceremonially reenacts the original sacrifice of Christ by eating of his body and drinking his blood. But Jung cautions "One might be tempted to explain the symbolism of alchemical transformation as a parody of the Mass were it not pagan in origin and much older than the latter."[28]

Atalanta fugiens is a unique alchemical text because it succeeds in orchestrating disparate expressive forms, emblems, epigrams, and fugues, into one powerful unit. One must surround oneself with its visual, verbal, and aural symbolic imagery to perform it; it must be performed in order to have its purpose fulfilled. Celebrating the ancient and divine mixing and uniting of opposite forces, *Atalanta* is a sort of prayer, a blissful and rejoicing one for the most part (even if the treatise is replete with images of sacrifice and loss). Its collection of musical "fugues" is three-voiced to correspond to the three necessary raw elements of alchemy: mercury, sulfur, and salt. Furthermore, the fugues align themselves with the repeated rejoicing of combined energies of "opposites," such as man and woman, by analogy. The word "fugue" means "the hunt or the flight of voices from each other," a meaning that echoes the Greek myth on which the very title of the work is based. Atalanta, the beautiful princess who could outrun all her suitors, was caught by Hippomanes when he tossed out three golden apples in her path. This powerful tension works in analogy to the symbolic opposing forces of man and woman, hunter and hunted. The building energy throughout the text moves toward a harmony fueled by the intense pull between polarities of not only the symbolic sexes, humans and monsters, and death and life, but also between disparate forms of musical, poetic, and visual arts.[29]

Like an alchemical text, the *America* encourages the same active role in its readers: it seems to build inexorably volume by volume, but accreting into an ultimate depiction of a degenerate and monstrous, even demonic, New World. Each image corresponds to captions of fantastic description. The text, building image upon image, leads its reader toward the mixing and uniting of disparate forces. For example, the image of cannibalism, undoubtedly one of the most transgressive and taboo of human practices – and a symbol of the tension between the forces of death and life – builds at the end of the *America* series, when the security of imposed boundaries of European society were likely to be at their nadir, and when wars of religion dominated the social scene. Eroding early modern European systems of classification and offering more fluid models both threatened

---

[28] Jung, p. 313.

[29] Hildemarie Streich, introduction, *Atalanta fugiens*, ed. Joscelyn Godwin, pp. 21–4, 33–5.

and renewed the controlling mindset of the age. Both *Atalanta* and the *America* flirt heretically with theological, political, and sociological systems by calling into question the often arbitrary divisions that fight to instill identification and difference in the period. Although the monstrous had purchase on the European consciousness since antiquity, it was an object both of extreme fascination and extreme abhorrence in the early modern period, perhaps abetted by the advent of printing, as a proliferation of treatises on monstrosity suggests.

Many historical forces likely played a part in this pervasive crisis of representation. Christianity had privileged mind over body, man over woman. The Bible had divided and enumerated its people, separated clean humans and animals from the unclean. Plagues, religious wars, witch hunts, and inquisitions wracked the continent, spreading a paranoia that not only shunned the outsider, but created her as such, pointed her out, hunted her down, and put her to death. Jean de Léry, the French Protestant missionary and travel writer of *History of a Voyage to the Land of Brazil*, witnessed barbarities in his own land as severe as any encountered in the Americas. Persecuted and besieged during the Wars of Religion (1562–1598), he watched his own people eat each other.[30] Europeans were shaped and ruled by thinking that was at once self-protective and destructive, thinking that required its proliferation for its survival. So a social consciousness persisted that sought order by means of rejection of that which appeared out of place. The Occident inscribed the monstrous as that which challenged the ordained divisions between entities. Those who challenged religious doctrines or societal norms were denounced as witches or heretics. Any bodily deformity was thought to be the result of a demon seed, for it evaded the anatomical rules, stepped over the boundary. Too many toes signified aggression against the divine; a deficiency or absence of features announced the subhuman or the decrepit. This was a time when the half-human half-animal "wild man" was believed to stalk the forests of Europe, wandering somewhere outside of civilization.[31] Predictably, Europe "discovered" this savage beast, both the divine predecessor and the evil aberration of humanity, in the New World: the so-called Indian.[32] Along with the wild man, behemothic monsters were thought to hunt the sea and stalk the land of the New World. Travel writers tell of monstrous sea dogs that are part fish, part bird, part mammal, amphibious creatures that chase after sailors until they are clubbed to death.[33] The depiction of these fantastic creatures in the *America* marks a European ambivalence toward a world that offered freedom from the boundaries imposed by their own culture. The dissolution of those boundaries evoked both horror and desire. As A. James Arnold suggests that it is difficult to categorize the monstrous, whence derives its

---

[30] Janet Whatley, introduction, *History of a Voyage to the Land of Brazil*, ed. Janet Whatley (Berkeley: University of California Press, 1990), p. xviii.

[31] Whatley, p. xxii.

[32] See Hoxie Neale Fairchild, *The Noble Savage: A Study in Romantic Naturalism* (New York: Columbia University Press, 1928).

[33] Bucher, p. 150.

monstrosity. Even New World cartography gives evidence of a fear of marginality: "Monsters lurked in the seas at the edges (liminal sites) of the known world as cartographers conceived them. Moreover, these monsters were logical projections of Otherness, within the discourse of European superiority. When actual monsters were not encountered by the explorers, monstrous traits were attributed to whatever Natives were at hand in order to justify branding them enemies of God."[34] Like cartography, alchemy also uses a spatial "map" in describing its process in images. These images often have their most revealing configurations in their margins, at their borders; one might note, for instance, the ruins in the background of a number of emblems of the *Atalanta* (1, 14, 16, 50), the obelisk and curious double obelisk forms, also echoed by church steeples (3, 4, 5, 6, 7, 8, 11, 27, 36, 37, 39, 40, 50), islands, ships, cubes, moons, all symbolizing stages of the process. In ancient and modern city planning, obelisks were used to mark significant historical events, but also significant locations and monuments; alchemical emblems in the *Atlanta*, by pushing these objects into the background, even though their significance might be central to the process, create a movement of attention between the central figures and the margins or the background. Similarly, the *Atalanta* explores the boundaries between male and female, human and animal, Both the *America* and the *Atalanta* signal a suppressed curiosity for the manipulation and reconfiguring of arbitrary boundaries between beings and objects. Different genders often blur into one sex, as the women of the New World are sometimes masculinized in appearance, the men often feminized, according to European ideals; there is also an obsession with New World sexuality, which is frequently portrayed as deviant. Different races can sometimes seem the same, for example, the depictions of the women of the New World according to a European mannerist aesthetic: blonde, long-legged, with short torso and small breasts. Different metals can be made to be the same. All of this signals a discomfort with sacrosanct categories.

The monstrous also threatens carefully wrought divisions between the sexes. Gender was socially constructed to empower the dominant sex; it was subverted, frequently by means of cross-dressing, to escape the oppression of such a system. Judith Lorber reminds us that:

> In early modern England, the state enforced class and gender boundaries through sumptuary laws that dictated who could wear certain colors, fabrics, and furs. Cross-dressing and wearing clothes "above one's station"… thus were important symbolic subverters of social hierarchies at a time of changing modes of production and a rising middle class.[35]

Those who were biologically of a mixed sex, hermaphrodites, or those who displayed social behaviors considered at variance with their sex, not to mention

---

[34] A. James Arnold, "Introduction," in *Monsters, Tricksters, and Sacred Cows: Animal Tales and American Identities*, ed. A. James Arnold (Charlottesville: University of Virginia Press, 1996), pp. 9–10.

[35] Lorber, p. 87.

those who engaged in same sex coupling, were generally considered abominations. Julia Kristeva explains the above phenomenon in terms of what she has called the abject, that which is rejected and distanced from the self to form the subject. Because the abject is both part of the self and of the other, the subject forever pursues and abhors the abject. Kristeva finds boundaries both psychologically constructed and permeable; the subject stands before the abject in terror and awe.[36] This production of Otherness sheds some light on Europeans' reactions to the indigenous inhabitants of the New World as well as its ongoing obsession with alchemy. Both experiences fulfill the ambiguous need for the clarification of the self and the exploration of the boundary between the self and the other. Of course, women have been associated with the monstrous since the ancient Greeks, as suggested by Aristotle in fourth book of the *Generation of Animals*:

> The first departure indeed is that the offspring should become female instead of male; this, however, is a natural necessity. (For the class of animals divided into sexes must be preserved, and as it is possible for the male sometimes not to prevail over the female, either through youth or age or some other such cause, it is necessary that animals should produce female young.) And the monstrosity, though not necessary in regard of a final cause and an end, yet is necessary accidentally.[37]

Not only did early modern Europeans cling to this assumption; they entrenched it in Christianity's Manichean dualism that assigned women to the inferior corporeal. And so, put simply, to feminize the masculine was to denigrate it, to contaminate the purer with the baser gender. We see in New World cosmography the ascribing of female gender qualities, that is, cultural markers of the feminine such as dress and tasks, to Native men in order to assign them to an inferior status. In alchemical images we also find this same "degrading" of gender, but here the dissolving of gender distinctions seems to be empowering. Similarly, the image of the Amazon, a third, subversive and empowered gender, has been the object of both persecution and reverence.[38] The ambivalence of hegemonic society toward those who evade classification, whether man or woman, or a third gender, or from a different culture, often results in either rabid persecution of what is deemed to be monstrous or romantic lionization. Women in sixteenth and seventeenth century Europe were even blamed for the birth of monsters, in the tradition of Aristotle. Paul-Gabriel Bouce tells of a popular midwifery manual that explains the cause of the birth of monstrous deformity:

---

[36] Julia Kristeva, *Powers of Horror: An Essay on Abjection*, trans. Leon S. Roudiez (New York: Columbia University Press, 1982), pp. 1–17.

[37] Aristotle, *Generation of Animals*, in *The Complete Works of Aristotle*, ed. Jonathan Barnes (Princeton, NJ: Princeton University Press, 1984) vol. 1, pp. 1187–8.

[38] Lorber, p. 89.

> The cause is both external and internal. The external one is the outside object on which the woman has cast her eyes; the internal one is the strength of the imagination, which, after receiving the impression of the outside object, communicates it to the informing faculty which then imprints it on the seed.[39]

In "A Weroans, or Chieftain, of Virginia" (*Admiranda narratio*, plate 3), engraved from the painting of the colonial artist John White, one cannot mistake the classical influence upon the figure of the "Weroan." He stands like a late medieval statue of the Virgin Mary or the Three Graces; one hand on hip, one leg splayed out, he appears to carry himself as does a European female, even if this stance is an imitation of that of the Apollo Belvedere, the exaggerated bend in the body feminizes the figure. So, although he is armed and displays superior physical condition and muscularity, he is tamed and feminized by his classic stance, literally put on display, in the way in which female beauties or curiosities would be. Although this mode of depiction was used primarily to represent the female body,[40] Vesalius and later anatomists used this pose for male figures as well (see Long, Figure 3.4).[41] This mode of representation of the body is also apparent in the first emblem of the *Atalanta*, which displays a pregnant man (see Long, Figure 3.5). The chieftain appears animal-like in his taxonomically displayed anterior and posterior views – an object of physical study, rather than a subject in his own right. A tail, supposedly that of a slaughtered animal, hangs between his legs, and shows his animality in not only his implied prehensile abilities, but also in his sexual prowess or even excess. His feathers look like horns, features which suggest the bestial or diabolical (a recurrent theme in the *America*); his tattoos resemble animal markings. Remarkably, his countenance has all the shape of that of a European, which reveals the European need to record difference, but not too much. At this point in European contact with the New World, language and behavior are enough to establish Otherness, but as difference began to erode, confronting Europeans with the abject mirror of their own excesses, the representations of Native peoples grew more demonic. In Thomas Hariot's report of Virginia, from which this illustration was taken, he states:

> Always ready to defend themselves, they carry a quiver made of rushes and in one hand hold a bow, in the other an arrow. So attired they go to war or attend their solemn feasts. They love to hunt… When the chiefs go to battle they paint their bodies in the most hideous ways they can think of. (p. 231)

---

39 Paul-Gabriel Bouce, "Imagination, Pregnant Women, and Monsters, in Eighteenth Century England and France," *Sexual Underworlds of the Enlightenment*, eds. G.S. Rousseau and Roy Porter (Chapel Hill: North Carolina University Press, 1988), p. 86.

40 See Jonathan Sawday, "The Realm of *Anatomia*," from *The Body Emblazoned: Dissection and the Human Body in Renaissance Culture* (London and New York: Routledge, 1995), pp. 183–229.

41 Andreas Vesalius, *De Humani Corporis Fabrica* (Basel: I. Oporini, 1543).

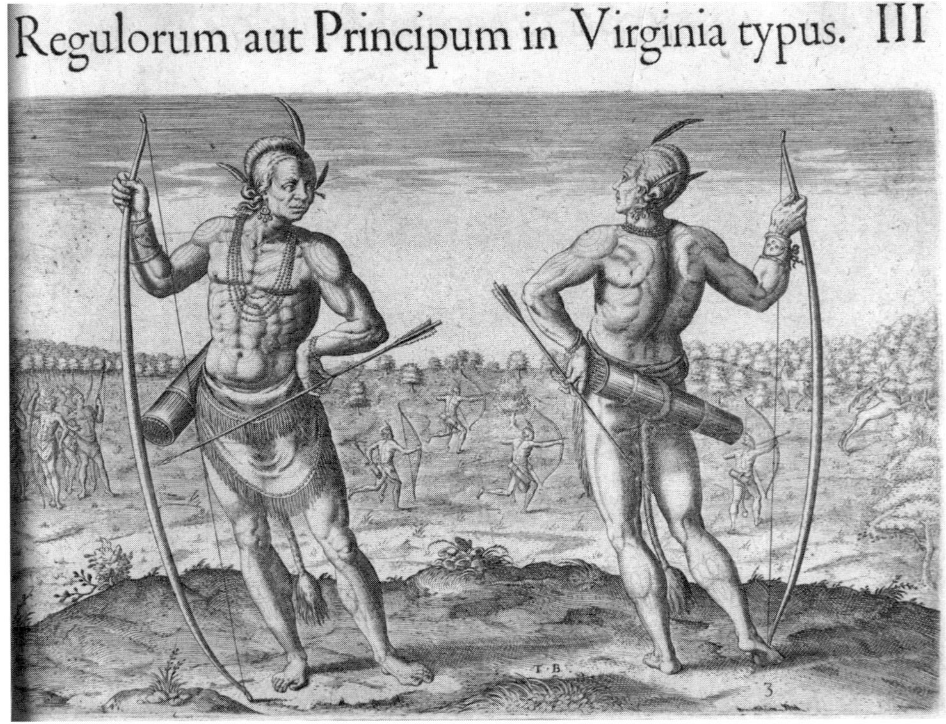

Fig. 4.6 A Virginian Ruler, from de Bry, *America, Brevis et fida narratio Virginiae*. Courtesy of the Division of Rare and Manuscript Collections, Cornell University Library.

The Weroan, like an animal, is always ready to fight. His lack of clothing and his use of the same attire for both war and peace mark him as a marginal animal-like being. Colonists even went so far as to say that American Indians had, like animals, a keen sense of smell: "They followed their enemies by scent, as dogs follow wild beasts" (p. 63). The above passage juxtaposes the hunting of animals for food with the "hunting" of humans for sport – war and feasts appear to be synonymous; the Native's hunting and feasting by smell provides a confused and repellent image of cannibalism. Also, because Europeans had long ago taken up agrarian lifeways (as had the Native Americans, but this aspect of their existence does not seem to have been recognized or at least fully acknowledged by early explorers), and hunted only for sport, Native traditions of hunting seemed clearly uncivilized, and even bestial.

In Merian's engravings of the alchemical text *Atalanta fugiens*, we see the monstrous commingling of human and animal traits as well. As part of an alchemical treatise, the images of *Atalanta* are meant to affect the reader on an almost preconscious level. They are to be meditated upon as symbolic embodiments of natural forces in the universe that can be tapped and manipulated, harnessed and put to rest. One such image celebrates the commingling of animal and human forces: Maier's second emblem, "Its nurse is the earth" (see Long, Figure 3.7), probably also engraved by Merian, a son-in-law of de Bry. As in the previous illustration, women are associated with animals, occupying a paradoxical position of great power as producer-nurturer and of unharnessed brutality as hunter-avenger. Here, humans are nursed not only by their own kind, but also by animals – both by grazers with cloven hooves and by predators with claws and sharp teeth. The alchemist attempts to harness the life-giving power of the living earth, with no regard to assigned differences. The earth and its animals overflow with life-giving spirit; in this economy or surplus or even excess, boundaries dissipate, for they are unnecessary. Those who occupy and nurse from both animal and human realms have acceded to a higher realm of being, beyond difference.

A last and subtler transgression of boundaries that would warrant early modern Europeans' condemnation of the monstrous has to do with human behavior itself, and its taboos. Complex behavioral codes become clear when we view our "sins" as an elaborate system of laws stemming from the myth of the Fall. According to this story, humanity was once innocent, but, for its arrogance, was condemned to slow corruption. Henceforth, our task has been to avoid temptation, to chasten the body in order to return to our original state. Therefore, actions that display a disregard for our corrupt state, such as wearing no clothing, are condemned not only as violations of social mores, but also are viewed as an insult to God. Cannibalism is another such insult. The taboos of nakedness and cannibalism can also be seen as transgressions of the subject-object distinction we struggle to uphold, as Kristeva would say. In the face of these violations, we are made painfully aware of what we have thrown out to uphold our divisions between self and other. And so nakedness and cannibalism become the behavior of the monstrous, pushed to the margins of our thought. Bernadette Bucher, in her study of the illustrations of de Bry's *America*, says cannibalism "appeared as a sort of antimatter, a phenomenon leading ineluctably, by a slow gradation of small differences, toward a dissolution of cosmic and social world."[42] But "dissolution" is a key step in alchemy. Through the careful dissolving of separate elements into one fluid and dynamic system, one is able to bring about an even higher order. Clearly, ancient cosmologies rooted in alchemy are aware of a deeper knowledge that Judeo-Christianity has perhaps forgotten. After all, what are we to make of Christ's nakedness and the ritual eating of his body and drinking of his blood? De Bry's illustrations of hermaphrodites, both in the *Atalanta* and in the *America*, invoke a similar nudity and cannibalism. Recall that the pictures include a spit, a burial scaffold, and a gurney – all used to prepare human bodies for transformation, allowing for the revival of life through death and life-in-death. The first and last steps of the alchemical process are those of *nigredo* and *rubedo*, the blackening and the reddening,[43] the killing and the resurrection, phases that demand the destruction of the thing before it can be moved to a higher state.

In viewing the illustrations of de Bry, we must systematically untangle the likenesses between his New World depictions and his alchemical images. His illustrations are complicated for several reasons. He had never been to America, and so de Bry compiled his *America* from those who had, by interviewing them, reading and editing their accounts, or obtaining their paintings and sketches, from which he made his engravings.[44] Many of his sources exaggerated their experiences, to say the least, some embellishing to such a degree that other cosmographers entered into ongoing battles for the true account of the New World. Stephen Greenblatt declares: "The authors of the anecdotes with which [*Marvellous Possessions*] concerns itself were liars – few of them steady liars, as it were, like Mandeville, but frequent and cunning liars none the less, whose position virtually required the strategic manipulation and distortion and outright suppression of the truth."[45] For example, Lery, a Protestant missionary, considered his account veritable and correct down to the utmost detail, and was archly opposed to the outrageous account of Thevet, a Catholic missionary given the title of "Royal Cosmographer."[46] Political and religious tensions interfered violently with "objective" accounts. Catholics claimed they had the Pope's consent to colonize America and that all Protestants seen in America should be wiped out, while Protestants sought refuge in America

---

42 Bucher, p. 82.

43 Jung, pp. 228–32.

44 See Bucher, pp. 3–12 and Lorant, pp. 30–31. Both sources claim that there is very little known about de Bry and his work. Although a goldsmith by trade, he and his family were to win fame for his illustrated series *America*, the first copperplate-engraved New World cosmography, published in Latin, German, English, and French. De Bry sought out those who had been to the Americas or who knew of written account or illustrations. He worked with the famous Richard Hakluyt, among others, and obtained from the widow of John White, the first English painter of America, many of the sketches that were to become his engravings of the Great Voyages. And it is believed that he at least in part illustrated alchemical treatises, such as the *Atalanta fugiens*, often using the same figures.

45 Greenblatt, *Marvelous Possessions*, p. 7.

46 Lery, xlv–lxii. See Roger Schlesinger and Arthur P. Stabler, eds, *André Thevet's North America* (Montreal: McGill-Queen's University Press, 1986).

from religious persecution and hoped to found new Protestant states. Protestants aligned themselves with the enslaved Native peoples of Peru, and so represented the Catholic Spaniards as wicked captors. Protestants, believing humans to be naturally given to spiritual corruption, claimed the souls of Native people to be at a deeper level of corruption, and so facilely imposed a religious hierarchy upon them. On the other hand, Catholics, holding that humanity has been stripped of its original gifts since the Fall, considered American Indians, like humanity in general, to be spiritually weakened.[47] These considerations are of value when one analyzes a text as ambiguous as the *America*, as well as in sorting out the *Atalanta* (since corruption is an important part of the alchemical process). As we know that de Bry compiled and engraved the *America* before participating in the project of the *Atalanta*, we could speculate that the former informed the latter in a number of ways. In fact, many of the images in the *Atalanta* are obvious revisions of the New World images, as we have seen. Was alchemy to affirm the observations of the New World or to validate in the new land that which it had celebrated? Or did alchemy seek out and project upon America all that it hoped to find? We could dismiss de Bry as a quack goldsmith who wanted to see monsters in both his texts, if it were not that the *America* draws on a wide range of sources and demonstrates an awareness of the diverse and disparate forms of knowledge of the times. So, perhaps the monstrous images de Bry both sought out and rendered repulsive reveal a greater European consciousness of the early modern period, a self-contradictory mentality that is hardly as simplistic as it might seem at first glance.

Entwined in de Bry's later volumes of the *America* are the reasons for his increasingly horrific depiction of the indigenous people. At times Indians appear to be decaying, their breasts sagging, their jaws gaping. In one engraving, Brazilians are shown gnawing on themselves. How could such an Edenic image shift to one of corruption and abysmal damnation? Perhaps the representations of the New World became increasingly more depraved as political and religious tensions mounted in Europe. De Bry, a Protestant of Flemish origin, takes incredible liberties in spreading the "Black Legend." In this New World myth, the Spanish conquest is demonized purely as a cruel and unrelenting search for gold with which to glorify European, particularly Catholic, culture in the name of Christ. But, while the conquistadors were probably more cruel to American Indians than other explorers, the French were often as exploitative. And the French were indeed in search of gold, and were willing to destroy Native populations to obtain it.[48] The French, in

---

[47] Bucher, p. 83.

[48] See Le Moyne's account of the French expedition to Florida in 1564 in Lorant's *The New World*, p. 48: "La Roche Ferriere returned to the fort and reported that all the gold and silver he obtained for us had come from the Apalacty Mountains and that the Indians from whom he had received these metals knew of no other place where they could be found." In Laudonniere's narrative in the same book, p. 64: "De Groutaut was anxious that I should ally myself to this chief in the belief that between us we could conquer all the adjacent tribes and clear the way to the Apalacty Mountains, which we wanted to reach. The chief himself sent me a flat piece of brass dug out of the mountains; from their base rises a stream rich in gold, though the Indians believe it to be brass."

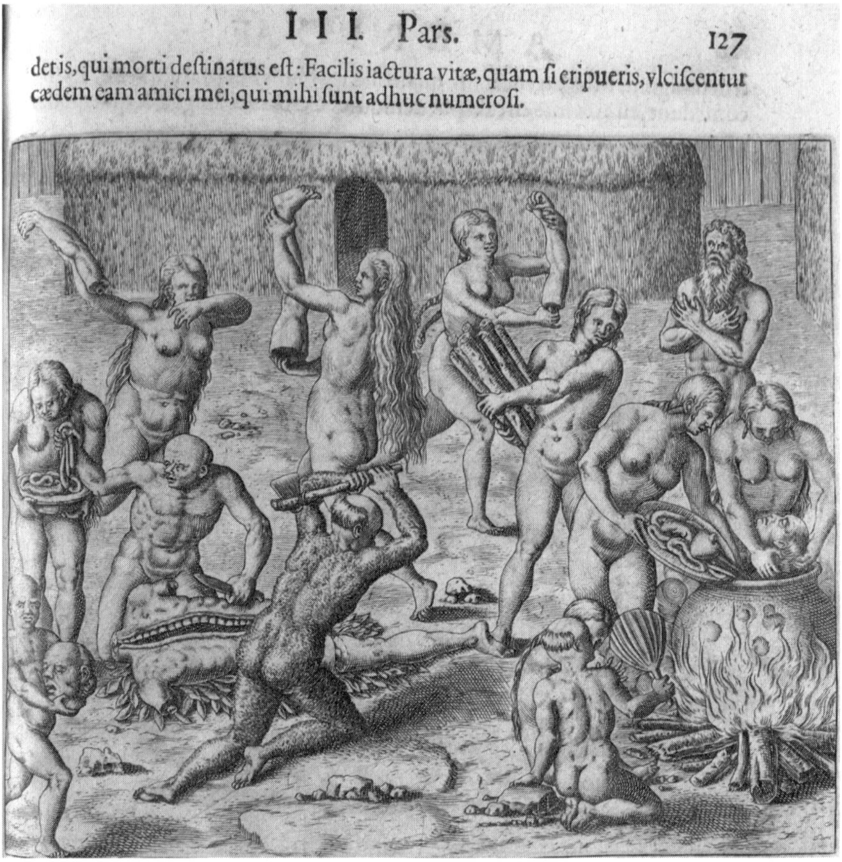
III. Pars. 127
detis,qui morti deſtinatus eſt: Facilis iactura vitæ,quam ſi eripueris,vlciſcentur cædem eam amici mei,qui mihi ſunt adhuc numeroſi.

Fig. 4.7 Cannibals Cooking and Eating Humans, from de Bry, *America tertia pars*. Courtesy of the Division of Rare and Manuscript Collections, Cornell University Library.

erecting their elaborate myth in order to justify the conquest of the New World, had to depict the Spanish as the devil in the myth of the Fall of Man.[49] It is true that the Catholic Spanish were more likely to be shaken by the prospect of cannibalism, because it was an act that, on the theological level, they condoned. In response, the French could say the Spanish had, by implication, both brought American Indians to this depth of corruption, and that they even partake of it themselves. In this system, French Protestants are not only vindicated, but called forth by God to bring American Indians into subjection. Native people, then, are assigned the ambiguous status of both innocent autochthon and cunning tempter. This applied

[49] Henry S. Bausum, "Edenic Images of the Western World: A Reappraisal," *South Atlantic Quarterly* (Autumn 1968): 677.

ambiguity fostered the labeling of Native people as monsters, dual beings whose appearance and behavior were deceptive or unstable. The portrayal of native people as anthropophagous concretized this depiction of them as monsters.

Kristeva would consider the image of cannibalism to be the ultimate abject confrontation; it combines both unbearable experiences of "food loathing" and the viewing of a corpse. Not only does one convulse before the borderless cadaver, but one must eat of it as if it were shit, for both are the refuse that the limited self has cast off to preserve itself: "There, I am at the border of my condition as a living being. My body extricates itself, as being alive, from that border. Such waste drops that I might live..."[50] A violent reaction to monstrous behavior catalyzes the objectification – indeed, the *abjectification* – of the people of the Americas, bringing on the onslaught of full-blown colonization. Bucher sees this process as the inner machinery of the New World myth.[51] As Europeans assimilated into the alien land, relying less and less on the theft of Native American food and on hunting for sustenance, learning the Native languages, living in Native towns, and marrying Native women, they reacted to this unacceptable intimacy by further distancing the Native Americans. Cannibalism became an image of this dangerous assimilation, this threat of absorption of the colonizer by the colonized, thus justifying annihilation of the other as defense of the self. How else does one justify the dispossession of lands belonging to rational human beings? Helen Carr explains: "if the Americans intended to establish an empire, and to legitimize the movement across the continent by which that empire could be achieved, they would have to re-invoke all the European assumptions of Indian otherness and savagery, their inferiority and deficiencies, which had earlier been used to justify colonization."[52] In the settler imagination, American Indians became more inhuman, more monstrous.

If we study the later engravings of the *America* that accompany the accounts of French missionaries in the land named "Brazil," we see the European fear of the loss of boundary between self and other – in the extreme.[53] For here, the Tupinamba devour that very boundary. We see, iconographically, the perverse anxiety concerning Europe's fate should it approach too closely the culture of the Other – it will simply be swallowed up. In Figures 4.5 and 4.7, we see the terrified Frenchman with beard and long hair, who seems to be pleading with the Indians to spare his life. A child plays with a severed head in Figure 4.7; thus the artist portrays the Natives as cruel by nature, from birth. In the same engraving, the children fan the flames; a woman in the upper left corner of the engraving

---

[50] Kristeva, p. 3.

[51] Bucher, pp. 13–23.

[52] Helen Carr, *Inventing the American Primitive: Politics, Gender and the Representation of Native American Literary Traditions, 1789–1936* (New York: New York University Press, 1996), p. 24.

[53] The figures alluded to in this argument, from de Bry's volume on Brazil, are also to be found in Bucher's book, *Icon and Conquest*.

is driven, in a frenzy, to gnaw her own flesh, her eyes squinting in a monstrous grimace. And who is the hirsute man wielding a club? Although de Bry had access to accounts that dispelled the myth of the hair-covered savage, long a figure on the European mythical scene, adding this figure to the depiction of the cannibals increases the anthropophagous mayhem. Léry states, in his account of the land of Brazil, that "… contrary to what some people may think, and what others would have one believe, they are by no means covered with hair; in fact, they are not by nature any hairier than we are over here in this country."[54] For, during this time, outlandish descriptions circulated depicting Native people to be covered in hair like the Savage Man or Wild Man of European lore. In comparison to de Bry's earlier illustrations, these are by far more decadent; also in figures 5 and 7, the faces of the female Indians are wrinkled, as if they were aged or rotting. The woman to the left of the circle appears engaged in an autoerotic and even autophagous fetish, the actions linking the sins of murder, lust, and gluttony. This engraving, with its body parts, suggests the European male's Orphic fear of woman as monster, as destroyer of man if she is left unfettered, as Native women were judged to have been. This movement into greater and greater monstrosity in the depictions of New World natives, from cannibalism to demonic possession to grotesque animalism, suggests a more and more problematic relationship with this world, once newly discovered, now largely destroyed (at least in terms of the native populations), and nonetheless resistant to control by Europeans, who themselves have fallen into animalistic behaviors.

The image of cannibalism as monstrous in the *Atalanta* problematizes those of the *America* because in the *Atalanta* it becomes an image of renewal and abundance. Perhaps the most frequent and powerful image in alchemy is that of the euroboros, that of the snake eating its own tail; a symbol of eternity but also of the self-destructive nature of the world. In this economy, cannibalism becomes the sacred practice of bringing renewal through consumption (or corruption), ingesting the component self to bring unity and harmony: "Time and again the alchemists reiterate that the *opus* proceeds from the one and leads back to the one, that is it is a sort of circle like a dragon biting its own tail."[55] How could the depiction of cannibalism in the New World, which presents the new land as a corrupt, fallen place where life feeds on itself into chaos be at such variance with the alchemical regenerative euroboros (Emblem 14)? The circular form of the dragon suggests the endless cycle of life; nature, by destroying itself, will be reborn. The caption reads: "The famished Polyps gnawed at their own legs/And hunger, too, taught men to feast on men." (p. 133) Does famine reduce humans to their true nature and teach them the secret way of the alchemist, the way to the prima material? This implication would fit well with the belief of the period that the American Indians were closer to the origin of humanity. Like the Americans, the euroboros needs the same treatment: "Subdue it by hunger, prison, iron, until/

[54] Lery, p. 57.

[55] Jung, p. 293.

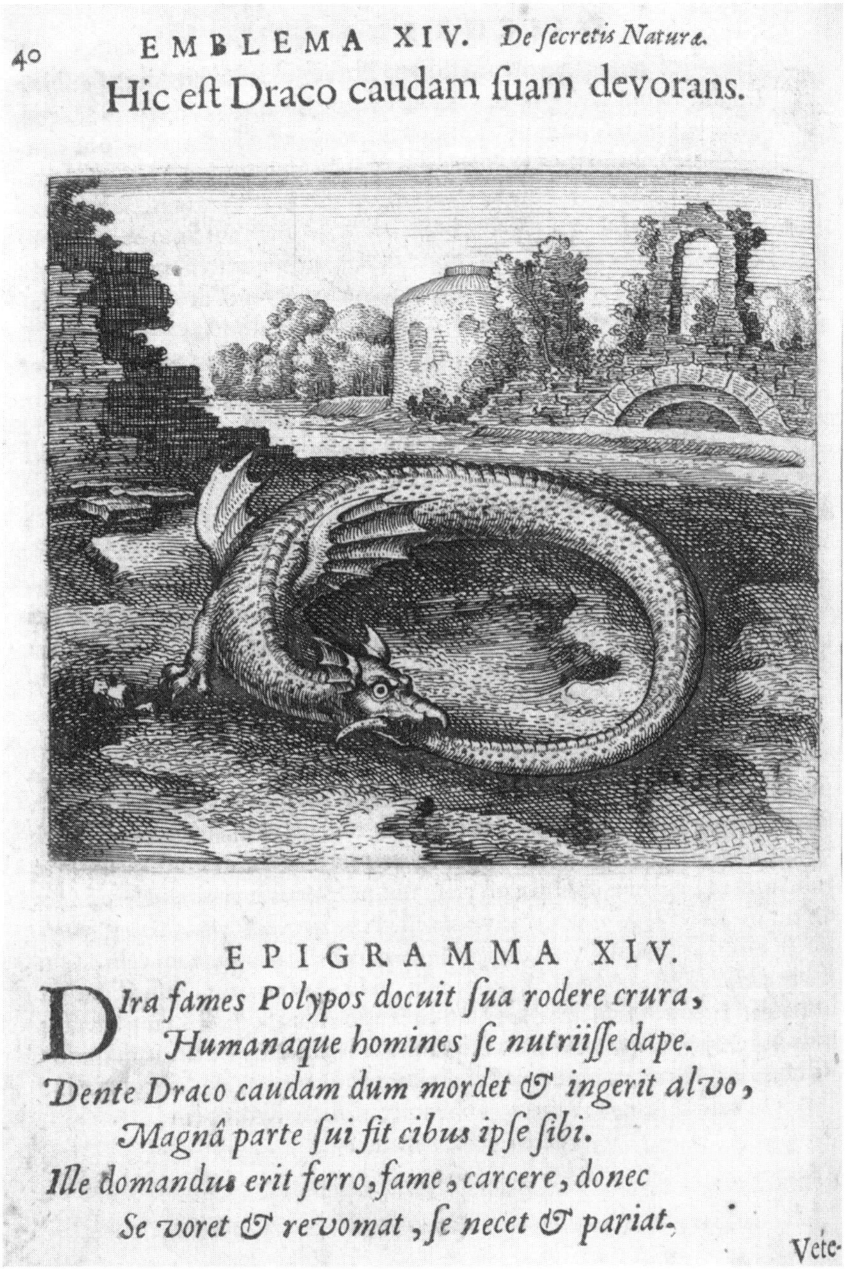

40 EMBLEMA XIV. *De ſecretis Naturæ.*

Hic eſt Draco caudam ſuam devorans.

EPIGRAMMA XIV.

Dira fames Polypos docuit ſua rodere crura,
Humanaque homines ſe nutriiſſe dape.
Dente Draco caudam dum mordet & ingerit alvo,
Magnâ parte ſui fit cibus ipſe ſibi.
Ille domandus erit ferro, fame, carcere, donec
Se voret & revomat, ſe necet & pariat.

Vete-

Fig. 4.8 "Here is the Dragon Eating its own Tail" (The Euroboros), Emblem 14, from Michael Maier, *Atalanta fugiens*. Courtesy of the Division of Rare and Manuscript Collections, Cornell University Library.

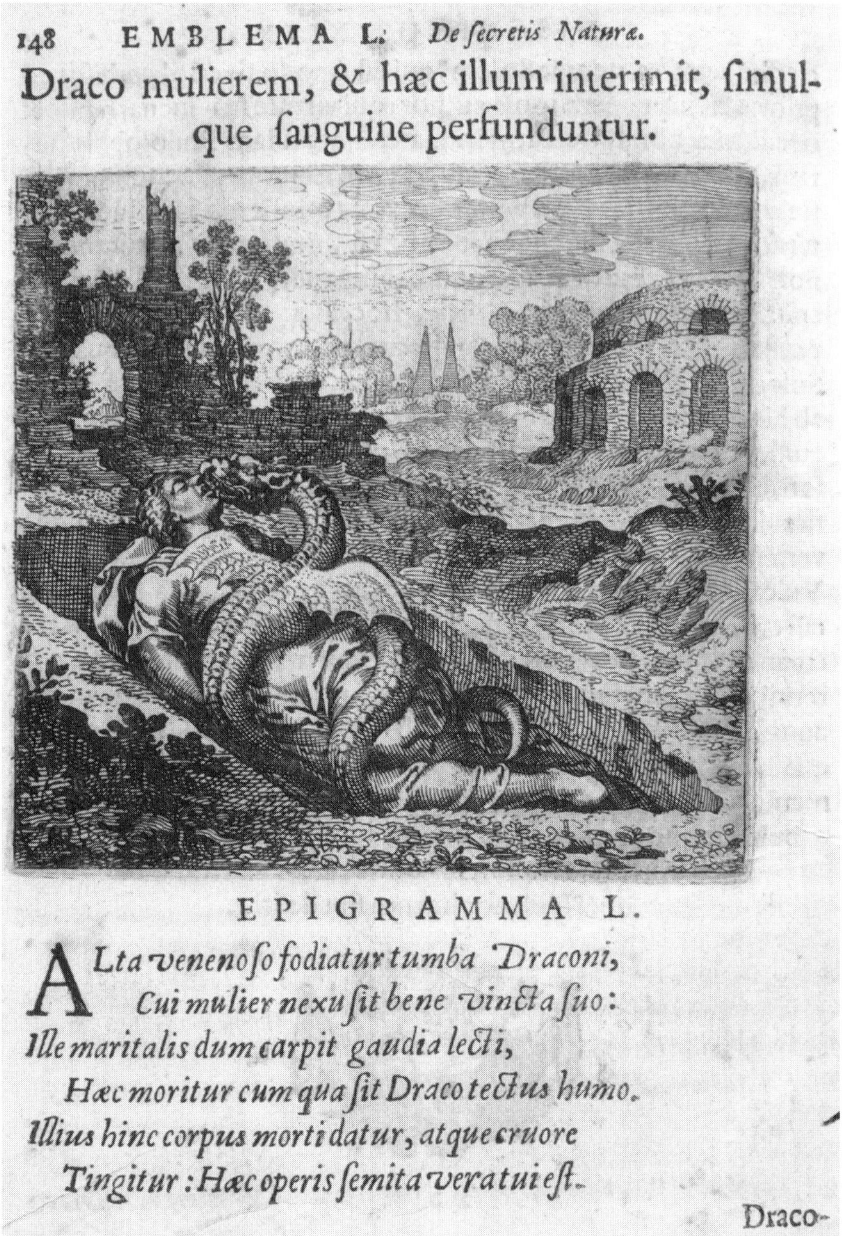

148 EMBLEMA L. *De ſecretis Naturæ.*

Draco mulierem, & hæc illum interimit, ſimulque ſanguine perfunduntur.

EPIGRAMMA L.

Alta venenoſo fodiatur tumba Draconi,
Cui mulier nexu ſit bene vincta ſuo:
Ille maritalis dum carpit gaudia lecti,
Hæc moritur cum qua ſit Draco tectus humo.
Illius hinc corpus morti datur, atque cruore
Tingitur: Hæc operis ſemita vera tui eſt.

Draco-

Fig. 4.9 The Dragon and the Woman Intertwined, Emblem 50, from Michael Maier, *Atalanta fugiens*. Courtesy of the Division of Rare and Manuscript Collections, Cornell University Library.

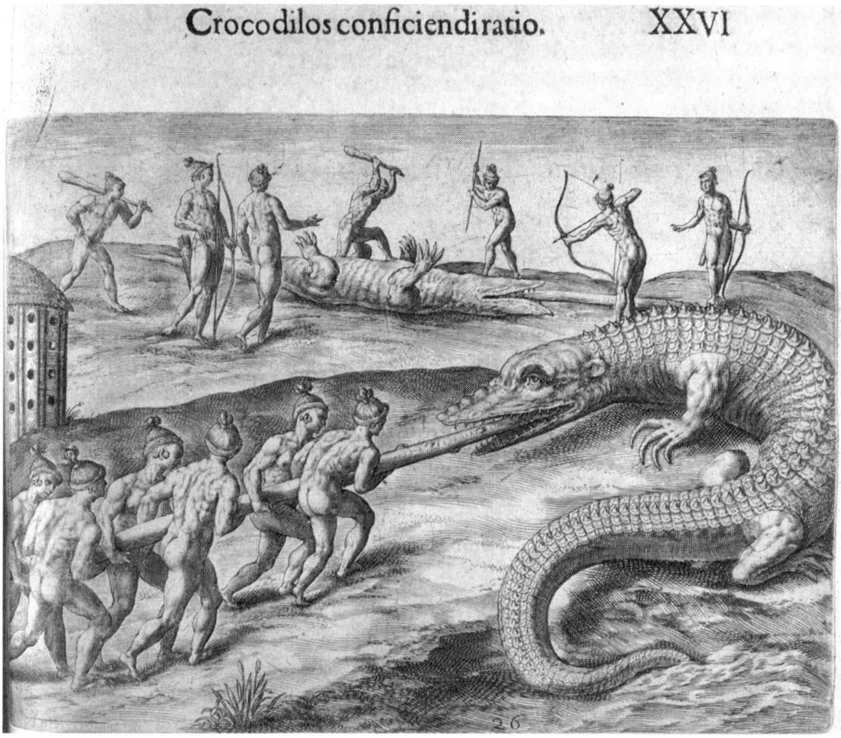

Fig. 4.10 "Cutting Up the Crocodiles" from de Bry, *America, Brevis narratio*... Courtesy of the Division of Rare and Manuscript Collections, Cornell University Library.

It eats itself, vomits, dies, and is born." (p. 133) Here again, the monstrous is both horrible and holy, because it dares to transgress the constructed boundary not only between self and other but also between life and death itself (Emblem 50). This figure of eternal death and renewal echoes, with its ridge of spikes running down its spine, the monstrous New World alligators (plate 26 in the *Brevis narratio*). Did images of this "New World" inspire alchemical representations of the monstrous, or were they themselves guided by cultural attitudes and longstanding images that had filtered down through alchemical lore? The give and take of these two sources is unmistakable. The Western world, ambiguously fascinated with the Americas, found in them the confirmation of its suppressed beliefs in the solubility of difference, a concept that was to flourish, somewhat protected, in alchemy.

In a time rife with a fear of the anomaly, a time obsessed with the scientific categorization of all things, the New World and alchemy offered a reviving if menacing retreat. The encounter with the Americas was to rock the social, religious, and political assumptions of the Europeans, and force the continent to reconsider the arbitrary distinctions made between man and animal, woman and man, European and American, normal and abnormal bodies, and behavior. As walls between actual and assumed worlds began to fall, Europeans struggled to uphold the boundaries they had established between different aspects of identity by constructing the myth of the savage, a myth that both worships and condemns the cultural Other. Freedom from such imposed difference would resurface time and again in the heretical texts of alchemy. But a "new world" would provide for Johann Theodor de Bry, his family, and his hopeful audience a pure realm in which to examine, manipulate, and even solve the problems of difference with the ideas inherent in alchemy. And so both the *Atalanta fugiens* and the *America* are imbued with the tortured impressions of "strangers in a strange land," as students of alchemy struggles with boundaries that are not there, trying, like the hungry euroboros, to make us new again.

Chapter 5
The Animal Within: Chivalry, Monstrosity, and Gender in Renaissance Spain

Simone Pinet

> Más hemos aprendido a vivir de los animales que de los hombres, más de los rústicos que de los doctos. Las artes de reinar que inventó la especulación hicieron tiranos, y antes derribaron que levantaron imperios.
>
> —Diego de Saavedra Fajardo, *Corona gótica*, prologue to the reader

Some 20 years ago, Paul Julian Smith opened his discussion of the body in Hispanic literature through the analysis of two emblems in Covarrubias' 1610 *Emblemas morales*, one of a siren, the other of a bearded lady. After pointing out the obvious monstrosity that the sexing and/or de-sexing of the figures entails, Smith reflects on the less obvious discursive effects of these images. In the second emblem, in particular, the verses bespeak the body's meaning itself, rendering the articulation of the corporeal and the rhetorical evident: "Soy hic, et haec, et hoc. Yo me declaro,/Soy varon, soy muger, soy un tercero,/Que no es uno ni otro, ni está claro/Qual destas cosas sea. Soy tercero/De los que como a monstro horrendo y raro/Me tienen por siniestro y mal aguero/Aduierta cada qual que me ha mirado,/ Que es otro yo, si viue afeminado." ("I am hic, and haec, and hoc. I declare/decline myself. I am man, I am woman, I am a third who is neither one nor the other, nor is it clear which of these things I am. I am a third such as those horrendous and rare monsters taken for sinister and ill-fortuned. Take note each who has seen me, that it/(s)he is another I, if living as effeminate.")[1] Here, Smith remarks, "biological categories are traced back to their grammatical equivalents," in a correspondence often invoked in early modern culture, allowing "freedom of movement between the bodily and the discursive (anatomy and grammar)," finding "one of its most potent allegories in the ever varied and contradictory figure of woman."[2] But the morality of the emblem does not reside in this declaration of the fact of ambivalence or ambiguity, but in the possibility that the spectator, after seeing this "neither

---

[1] All translations are mine unless otherwise noted. I would like to thank Kathleen P. Long for her suggestions and careful reading.

[2] Smith, p. 16.

and both," as the motto declares in a banner above the figure of the lady, might consider that same ambiguity within him or herself.[3]

As the Middle Ages wore out the once clear distinctions between species, increasingly defining humanity through action and not through essence, there arose a need to establish a limit between the human and the nonhuman based on different parameters. Language itself became one of the distinctive traits that marked off this difference, in the specific sense that it made it possible for humans, and for humans alone, to distinguish between good and evil. The renewed emphasis on the linguistic sciences exercised by humanists such as Antonio de Nebrija, though following a long medieval tradition initiated by Isidore of Seville in his *Etymologiae*, is multiplied in the period in dictionaries, vocabularies, glossaries. At the turn of the sixteenth century, Nebrija and other figures such as Alonso de Palencia and Fernández de Santaella construct an elaborate taxonomy of language, which both brought language into scientific discourses of the early modern period and unabashedly infiltrated the sciences with rhetoric, which by the mid-sixteenth century became central to Spanish culture, cultivated by figures such as Juan Luis Vives, Benito Arias Montano, Francisco Sánchez de las Brozas, Huarte de San Juan, Fray Luis de Granada, and others. Intrinsic to this emphasis on rhetoric was a language's capacity for ambiguity, exploited productively but also seen with suspicion. Etymology in Nebrija, for instance, serves both as the definition of the hybrid or the monster by cutting the word itself in parts and explaining them, and via false etymology, as procreator of new monsters.[4] In literature this ambivalence is figured early on in Fernando de Rojas' *La Celestina* (1499), where Celestina's in-between-ness defines not only her profession or the multiple layers of cultures that shape her character, but also her language. As a characterizing trait, Celestina's language is both a part of her humanity at its most basic, and a part of her more suspicious qualifications as procuress, sorceress, monster, or witch. Her speech and its nuances, tones, levels, and functions link her and her actions to alchemy

---

[3] For an analysis that looks at medical discourses to discern literary types (in this case, Cervantes' "mujer varonil") see Sherry Velasco, "Marimachos, hombrunas, barbudas: The Masculine Woman in Cervantes," *Cervantes: Bulletin of the Cervantes Society of America* 20.1 (2000): 69–78.

[4] Juan Casas Rigall goes on to explain that "this philological competence will allow Nebrija to avoid one of the most curious causes of deformation and even the genesis of medieval monsters: false etymology," ("Las razas monstruosas según Nebrija," in *Fantasía y literatura en la Edad Media y los Siglos de Oro*, ed. Nicasio Salvador Miguel, Santiago López Ríos and Esther Borrego Gutiérrez, Madrid: Iberoamericana/Vervuert, 2004), p. 136. For more on Nebrija's engagements with language see James M. Murphy, "Antonio de Nebrija in the European Rhetorical Tradition," *in Antonio de Nebrija: Edad Media y Rencimiento,* ed. Carmen Codoñer and Juan antonio González Iglesias (Salamanca: Universidad de Salamanca, 1944), pp. 447–56. For a general discussion on the relations between monstrosity, language and image see chapter 5 in Claude-Claire Kappler's classic study, *Monstres, démons et merveilles à la fin du Moyen Age* (Paris: Payot, 1999 [1980]), pp. 187–204.

and medicine, to prostitution and the market of the flesh, to a dexterity of words that is both masterful and monstrous, an ambiguous nature within language as the defining trait of the human.[5] At the end of the fifteenth century, Celestina's language illustrates the interiorization of divisions one perceived outside the limits of the body:

> By the late Middle Ages, the animal that prowls within each of us became increasingly evident. Thinkers moved more closely to the Greco-Roman view that saw humans along a continuum with animals, with the potential of lowering themselves to the bestial level by their actions. This view that we can see emerging in the twelfth century dominated Renaissance thought.[6]

In terms of poetics, of literature or art in general, humanity is progressively characterized by the ability to distinguish between lies and truth, between the fake and the real, and moreover, by the capacity of fiction – which proves itself through the second-degree ability to fake that one is faking. That is, humanity is characterized by its capacity for setting up artifices, for the fictionalization of fiction. It is this capacity for constructing artifices that will unite politics and poetics through the figures of monstrosity in sixteenth-century Spain, in a time and place that sit both at the origin of the absolutist State in Europe, and thus at the beginning of modern empires, and at the center of an artistic production known as the Golden Age, with effects that can still be perceived today.

---

5 James F. Burke reads the plot itself of *Celestina* as mirroring alchemy's principle of joining opposites (Calisto and Melibea) through a mediating quintessence, Celestina herself. As he points out, the result is destruction, not creation. Burke first insightfully surveys critical work on change and metamorphosis as essential to Celestina's plot (pp. 129–35), while devoting the second part of the article to detailing alchemical allusions in the work, specifically referring to the process noted in the prologue and to Calisto's transformation ("Metamorphosis and the Imagery of Alchemy in *la Celestina,*" *Revista Canadiense de Estudios Hispánicos* 1.2 (1977): 129–52. While Burke argues that it is a certain popularity of symbols and imagery of alchemy that find their way into Rojas' work, the intermixture of science, hermetic thought and medical discourse was present in literary texts preceding *Celestina*. Alchemy will progressively and rapidly lose legitimacy, to the point that in *Don Quijote* it is used as an ungendered synonym for trick or fraud, but in *Celestina* itself it is curious that in its association with the character of Celestina, alchemy is gendered and already portrayed as deceit, "una burla." See also Erica Morgan, "Rhetorical Technique in the Persuasion of Melibea," *Celestinesca* 3.2 (1979): 7–18; Malcolm K. Read, "The Rhetoric of Social Encounter: *La Celestina* and the Renaissance Philosophy of Language," in *The Birth and Death of Language: Spanish Literature and Linguistics. 1300–1700* (Potomac: Studia Humanitatis, 1983), pp. 70–96; and the more general and influental Francisco Rico, "Brujería y literatutra," in *Brujología: Ponencias y comunicaciones del primer congreso español de brujología celebrado en San Sebastián, septiembre de 1972* (Madrid: Seminarios, 1975), pp. 97–117.

6 Joyce E. Salisbury, *The Beast Within: Animals in the Middle Ages* (New York: Routledge, 1994), p. 167.

For if the Middle Ages built around the distinction between human and animal the possibility for knowledge, as the distinction became internalized and self-knowledge became the goal, to the effect that humans began to perceive their own animalhood, then the distinction increasingly had to rely upon politics. In other words, with the notion of human entailing its part of bestiality, the fundamental distinction now became that between the *political* animal and the animal per se in a partial return to Aristotle's *Politics*. This is, of course, a question at the core of any political gesture to this day, as Giorgio Agamben reminds us in *The Open: On Man and Animal.* Such a delimitation, in the centuries following the articulation of a nation-State in Spain, became key to the interrogation of the nature of political power and the legitimization of sovereignty across Western Europe, including its relation to its transatlantic territorial claims. Once it was no longer possible to find a source for power or its legitimization through the divine, power was made to rely upon a human covenant. The distinction between what is human and what is not was thus displaced to an imagined frontier between the state of nature and civil society, which is similar but not identical to the division between nature and culture. In those debates about sovereignty in political texts, we thus find that monstrosity, at the heart of power, stands as a symbol, if not also as a symptom.

Books of chivalry, as one of the key *fictional* genres of political ideology produced in the nascent Spanish empire, illuminate a pivotal stage in monsters' itinerary towards their central place in Thomas Hobbes, where they are presented as sovereignty itself. Replete with beasts coming from diverse medieval literary and artistic traditions, chivalric literature made of monsters a *topos* put in place to signify the instability of the power of kings and emperors.[7] In the many kingdoms that knights errant see on their travels, monsters appear as the imminent danger, as the threat of chaos or even as the impasse that must be overcome in order for monarchy to be able to establish itself. In this way, they make the presence of something or someone other than the figure of the absolutist king – something that is to be pushed *beyond* the limits of statehood – an essential element for the cohesiveness of the State itself. Monsters are there to be defeated, negatively mirroring the characteristics of the knight and counterbalancing monarchic power in the process; monsters, however, are precisely what bring together and separate, what lie across and within the distinction between the political animal and the animal as such. Texts such as the chivalric, which in this sense can be read as part of the debates on monarchy, include monsters as the return of the repressed:

[7] María Carmen Marín Pina, in "Los monstruos híbridos en los libros de caballerías españoles," offers an extensive catalogue of monstrous figures in the genre. The discussion centers on "hybrid monsters" such as the Endriago and Patagón, considered later in this article, on their genesis, their form and the combat with the hero. Being a brief, general overview, if generously documented, the article does not consider specific interpretive possibilities.

a reminder that we too are animals, or alternatively, that it is only the knight who can overcome the animal within.[8]

The discourse on monstrosity in the book of chivalry is thus negotiating the move from a political order as defined through divine power to a political order as defined by covenant, whether between knighthood and monarchy, or among the increasingly differentiated noble classes. What is ambiguous in the book of chivalry is the legitimization of this sovereignty, which tests the boundaries of political order through battles that take place precisely on its limits, right at the origin of the absolute State.[9] The debate over the status of fiction in the manifold contemporary discussions on poetics, particularly for their interest in books of chivalry and their "fantastic" presentation of monsters, can thus also be read as a debate within political discourse.

Spain's sixteenth-century discourse on monstrosity falls within two major categories. The first, in consonance with the scientific developments in the rest of Western Europe, comes from medical treatises inspired by Aristotle and Galen, and the second, from a variety of literary genres, from romance to literature of travel, didactic literature and bestiaries. These latter works are embedded in the chivalric genre in Spain, which specifically reworked a medieval tradition that imbricated romance's interest in the marvelous with the era's renewed interest in the monstrous races and the monstrous in general in a new scientific perspective. Following the publication of Hartmann Schedel's *Liber chronicarum* in 1493, which included numerous illustrations of strange beings – among them, to the left and on the verso of a mappamundi woodcut, the monstrous races believed to inhabit the margins of the world –, there was a general scientific interest in these phenomena that culminated in the work of natural philosophers such as Huarte de San Juan, who linked physiology, psychology, and eugenics in his *Examen de ingenios para las ciencias* (1575) and Ambroise Paré's treatise on surgery, first published in 1573, which included the work known as *Des monstres et prodiges*,

[8] For the chivalric as/within debates on monarchy, *La caballería castellana. Textos y contextos*, ed. Carlos Heusch and Jesús Rodríguez Velasco, (Montpellier: Equipe d'études ibériques, latinoaméricaines et du monde lusophone, Université de Montpellier III, 2000) and also Rodríguez Velasco, "Teoría de la fábula caballeresca," in *Libros de caballerías (de "Amadís" al "Quijote")* (Salamanca: SEMYR, 2002), pp. 343–58, where he analyzes the ideas of nobility inherent to chivalry and to monarchy through what he terms the *chivalric fabula*.

[9] I refer here to liminality not only in a metaphoric sense, but to the actual frontiers of medieval sovereignty and its territorial binds. If historically these limits were questioned through the continued exploration of the African coastlines and subsequently through the encounter with the New World (see P. Russell, "El descubrimiento de las canarias y el debate medieval acerca de los derechos de los príncipes y pueblos paganos," *Revista de Historia Canaria* 36, 171(1978): 9–32), literature also represented these political explorations at the margins of legitimate power through encounters often spatialized upon islands, to be dominated or given as royal gifts (see S. Pinet, *Archipelagoes*, Minneapolis: University of Minnesota Press, 2010).

linking monstrosity and reproduction. The book of chivalry thus emerges in the transition between the consideration of the monster as marvel and the naturalistic approach to the origin of monstrosity.

The scientific texts most prone to refer to monstrosity are treatises on women and gestation and/or birth, and they display the general traits that Marie-Hélène Huet has pointed out for the relations between gender and scientific discourse in the first part of her book *Monstrous Imagination*.[10] As Elena del Río Parra has amply documented and studied, the transition of the sixteenth to the seventeenth century is inhabited both by translations of old manuals and the production of new materials that include treatises on surgery, medical or natural philosophy publications, even essays on aesthetics or entertainment literature that do not cohere into a genre as they did in other European countries.[11] Spain's discourse on monstrosity does not substitute a new approach or explanation for the old models, but proceeds by accumulation, even when contradiction between these different positions is obvious. Del Río Parra identifies three main theories that circulate on a par by the seventeenth century. A first, Aristotelian attitude identifies monsters as abominable errors or games of nature that are outside nature; foreign to the universal project, they are thus morally suspect. A second attitude perceives monsters as an exception to the rule but within nature, and a third one sees them as a rare thing or a "singularity."[12] Spanish discourse on monstrosity, writes del Río Parra, is characterized not by a much hailed (and suspect) scientific underdevelopment in the Iberian Peninsula, or a particular emphasis on religiosity, but by the coexistence of many approaches to monstrosity. If Michel Foucault argued that the classificatory drive of the eighteenth century revealed the analytical, enlightened need to catalogue knowledge, then "in the Spanish seventeenth century this cataloguing is not due to differentiated disciplines (law, religion, medicine, surgery) but to a fluidity between the areas of knowledge that turns the object of study in a cumulative and pluriform tale: the monster is not the distinct object of every discipline but a sum of what is known, including the speculation on what is still unknown" (p. 45). Bridging the scientific and the literary, the numerous "periodicals" that account for real and imagined monstrous beings bear witness to this manifold discourse, encompassing their traditional interpretation as omens,

---

[10] Cambridge, MA: Harvard University Press, 1993.

[11] *Una era de monstruos. Representaciones de lo deforme en el Siglo de Oro español*. (Madrid: Iberoamericana/Vervuert, 2003), pp. 34–5. See a list of the main examples of translated works in note 11 to page 37 in del Río Parra, and note 13 for less known references. Del Río Parra focuses on four texts in her first chapter, the 1585 translation of Boaistuau's *Historias prodigiosas y maravillosas* with its continuations, J. Rivilla Bonet y Pueyo's *Desvíos de la naturaleza. O tratado del origen de los monstruos* of 1695, J.E. Nieremberg's *Curiosa filosofía* of 1630 and its continuation, and A. de Fuentelapeña's *El ente dilucidado* (1628–1702), the latter two being the most influential texts of the period.

[12] Del Río Parra, pp. 42 and *passim*.

increasingly tied up with political discourse.[13] But perhaps what is most productive for the thought on the monstrous in literary discourse are its links to or even its identification with rhetoric, through metaphor as the definition of the mimetic process central to the period.[14]

Finally, the changing articulation of an ill-fitting class of knights in chivalric literature, from a merit-based society to the figure of the knight as diplomat, takes us to the genre's function as a manual of courtesy – of self-fashioning – as occurred with Herberay des Essarts's translation of the *Amadís* into French.[15] The chivalric is based on the binome love/war, and much has been said about the role of women and the courts in the articulation of the love component in this tension. However, for the field of military exploits, the role of women appears to be less visible: duels, tournaments and wars are waged among men, even if the sporadic Amazon makes an appearance and damsels serve as witnesses or pretexts.[16] Here

---

[13] See *Les* Relaciones de sucesos *(canards) en Espagne (1500–1750). Actes du premier colloque international (Alcalá de Henares, 8, 9 et 10 juin 1995)* (Alcalá: Universidad de Alcalá de Henares/Publications de la Sorbonne, 1996), especially Victoria Campo, "La historia y la política a través de las relaciones en verso en pliegos sueltos," 19–32; Mercedes Fernández Valladares "Historia y política en las relaciones góticas de la Colección Medinaceli (Descripciones: segunda parte)," pp. 133–56; Juan Carlos Izquierdo "El Luteranismo en las relaciones de sucesos del siglo XVI," pp. 217–26; and Augustin Redondo "Los prodigios en las relaciones de sucesos de los siglos XVI y XVII," pp. 287–304.

[14] See Severo Sarduy, *Ensayos generales sobre el Barroco* (México: Fondo de Cultura Económica, 1987) for metaphor and rhetoric in the Baroque. Del Río Parra also references Sarduy; Roland Barthes's *Le Degré zero de l'écriture* (Paris: Seuil, 1953) for the suggestion of the monstrous as the essentially poetic; and R.W. Lee's *Ut Pictura Poesis: the Humanist Theory of Painting* (New York: Norton & Company, 1912) for a concept of mimesis in the sixteenth century.

[15] For a reading of the knight as absorbed within the administration of monarchy, see Axayácatl Campos García-Rojas, "'Ser muy bien hablado en diuersas lenguas': el poliglotismo como arma cortesana en los libros de caballerías (Claribalte)," en *Actas del Congreso Internacional X Jornadas Medievales* (México del 20 al 24 de septiembre del 2004), Concepción Company, Aurelio González Pérez and Lillian von der Walde Moheno, eds. (Mexico City: UNAM/ El Colegio de México/ UAM-Iztapalapa), pp. 17–30.

[16] See María Carmen Marín Pina, "Don Quijote, las mujeres y los libros de caballerías," in Kurt Reichenberger, ed. and prologue and Darío Fernández-Morera, ed., *Cervantes y su mundo II* (Kassel, Germany: Reichenberger, 2005), pp. 309–40; and "Aproximación al tema de la virgo bellatrix en los libros de caballerías españoles," *Criticón* 45 (1989): 81–94; also María José Rodilla, "La caballería de las damas: Un acercamiento a la mujer en el 'Amadís,'" in Serafín González and Lillian von der Walde, ed. and preface, *Palabra crítica: Estudios en homenaje a José Amezcua* (Mexico City: Universidad Autónoma Metropolitana, Unidad Iztapalapa--Fondo de Cultura Económica, 1997), pp. 285–94. For the translation into French, see the collection *Les Amadis en France au XVIe siècle* (Paris: Editions Rue d'Ulm/Presses de l'Ecole Normale Supérieure, 2000); as manual for self-fashioning see E.B. Place, "El *Amadís* de Montalvo como manual de cortesanía en Francia," *Revista de Filología Española* 38 (1954): 151–69.

monsters are the extreme version of both evil and the power of human capacity, as the supernatural finally succumbs to the virtuosity and valor of the knight.

In the history of these monsters of chivalry, scientific discourse often comes into play: the genre's affiliations with travel literature link it to natural histories and their chapters on monsters, and as the genre develops there appear more anthropological observations, linguistic precisions, or archeological remarks. Gender, as is to be expected, often plays a crucial role in the presentation of these monsters, either in their conception or in their gestation, with monsters being created from a deviant desire that requires the presence of a female. In books of chivalry of sixteenth-century Spain, the construction of monstrosity follows a series of behavioral patterns that are attributed to women, patterns that can be traced back to the surge in debates on the virtue of women or to the misogynist literature that enjoys much special attention in the fifteenth century, and which achieve confirmation through science in the shape of medical treatises in the following decades.[17] In this way, chivalric monsters capture, for the education of a class, a sideways glance to the feminine, wary of the dangers of the female body and desire, and articulated as a politics for the emergent state that paradoxically will have been *engendered* by a woman: Queen Isabella.[18] In the construction of monsters within the genre, gender is yet another ambiguous and problematic boundary. Its status, as derived from the relation between political animal and animal, especially at the birth of an empire with a queen at its center, will be a point of constant return for my analysis of monstrosity in the following pages.[19]

If all political order needs some exclusion, this exception to nature can be placed in the period in its own particular space. This location, though, will not be exactly coincidental with feminine space but rather with that of the recently discovered

[17] The extensive literature addressing the behavior of women ranges from the popular and cultivated texts circulating in the medieval period, sapiential and exemplary texts, translations, and discourses embedded or inherent to different genres, such as sentimental fiction and courtly romance in general, to later works such as the fifteenth-century *Castigos y doctrinas que un sabio daba a sus hijas* (fifteenth century) and Juan Luis Vives's well-known *Instrucción de la mujer cristiana*. For the medical texts, consider Francisco Núñez, *Libro intitulado del parto humano* (1580), Damián Carbón, *Libro del arte de las comadres o madrinas y del regimiento de las preñadas y paridas* (1541), and the anonymous *Traducción del Compendio de la humana salud de Johannes de Ketham (c. 1400–1500),* all edited by María Teresa Herrera and María Estela González de Fauve (Madison: Hispanic Seminary of Medieval Studies, 1997).

[18] For literary and political gender relations in Isabel's court, see Barbara Weissberger, *Isabel Rules. Constructing Queenship, Wielding Power* (Minneapolis: University of Minnesota Press, 2004).

[19] For a succinct summary of female sovereignty in Iberia and its distinct legal context, see Sharon L. Jansen *The Monstrous Regiment of Women. Female Rulers in Early Modern Europe* (New York: Palgrave, 2002), esp. pp. 7–23: for case studies see *Queenship and Political Power in Medieval and Early Modern Spain,* ed. Theresa Earenfight (Burlington, VT: Ashgate, 2005).

Americas, which in many cases bring back the names for these "monsters" from books of chivalry, with Patagonia and California as well-known examples.[20] Furthermore, one of the fundamental exclusions will serve as a reminder of the fact that all political order is based on the order of a nature that has been erased – the erasure of our own animalhood, one which will be attributed, if only as a tendency or as more prone to being its victim, to women.

Internal Excess

Monstrosity in the book of chivalry is not the result (or not only) of excess, either of pure physicality or pure behavior.[21] There must be a combination of physical and moral elements, and there must be something beastly about the semblance as well as something vicious about that immorality, something unchangeable, unconvertible about it for there to be monstrosity. That is why giants are not monstrous in chivalric literature, and even though their presence is pervasive throughout the genre, they are usually not there to signify the absolute otherness of the monster but more often than not as mere hyperbolic mirrors of the knight's heroism.[22] They are there simply as an inflated humanity – in its inclusion of animalhood – as a sort of overflowing humanness that serves as reminder for the desire of limits, of propriety, of containment. As such, the giant is the opposite of the epic hero as personified in the Cid's characteristic trait, *mesura*, which connotes temperance,

---

[20] A general account of books of chivalry and the Americas can be consulted in Javier Roberto González, "Libros de caballerás en América," in *Amadís de Gaula 1508: Quinientos años de libros de caballerías* (Madrid: Biblioteca Nacional de España/Sociedad estatal de conmemoraciones culturales, 2008, pp. 369–82). For extensive accounts on Patagonia, see Javier Roberto González's *Patagonia-patagones: orígenes novelescos del nombre* (Rawson, Argentina: Subsecretaría de cultura de la Provincia del Chubut, 1999); for California, all relevant texts and maps are to be found in Miguel León Portilla, *Cartografía y crónicas de la antigua California* (Mexico City: Universidad Nacional Autónoma de México, 2001).

[21] Medieval typologies of monstrosity roughly followed those established by Isidore of Seville's: 1) hypertrophy, 2) atrophy, 3) excrescence of bodily parts, 4) superfluity of bodily parts, 5) deprivation of parts, 6) hybrid, 7) animal births by human women, 8) mislocation of organs or parts, 9) disturbed growth (being born old), 10) composite beings, 11) hermaphrodites, 12) monstrous races." See David Williams, *Deformed Discourse: the Functions of the Monster in Medieval Thought and Literature* (Montreal: McGill-Queen's University Press, 1996), p. 107.

[22] Jeffrey Jerome Cohen's study of giants in medieval English romance offers a striking analysis of the role of gender in the construction of nationhood, especially through psychoanalysis. One would be hard pressed to make use of his insights for the Spanish context, as the overt focus of the book is English literature and its ties to French materials. The only mention of a Spanish character is, curiously, the Patagones, which Cohen makes part of the giant's progeny in the introduction, with which, however, neither the Patagón nor its ancestors have any relation. See *Of Giants. Sex, Monsters and the Middle Ages* (Minneapolis: University of Minnesota Press, 1999).

containment, balance, and propriety. It is curious that Spanish epic does not present giants as potential contenders for its heroes, as the French *chanson de geste* often does, from the ferocious Loquifer to Ferragus to the controversial Rainouart. As is well known, Arthurian romance took the character from epic into Chrétien's *Yvain*, where he appears as the evil Harpin de la Montagne, and from then onwards the giant, both in its foundational and in its folkloric traits would become a typical presence in chivalric fiction.[23] In the book of chivalry, the monster emerges when this uncontained physicality is duplicated into a transgressive morality. This excess inevitably takes shape though sexuality: excessive desire, frequently incest, and especially zoophilia, which brings to mind interesting echoes from the news of fabulous fauna that reached the Peninsula from the Americas and sparked the renewed interest in natural history. Both characteristics must be present, excessive form and deformed morality, as if excessiveness had to occur at least twice for the monstrous to appear.

I will look here at two particular cases, the most famous being engendering of the Endriago, lord of the Ínsula del Diablo, with an excursus on Andandona, both in the *Amadís de Gaula*; and that of the Patagón, the notable monster of the *Primaleón*, after which I will return to the politics of gender, the rhetoric of monstrosity, and a discussion on the nature of power through the monstrous.

Love of Family (or Narcissism 1)

The encounter with an absolute Other in the *Amadís* takes place upon an island, ruled over by a monstrous beast, the Endriago.[24] The arrival upon this island is mysterious, framed by a sudden change of wind, a fierce sea contrary to both ship and the knowledge of sailors, a dense rain and onerous skies that land them roughly after 8 long days. Upon recognizing their whereabouts, the sailors turn desperate and wish for the ship to be thrown back into the sea.[25] The sailors' relief is turned upon arrival into premonitions of death. The realm of the monster, whose name is Endriago, is identified, and fear of it supersedes anything the sailors have just gone through. The island is described as uninhabited and some paragraphs later, Elisabad, the character in charge of chronicling the events, tells the story of the place. We are told that the island once belonged to a terrible giant called Bandaguido who ruled over other giants with territories around his

[23] The possibility of conversion in the giant is, of course, a most relevant difference between it and the monster, for which conversion is unthinkable.

[24] For an analysis of the episode as one of the most gratuitous and fantastic of all the romance, see Cacho Blecua, *Amadís: heroísmo heroísmo mítico cortesano* (Madrid: Cupsa Editorial, 1979), p. 281 and ss. For an opposite argument in terms of its conception as a key episode in Montalvo's recantation, see Juan Manuel Avalle-Arce, *Amadís de Gaula: El primitivo y el de Montalvo* (Mexico City: Fondo de Cultura Económica, 1990,) chapter 7, especially pp. 290–95.

[25] Garci Rodríguez de Montalvo, *Amadís de Gaula*, Juan Manuel Cacho Blecua, ed. (Madrid: Cátedra, 1987–1988), pp. 1129–30.

realm. Bandaguido married a giantess, gentle and kind, whose pity balanced her husband's cruelty to Christians. Their daughter, Bandaguida, turns out to be a most beautiful giantess, in fact more beautiful than any of her blood and size, "mas como la gran hermosura sea luego junta con la vanagloria, y la vanagloria con el pecado, viéndose esta donzella tan graciosa y loçana, y tan apuesta y digna de ser amada de todos, y ninguno, por la braveza del padre, no la osara emprender, tomó remedio postrimero amar de amor feo y muy desleal a su padre" ("but as great beauty is to be accompanied by vanity, and vanity with sin, the damsel, seeing herself so graceful and exuberant, and so handsome and worthy of being loved by all, and by none, for no one would dare because of the fierceness of the father, took as a remedy to love her father with an ugly and most unloyal love," book III, ch. 73–4). Incest, by way of excessive beauty that in a concatenation of sins leads to vanity and a sense of entitlement that is coupled with sexual need, is introduced as a prelude to the story of the monster itself. It is also the result of a *crescendo* of other smaller sins: the cruelty of the father against Christians, emphasizing religious difference and thus the marginality of these giants and their kingdoms; the vanity of the daughter in a causal relationship with her beauty; and the solution the daughter Bandaguida must find because any possibility of a suitor is trumped by the fierceness of her father. Bandaguida is, in a way, a victim of both her beauty and her father's zealous and "effective" protection of her. As Rafael Mérida has noted, Montalvo here could have made use of the episode to condemn female vanity, allying himself with the contemporary clerical misogynist discourse and fifteenth-century debates on female virtuosity. Instead, Montalvo inserts a moral excursus where he makes clear that guilt lies in the father – or in fathers and men in general – for men should take care to distance themselves from the possibility of this sort of deviant desire.[26] Before the Endriago can come into being – the monster, for these giants are not yet monstrous – another sin is accumulated upon incest, that of homicide, as father and daughter devise to murder the kind giantess, wife and mother. After the deed is done and the mother lies deep inside a well, the giant takes his daughter as his wife. This, however, is not the first time that we have stumbled upon vain giants in the narrative.

Just eight chapters before (III, 65), and as a grand opening for Book III, as Amadís sails from his Ínsula Firme towards Gaula, and after just 5 days of alternating good and bad weather, they find themselves near an apparently beautiful island, covered with trees. Bruneo de Bonamar and Amadís decide to disembark in search for adventures, but a master warns them against it, telling them that the place in question is the Ínsula Triste, the kingdom of Madarque, most cruel of giants.[27] This is certainly not the first or the last encounter with giants

---

26 Rafael Mérida, "Tres gigantas sin piedad: Gromadaça, Andandona y Bandaguida," in *Literatura de caballerías y orígenes de la novela*, Rafael Beltrán ed. (Valencia: Universitat de València, 1998), pp. 219–33 (pp. 224–5).

27 For the Castilian *Tristan* as a source for the Ínsula Triste, see Martin de Riquer, "Agora lo veredes, dixo Agrajes," *Estudios sobre el Amadís de Gaula* (Barcelona: Sirmio,

or their relatives, as they are very popular in our romance. From Gandalaz to Famongomadán (giant of the Lago Ferviente and the Ínsula de Mongaça) and his wife Gromadaça; Madanfabul (giant of the Ínsula de la Torre Bermeja); Cartadaque de la Montaña Defendida; Albadançor; Gadancuriel; Ardán Canileo el Dudado; Balán; Bravor; Basagante; Dandasido; Madarque (giant of the Ínsula Triste) and his sister Andandona; Cuadragante; Lindoraque; Andaguel; Madasima (who is of giant lineage but who retains none of the traits, either physical or possibly moral); Barsinán (lord of Sansueña) are just some of them, and sometimes it is hard to discern just how much of giant there is still in some of the characters, as marriages between giants and smaller humans are common in the romance. Often the only sign of their gigantism is a nominal aggregation, as if size were corresponded linguistically in a name. Some of these giants, barely bordering the marvelous, are good, some bad, some gentle and kind, some horribly cruel, some beautiful and some particularly ugly. A great many of them rule over their own kingdoms, which brings in the political element. Their characteristics –their moral nature – will be revealed contextually. When the *jayán*, the common appellative for giant, who kidnaps Galaor is characterized as "dessemejado," what provokes fear (in the spectators of the scene, but also in the reader) is not precisely his appearance, contrary to what many critics assume, but the fact that the parents of the young prince cannot do anything to help their child. Afterwards, we see how Gandalaz, the giant, raises Galaor appropriately and, leaving him with a hermit, sees to his knightly apprenticeship through books.

Returning to our heroes approaching the giant Madarque's kingdom, it is not without fear that Bruneo and Amadís take up the challenge to go in search of the giant. Suddenly, they see Amadís's dwarf, Ardián, come running towards them, urging them to save Galaor and king Cildadán, who are fighting a giant's men. There follows a brief digression on pride, built upon the Babel episode and the mention of Nembrot, the proud giant builder of the Tower.[28] The defeat of pride,

---

1987), pp. 7–54. See also Rafael Ramos, "El *Amadís* de Juan de Dueñas: 'La ínsola del Ploro'," in *Actas del III Congreso de la Asociación Hispánica de Literatura Medieval*, ed. María Isabel Toro Pascua, (Salmanca: Biblioteca Española del siglo XV. Departamento de Literatura Española e Hispanoamericana, vol. II, 1994, pp. 843–52), who argues that the Ínsula Firme "may have had at some point of its complex textual life the name of *ínsola del Ploro*" based on the analysis of Juan de Dueñas's verses (p. 852).

[28] For more on giants and the Tower of Babel in the Spanish tradition, see Cacho Blecua, "Introducción al estudio de los motivos en los libros de caballerías: la memoria de Román Ramírez," *Libros de caballerías (de "Amadís" al "Quijote),"* (Salamanca: SEMYR, 2002), pp. 27–53, especially pp. 42–3, and Simone Pinet, ""Babel historiada: un episodio del *Libro de Alexandre*," in *Literatura y conocimiento medieval. Actas de las VIII Jornadas Medievales*, ed. Lillian von der Walde, Concepción Company, Aurelio González, (Mexico City: Universidad Nacional Autónoma de México, Universidad Autónoma Metropolitana, El Colegio de México, 2003), pp. 371–89. For more on pride in books of chivalry, see Winston A. Reynolds, "Los caballeros soberbiosos del Amadís," in *Cuadernos Hispanoamericanos* 350 (1979): 387–96.

whether embodied by men or their hyperbolic mirror figures, such as giants or dwarfs, male or female, is a *topos* of the knight's combats in chivalric literature as much as a recurrent motif in medieval Castilian literature which flows into the early modern period, and as such is part of the construction not only of gigantism but of monstrosity in general. All four knights then marvelously defeat men and giant, but the giant's life is pardoned because 1) he is the father of Gasquilán, King of Suesa, whom Cildadán loves dearly; and 2) because Amadís makes him promise he will become Christian and build churches and monasteries, in a doubly bound motif, as it is a *topos* of Arthurian romance to have the knight fight against "mauvaises coutumes," and as the motif of conversion will become prevalent in posterior books of chivalry, mirroring the colonial politics of the Spanish empire.

As the knights prepare to leave, they stop by to see how the giant is recovering from his wounds. He is being looked after by Andandona, his older sister by 15 years who presents a peculiar physiognomy: she is covered with white, rough hair which cannot be brushed, her face ugly to the point she resembles a devil. She carries bow and arrows, is dressed with the skin of animals she kills, and is a fierce enemy of Christians. She presents paradoxical qualities, such as being extremely large but also extremely light, while she also has the ability of taming all animals and being able to mount all horses, no matter how savage they are, reinforcing her closeness to animalhood but also a connection to nature itself.[29] She is on many occasions confused with or called the devil. Three chapters later, she encounters death in the hands of Gandalín. Trying to kill Amadís, she fails, flees with Gandalín after her, in her hurry she makes her horse rise and she falls under it, Gandalín in turn runs her over and decapitates her.

Andandona thus bears different traits that approximate her to the monstrous, which we do not really encounter until we have read the following description of the Endriago:[30]

> Tenía el cuerpo y el rostro cubierto de pelo, y encima havía conchas sobrepuestas unas sobre otras tan fuertes, que ninguna arma las podía passar, y las piernas y pies eran muy gruessos y rezios, y encima de los ombros havía alas tan grandes,

---

[29] For wild beings, see Richard Bernheimer's classic, *Wild Men in the Middle Ages: A Study in Art, Sentiment, and Demonology*. New York, Octagon Books, 1970 [1952]. For an exhaustive Spanish context for the figure see Santiago López-Ríos, *Salvajes y razas monstruosas en la literatura castellana medieval* (Madrid: Fundación Universitaria Española, 1999); also A. Deyermond, "El hombre salvaje en la novela sentimental," *Actas del Segundo Congreso Internacional de Hispanistas* (Nijmeigen: University of Nijmeigen, 1967), pp 265–72.

[30] Cacho Blecua in *Amadís: heroísmo*, "La génesis del monstruo," pp. 31–7, François Delpech, "Fragments hispaniques d'un discours incestueux," *Autour des parentés en Espagne au XVIe et XVIIe siècles. Histoire, mythe et littérature*, ed. A. Redondo (Paris: Publications de la Sorbonne, 1987), pp. 77–128 and Gracia, "La bestia ladradora," put the Endriago in relation to the Arthurian motif of the Barking Beast, the *Beste Glattissant* from the *Suite du Merlin* to the Castilian *Baladro del sabio Merlín* and the Castilian and Portuguese *Demandas*.

> que fasta los pies le cubrían, y no de péndolas, mas de un cuero negro como la pez, luziente, velloso, tan fuerte que ninguna arma las podía empeçer, con las cuales se cubría como lo fiziesse un hombre con un escudo. Y debaxo dellas le salían braços muy fuertes assí como de león, todos cubiertos de conchas más menudas que las del cuerpo, y las manos havía de fechura de águila con cinco dedos, y las uñas tan fuertes y tan grandes, que en el mundo podía ser cosa tan fuerte que entre ellas entrasse que luego no fuesse desfecha. Dientes tenía dos en cada una de las quixadas, tan fuertes y tan largos, que de la boca un codo le salían, y los ojos, grandes y redondos, muy bermejos como brasas, assí que de muy lueñe, siendo de noche, eran vistos y todas las gentes huían dél. Saltava y corría tan ligero, que no havía venado que por pies se le pudiesse escapar; comía y bevía pocas vezes, y algunos tiempos, ningunas, que no sentía en ello pena ninguna. Toda su holgança era matar hombres y las otras animalias bivas, y cuando fallava leones y ossos que algo se le defendían, tornava muy sañudo, y echava por sus narizes un humo tan spantable, que semejava llamas de huego, y dava unas bozes roncas espantosas de oír; assí que todas las cosas bivas huían ant'él como ante la muerte. Olía tan mal, que no havía cosa que no emponçoñasse; era tan espantoso cuando sacudía las conchas unas con otras y hazía cruxir los dientes y las alas, que no pareçía sino que la tierra fazía estremeçer. Tal es esta animalia Endriago llamado como vos digo. (pp. 1132–3)

> (Its body and face were covered by hair, and on it shells overlaid one upon the other so strong that no weapon could pierce them, and its legs and feet were thick and strong, and upon its shoulders it had wings so large that covered it to the toes, and not of feathers, but of a leather pitch black, lustrous, hairy, so strong than no weapon could hurt them, with which it covered itself as a man with his shield. And under them very strong arms came forth like a lion's, all covered with shells smaller than those of the body, and hands it had like an eagle with five fingers, and nails so strong and big that in the world there was not a thing so strong as to come between them without becoming torn. Teeth it had two in each jawbone, so strong and long that from the mouth like an arm they protruded, and the eyes, big and round, very red like hot coals, so that from afar, at night, they were seen and all people fled. It jumped and ran so lightly that there was no deer that could escape it; it ate and drank few times, and sometimes, not at all, feeling no need to. All its pleasure was to kill men and other live animals, and when it found lions and bears who resisted it some, it became very angry, and yelled in deep screams horrible to hear; so that all live things fled him as death. It smelled so bad there was nothing it did not poison; it was so horrible when it shook its shells one against the other and crushed its teeth and wings that it seemed to make the earth tremble. Such is this animal called Endriago as I tell you.)

For sure, there are some similarities with Andandona, such as the lightness with which it can run, and the giant relatives. But the Endriago itself is no giant. It is a monster, covered with hair, scales, and wings (notice that the wings are covered in leather and not in fathers, as angel wings would), has parts of lion and eagle, and it blows smoke out of its nose. Not only is its appearance horrifying, but even the noises it produces make all things alive fear it like death, it also smells terrible and can make the earth tremble. All these characteristics in fact add up to a description of the Endriago as a machine of war, as Juan Manuel Cacho Blecua has suggested.

Its lightness, its meanness, all its physical power and, most of all, its indifference to lack of food or water or rest make it apparently invincible. That is, until it faces the heroic knight.

Amadís's victory is not only a victory over ugliness, following Ulrich of Strassburg's dictum in his *Summo Bono* that ugliness is the triumph of chaos over order, a victory that would be the restoration of order in the world, perfectly coherent with all other activity of our hero.[31] It is also a triumph over sin. For, as the text carefully informs the reader, the Endriago is the result not only of incest and homicide but, as a book kept by the emperor of Constantinople tells, the Endriago's traits are also the result of a cult of idols: one in the shape of man, who gives the Endriago reason, "yo le di de mi semejança en hazer conforme al alvedrío de los hombres, de que todas las bestias careçen" (p. 1132, "I gave him the ability to do as men's free will allows them, which all beasts lack"), which emphasizes the interiority of monstrosity within the human; another in the shape of a lion, who gives the Beast courage and fortitude; while the third, in the shape of a griffin, gives it wings and nails and lightness. The participation of devils in the conception of the Endriago is explicit: "aquella malaventurada noche fue engendrado una animalia por ordenança de los diablos, en quien ella y su padre y marido creían" (p. 1132, "that unfortunate night an animal was engendered by order of devils, in which she and her father and husband believed"). The four women who are there to raise the monster upon its birth are killed by the Endriago; all except for the fourth, who does not offer the beast her breast but feeds it cow milk for a year. When mother and father of the Endriago come to see it for the first time, the beast kills its mother and Bandaguido accidentally kills himself, while the Endriago flees out the door, "and not a long time went by that some were killed by it, and those who had ships and boats fled through the sea, so that the island was uninhabited, and it has been so for over forty years."

Ultimately, the association of ugliness and depravity or sin was a commonplace, as Harriet Goldberg remarks, and takes its authority from the Bible (Leviticus 21: 17–23, where the deformed are forbidden to approach the altar from profaning the holy sanctuary) and from a campaign linking historical events to the birth of monstrous children from incestuous relationships.[32] By the end of the twelfth century, writes Georges Duby, it was necessary to provoke the anxiety present in the population through the threat of teratological effects of sexual relations with blood-relatives, necessary because the simple prohibition was not doing much to stop these relationships.[33] This campaign in the Iberian Peninsula took shape, among other elements, in the printing of the *Libro del Anticristo* in the same years

---

[31] Quoted in Harriet Goldberg, "The Several Faces of Ugliness in Medieval Castilian Literature." *La Corónica,* 7 (1979): 81. For an analysis in opposite key, see Sylvia Roubaud-Bénichou, "Corps en beauté, corps à l'épreuve: le héros du roman de chevalerie," in *Le Corps dans la societé espagnole des XVIè et XVIIè siècles*, A. Redondo, ed. (Paris: Publications de la Sorbonne, 1990), pp. 253–66.

[32] Ibid., p. 84; Gracia, "El 'Palacio Tornante'y el bizantinismo del *Amadís de Gaula,*" p. 92.

[33] Quoted in Gracia, "El Palacio," p. 75.

Montalvo composed his *Amadís*, which takes the incest motif to the conception of the Beast itself, the Antichrist, due to the sexual encounters of a father with his daughter and the participation of devils in the conception of the Beast.[34] "The Endriago, like the Antichrist, obviates the misfortunes that illicit desires entail and which are associated generally with the idea that sins reproduce themselves into new crimes," writes Paloma Gracia, "for in general, sexual passions among family members lead to the homicide of direct relatives: in this way the Endriago of *Amadís* is a model as the Antichrist himself is, not only because its conception takes place after the parricide committed by its mother, but because in itself – its condition, or its appearance – it is a perfect example of both beast and devil."[35] Thus, its appearance is that of *absolute* ugliness, according to Goldberg's classification, and this is what distances the Endriago from all other beasts, "animalias," of evil beings in the romance. The most common form of ugliness in medieval texts is exaggeration – such as being a giant or a dwarf, a question of size – but it is also distortion or deformity: "Very flat noses, or long hooked ones were ugly as were sunken deep-set eyes either large or small. Frequently, ugly features were presented in animal terms – horse-teeth, rat's eyes, donkey's ears, dog's snout, so that along with deformity we can add the element of inappropriateness – the juxtaposition of the human and the bestial."[36] The link with the bestial also brought with it the characteristics or traits commonly assigned to the animal in bestiaries, providing a moral dimension to the physical. In *Amadís*, the example of Ardián Canileo, a giant who presents the ideally ugly portrait (thick neck, flat wide nose, snout like a dog's – which gives him his name – reddish freckled skin, thick lips and hair and beard so curly he couldn't comb it, heavy and bony) is an excellent example of this overlap, which could already be seen in Andandona.

Goldberg argues that along with the expected sensation of fright these descriptions produced in the reader, she or he experimented also a "*frisson* of delight," provoked by a relief and feeling of pride from surviving, vicariously, a perilous encounter, which with the intensity of the ugliness produces, at the same time, beauty. The popular motif of the comparison between beauty and beast – in the episode of the Endriago alluded to only by Amadís's invoking of Oriana – is a common situation in which one finds the ugly, providing us with another interesting scenario: "The nature of the sexual fantasy inherent in the encounter of innocent, vulnerable beauty with an ugly, lascivious, unrestrained creature is evident,"[37] Goldberg points out,

---

34 Ibid., p. 93. María Isabel Toro Pascua notes that the conception of the Antichrist as the result of an incestuous relation had already been presented in the peninsula by Francesc Eiximenis in his 1404 *Vida de Jesucrist*, and would continue to figure as essental to the Antichrist origins throughout the sixteenth century, as in Nicolás Díaz's 1588 *Tratado del Juicio Final* or the seventeenth-century *El Anticristo* by Juan Ruiz de Alarcón. ("*Amadís de Gaula* y la tradición apocalíptica medieval," in *Amadís de Gaula: quinientos años después. Estudios en homenaje a Juan Manuel Cacho Blecua*, Alcalá de Henares: Centro de estudios cervantinos, 2008, pp. 769–85.

35 Ibid., p. 94.

36 Goldberg, p. 82.

37 Goldberg, p. 82.

and these situations usually provide two solutions, one through moralizing, another one through humor, as we saw in the case of Andandona.

There is, finally, the link with the demoniacal, as the Endriago is said to contain within himself, even suggesting a double engendering, the devil itself. It is due to the force of incest that the devil entered in, which exits the monster's mouth before the soul does after it is killed by the hero: "before the soul came out of it, the devil came out of its mouth, and there was a great thunder in the air." The defeat of the Endriago is duly labeled not only marvelous, but miraculous, strengthening the episode's links with hagiography: "Certainly, sir, this is a miraculous thing, for I never heard of a mortal person fighting the devil, if it were not for those saints with their spiritual weapons," and, as is common in the *Amadís*, the event is inscribed into the landscape in the form of architecture, in this case, statues and a monastery that the emperor of Constantinople orders to be erected along with the dutiful writing down of the battle on a book – the book from which Elisabad tells us the story.[38]

The episode is structural to the romance. It is the most spiritual of Amadís's adventures, and the most difficult for him to achieve. In between the empires of Constantinople and the kingdom of Lisuarte de Grecia in Britain, Amadís defeat of the monster is a confirmation of monarchy.[39] He acts in the name of Lisuarte, but does so by liberating a territory belonging to the emperor of Constantinople, summarizing the military and diplomatic needs chivalry as a class fulfills for the nascent State. But Amadís's actions also place the hero and his claims for a class in a precarious borderline, both affirming monarchy and denying it absolute power, making it simultaneously universal and reliant upon this motivated, independent, and at times even stateless class. Decidedly ambiguous in the power he holds, the hero's subjection to a strict moral code is the sole guarantee of the knight's action in the name of his king. It is precisely this ambiguity that brings together monster and hero at the limits of statehood through a figure of morality that is ultimately a reflection on power: if monster and hero are but two sides of the same gesture, the key to the knight's positive sign is simply that of fidelity.

Love of Animals (or Narcissism 2)

The case of the Patagón presents interesting differences, which may be attributed to the book's inhabiting different political imaginaries, one tending towards the medieval, the other to a full-fledged Renaissance. In chapter 133 of the *Primaleón* (Salamanca, 1512) – the second book in the *Palmerín* cycle, we are told that Primaleón orders his men to leave the island of Címtara, where the adventure with

---

[38] The hagiographic links of the episode were first pointed out by John K. Walsh, "The chivalric dragon: hagiographic parallels in early Spanish romances," *Bulletin of Hispanic Studies* 54 (1977): 189–98.

[39] Toro Pascua, cited above, reads the episode as bringing together folkloric and apocalyptic materials. In light of the apocalyptic tradition especially, in the last pages of an insightful article, she links the episode to the messianic atmosphere that surrounded Ferdinand's figure, thus allowing for a historically grounded political reading of the Endriago episode (see esp. pp. 783–5).

the giant Gatarú has been finished by don Duardos. They have no provisions to stock the fleet, but Primaleón wishes to depart immediately without asking for help, and after 3 days they arrive at a much larger island, with a population spread out in cities and villages along the coasts. Received by the lord of the island and looked after by his sons, Primaleón inquires about the size and population of the island. Palantín, one of the sons, explains that the population is concentrated along the coastline because the central part of the island is of difficult access due to its high mountains. In these mountainous areas, in recent years, a strange people have come to live. They wish no contact with other people and live like animals, wild and solitary and eating what they hunt raw. Their dress, unseemly, is made of the skins of those animals they hunt but none of this compares to a man among them called Patagón: "Mas todo es nada con un hombre que agora ay entr'ellos que se llama Patagón" ("But it is nothing compared to a man now among them called Patagón").[40] Engendered by another mountain animal, one of the most horrible in the world except for its exceptional understanding and friendliness or attraction towards women, the Patagón is the result of zoophilia, committed by one of the savage women, called "patagones" because of their wildness, with the animal in question (a monstrosity anticipated by Pliny). It is only Fernando Bernal, the author of *Floriseo* (Valencia, 1516) who tells us that the patagones as a race, have their origin in even another previous case of zoophilia, this time between a man and an animal from whom a figure of man with animal skin resulted, who then would have had offspring by some woman thus engendering the patagones as a race. The sin, the moral *desmesura* is here, again, zoophilia. Duplicated, having its first occurrence as coming from a man, not a monster, not even a giant or dwarf or as the result of malefic enchantment; the second time as the enactment of lust of a (horrible but intelligent and friendly) animal on the body of one of these wild women. Patagón's composite body renders visible the duplicate sin at its conception and is, in fact, proof of it: "y que aquel animal engendró en ella aquel fijo; y esto tiénenlo por muy cierto según salió desemejado, que tiene la cabeça como de can y las orejas tan grandes que le llegan fasta los hombros, y los dientes muy agudos y grandes que le salen fuera de la boca retuertos, y los pies de manera de ciervo y corre tan ligero que no ay quien lo pueda alcançar" ("and that animal engendered in her that son; and this is certain because of how unseemly it is, having a dog's head and ears so large that they reach its shoulders, and teeth so pointed and long they come out of its mouth, and deer's feet and it can run so lightly that no one can catch it," p. 321).The Patagón only kills men that are not from its region, the mountains, and even when the men have jointly attempted to kill it they have been unable to hurt it. They have ceased to attempt fighting it or the race of patagones that come to its aid when the Patagón sounds its horn. The men have left it up to God to remove the Patagón from the world and thus satisfy a need that they are unable to fulfill for themselves, "for its death is very necessary to us" (p. 322). Primaleón will be the one, of course, who under the surname of

[40] María Carmen Marín Pina, ed., *Primaleón* (Alcalá: Centro de Estudios Cervantinos, 2001), p. 321.

Knight of the Broken Rock will achieve this: "Oh, Knight of the Broken Rock – said Palantín –, what grace has God given me that I never thought I would see so good a knight! Not all of those on this island could do what you by yourself have done!" (p. 324).

The Patagón resembles Andandona in eating habits, in activity (hunting, with the help of two lions), and in dress (skins of hunted animals), as well as in the lightness that enables it to flee or outrun anyone, along with a certain intimacy or understanding with animals (Patagón has two trained lions with him). He also carries the same weapons, the bow and arrows (he is also seen later using a knife). The resemblance with the Endriago, on the other hand, is mostly due to a sinful genealogy made visible through physical deformity, for even if the Endriago is also characterized by lightness, the monster of *Amadís* does not need dress, does not hunt with arms but kills with its own teeth and claws. Like the Endriago, the Patagón kills men and is responsible for a certain depopulation, while also being characterized as a sort of devil ("it is better to see the devil than to see it," p. 322, "we will take this devil prisoner," p. 323, and in Gridonia's words on p. 336, "This is the devil or its doing." It also shares with Andandona the gift of language, even if it is one that others – non-patagones – cannot understand.

Linguistic ability and deficiency are particularly interesting features, and they turn up on two occasions. First, when the Patagón, terribly wounded by Primaleón and chained – for the hero, finding it such a strange thing to look at, takes it prisoner so Gridonia may see it – bellows so fiercely that two patagones come to its aid. Upon seeing Patagón, they seem frightened and exchange many words: "ellos, cuando tal vieron a Patagón, fueron muy espantados y muchas cosas dezían, mas Primaleón no las entendía" ("when they saw Patagón in this way they were very frightened and said many things, but Primaelón could not understand them," p. 323). Primaleón kills the enemies, and his men take the monster back to be healed so that it can survive the trip to be exhibited in front of Gridonia. Patagón, wishing death upon itself, does not allow the wise men near it. At this point, another element, which was already present, if minimally, in the Endriago episode, makes its way into the narrative in an innovative and, as we will see, transformative way. Selvida, the only daughter of the lord of the island, comes to see the monster out of sheer curiosity. She is frightened at the sight of the Patagón, but the monster reacts by becoming tame, the result of a natural tendency, inherited from its beastly father, to be pleased by women – especially those as beautiful as Selvida.[41] As everybody becomes aware of Patagón's weakness in front of women, Selvida becomes instrumental in its healing and, in a way, in the monster's forfeiting its

[41] "Y sabed que él avía aquella condición, ansí como el animal que lo engendró, de ser muy ledo contra las mugeres y ansí lo fue Patagón contra Selvida que no pudo negar su natural, especialmente con aquella que le parecío estrañamente fermosa como ella lo era" ("And know that he was of the same nature, as was the animal who engendered him, of being very attracted to women and so was Patagón attracted to Selvida that he could not deny his nature, especially with one who seemed to him as strangely beautiful as she did," p. 325).

death wish. She persuades Patagón through language, more specifically through flattery: "començólo de falagar con dulces palabras, y rogávale que se dexase curar y él lo entendió bien, mas no lo quiso fazer porque él mesmo se entendía de curar. Y sacó la lengua muy grande y bermeja y començó de lamber las feridas y dezíale que aquello le bastaría, mas el su lenguaje ella ni otro no podían entender" ("she began to flatter it with sweet words, and she begged it to allow the men to heal it and he understood it well, but did not wish to for it could heal itself. And it stuck out a large red tongue and began to lick its wounds, and it told her that would be enough, but its language neither her nor any other could understand," p. 325). From the lips of this woman surge forth multiple perspectives on language: first there is flattery, characterized by the sweetness of the words, which often is the adjective used to refer to rhetoric itself, here intended as tone of voice, buttressed by the pleading characterization that follows. This flattery is intended to persuade the Patagón to allow them to look at its wounds. The Patagón *understands* this complex rhetorical game, but does not concede because it *knows* how to heal itself. The word *understand*, *entender*, here renders both comprehension and knowledge, understanding the language of Selvida and knowing how to heal itself are rendered through the same verb. Moreover, the instrument the Patagón uses to heal its wound is its tongue, the same tongue it uses to tell Selvida it will be fine in a language, however, that neither Selvida nor any other will comprehend. Patagón is capable of understanding the words Selvida says to it, but *its* words nobody understands. Some chapters later, on p. 138, Primaleón brings the Patagón for Gridonia to see and the *frisson of delight* that the hero had experienced in anticipation of the encounter of the monster is here reiterated:[42] "Primaleón ovo estraño plazer en ver a su señora con tanto miedo, que lo tenía abraçado y no lo dexava y d'esto folgó él mucho y díxole: -Mi señora, no ayáis miedo, que este que aquí veis es hombre umano y fará vuestro mandado. Y pídovos por merced que vos lleguéis a él y lo falaguéis y veréis cuán manso torna que lo podremos sacar de aquí y vello han todos" ("Primaleón felt a strange pleasure in seeing his lady so afraid that she held on to him and would not let him go, which he enjoyed very much, and said to her – My lady, do not be afraid, for this you here see is a human man, and will do what you want. And I ask you that you go to him and flatter it, and you will see it will become so tame we will be able to get it out of here, and all shall see," p. 336). Primaleón describes the Patagón in its *humanity*, emphasizing it as that which the lady's flattering words will tame and claim for obedience. Later on, while Patagón is being exhibited in the palace, Gridonia's lion, her personal guard, attacks it, ripping off its extant hand and badly wounding it. Primaleón threatens the lion and it backs down, allowing the hero to take its leash and to lead him back to Gridonia's chamber. The Patagón is thus fully transformed, this

[42] "Primaleón hovo muy gran sabor de reír y dio tanta priessa que luego se armaron y bien veinte cavalleros fueron a caça …" ("Primaleón really wanted to laugh, and hurried them all so much that they were armed fast and as many as twenty knights went out on the hunt," p. 322).

time through gratefulness at the kindness and courage of Primaleón: "Y desde aquella ora Patagón conoció el bien que Primaleón le fizo y desde allí adelante él le fue muy mandado y él mesmo se curó las llagas como fizo las que Primaleón le fizo" ("And from that moment Patagón knew the good that Primaleón had done for him and from then onward it was obedient and healed its wounds it had done with those that Primaleón had given it," p. 337). By now unable to attack, Patagón is unchained by Primaleón and assimilates into the community, devoting special attention to Zérfira – yet another beautiful lady.

There are three captivating elements to the composition of this narration: language, the beauty and the beast motif, and the emphasis on the monster's humanity, all interrelated. For beauty's humanizing powers are a *topos* that in this particular context anticipate what probably is Golden Age theater's most famous character, that of Calderón's Segismundo and the surrender of its bestiality when faced with Rosaura's beauty. Inevitably linked to femalehood, beauty is for the Patagón an indispensable condition for interaction with the community, for the human in the monster to come out. It is in fact almost lured out, as language becomes key in the process of transforming monstrosity through those sweet, flattering words that pacify the beast. But language is also part of the monster, it is not something that pertains solely to the human, and the idea of a misunderstanding or ignorance on the part of what is not monstrous is contemplated. In fact, language seems to be present in the monster in a much wider spectrum than in the other characters, for it can understand the others, but the others cannot understand it. Primaleón's characterization of the Patagón as human explicitly formulates monstrosity as an inhabitant of the self, as a possibility within all of us, as the sign of something that requires domination, control, suppression sometimes, though here merely meriting persuasion. However, the integration of the monster within the community does not entail – nor require – its understanding. The overcoming of the monstrous in the *Primaleón* passage is thus quite an interesting variation on *Amadís's* account of monstrosity: while there the knight's political necessity is made clear in the confrontation with the monstrous, Primaleón does not need to annihilate the monster since it seems more fruitful to turn this victory into a spectacle: the spectacle of chivalric power, based on virtue, which intersects with the ongoing discussion on the nature of nobility.[43] On the other hand, in terms of gender, this episode also becomes quite more interesting with the location of knighthood in the theater of political power, as female beauty becomes crucial for the spectacle of chivalry and thus for the victory over the monstrous to be truly

[43] Jesús Rodríguez Velasco argues that the discussion on nobility is at the core of what he calls the "chivalric fable," and brings together contemporary politico-juridical discussions, such as Dante's and Sasofferato's, to show how literature enacts a theory on knighthood that will have consequences in practical, historical terms ("Teoría de la fábula caballeresca").

functional.[44] It is woman as beauty that must first persuade the beast for it to survive, to then convince it to overcome its bestiality to enter the community. In a way, this is a strategy of conversion, of encapsulation, both domination and repression of the other without requiring understanding, where the interdependence of gender functions is vital for the success of the political enterprise being suggested.

In the case of *Primaleón*, gender becomes a central issue again outside of the text. The verses dedicated to the reader at the end of both the first and this, the second book of the cycle, indicate that the author of both books is a woman, identified with the pseudonym of Augustobrica, the Latin toponym for Ciudad Rodrigo.[45] The authorship of the *Primaleón*, which remains confusing to this day, if attributed to a woman such as Beatriz Galindo, Juana Contreras, María de Pacheco, Isabel de Vergara, Lucía de Medrano, or anyone in this group of cultivated women active in Isabella's court, would be "an early example of female authorship in Spain's Golden Age literature, predating Beatriz Bernal, Feliciana Enríquez de Guzmán or María de Zayas."[46] Beyond the attribution, Marín Pina argues that from 1511–1512 female authorship was used as a marketing strategy, and cites Francisco Delicado's prologue to the Venetian edition of *Primaleón* as example: "note that what follows is *more delectable because* it was composed by a woman."[47] Whether or not we consider a woman as its author, the question of books of chivalry as a genre particularly oriented to the explication and refunctionalization of a class in the context of the birth of the absolutist State in the figures of Isabella and Fernando, finds in *Primaleón* a gender component intimately related to the monstrous that is radically different from what medical treatises and scientific discourse in general presented.

The influence of the Aristotelian model both in the differentiation of species and of causality is central not only to the work of sixteenth-century philosophers such as Fray Luis de Granada, Francisco Sánchez, Juan Huarte de San Juan, and Juan Ginés de Sepúlveda, but also to humanists such as Antonio de Nebrija himself or Antonio de Torquemada – as is to be expected, though the Foucauldian assertion that one can see both elements (differentiation and causality) only from

---

44 While in most adventures Amadís' remembrance of his lady Oriana will strengthen him and thus guarantee his victory over his enemies, in the Endriago episode the moment when he remembers his lady before the combat with the monster is qualified as a weakness, a debility noticed by the monster who takes advantage of it. Love and woman in the episode thus take on well-known traits as debilitating forces.

45 "En este exmaltado y muy rico dechado/ van esculpidas muy bellas lavores/ de paz y de guerra y de castos amores/ *por mano de dueña prudente labrado*;/ es por exemplo de todos notado/ que lo verisímil veamos en flor,/ es de Augustobrica aquesta lavor/ que en Salamanca se ha agora estampado" ("... *by the hand of a prudent lady worked*;/it is for example of all noted/that the verisimilar we must see in bloom,/from Augustobrica is this work/ that in Salamanca has been now printed," *Primaleón,* p. 538).

46 Marín Pina, ix–x.

47 Cited in Marín Pina, x, my emphasis.

the seventeenth-century onward, as Strosetzki remarks, is countered by these Spanish early sixteenth-century figures.

Primaleón itself sets the distance between its discourse on monstrosity and those of medical and gestation/birth treatises or manuals. The book's anonymous dedication to Luis de Córdoba (but attributed to Augur de Trasmiera, author of the Latin verses that end the *Palmerín de Olivia*, who also attributes the work to a woman: "Femina composuit; generosos atque labores/filius altisonans scripsit et arma libro")[48] begins with a reference to Nature's mistakes, which result in monsters, some of which can be seen – a clear reference to a monstruous birth contemporary to the writing of the prologue: "Because if Nature once engendered a man with two heads or a hand with six fingers or, what we have seen in past days, a head with two bodies, this was contrary to its intention and without thinking" and insists some lines later that "If at times brute animals and plants degenerate and do not respond to their species, it is so against nature in the same manner that a man born with two heads or for a calf to be born to a woman or a lamb to a cow. For the intention of nature is to keep its norm, and if it is able to, to not mix castes" (p. 2). From monstrous births as a freak of nature's ordered habits, the idea of purity of lineage is underlined and thus the discussion on nobility's essence is staked out from the start. The dedication goes on to ask the young Córdoba – and its potential audience – to read this work in historical key, not as a fictionalized account of historical events and people, but as the enactment of a political theory at work already, if only in part, in the Catholic Kings' territorial policy, on dynastic rights, the victory over Granada, the fight for Africa, and the ongoing problems with *mudéjares* and Turks.[49]

The intricate relations between the chivalric genre and historicity have been well discussed and need not be retold here. As a genre that articulates a politics where a class, knighthood, is presented as a necessity in a role that moves progressively from the military to the courtly to the diplomatic, a role that is repeatedly emphasized in the antagonism with the monstrous, *Primaleón* weaves in the need for women as part of the process. Whether one is to consider beauty as the key element, that is, aesthetics as a female function in conjunction with male military *ingenio* (both physical power and savvy or wit), or one includes the language of persuasion, or rhetoric, as part of that female role, the prominent political position that women are given in this book is to be regarded not only as a feat of political theory but as a radically different view of the ties between women and monstrosity contemporary to the misogynist presentations common to scientific discourse.

In terms of poetics, as the century wore on and as numerous critics used the same arguments again and again against books of chivalry, commonplaces that have been catalogued by Elisabetta Sarmati, one that stands out – because it moves structure to metaphor, from the theory of literature to a practiced poetics

---

48 Cited in Marín Pina, ix.

49 For more details see Marín Pina, introduction, xi–xii.

in *Don Quijote* – is the characterization of the book of chivalry as monstruous: "No he visto ningún libro de caballerías que haga un cuerpo de fábula entero con todos sus miembros, de manera que el medio corresponda al principio, y el fin al principio y al medio; sino que los componen con tantos miembros, que más parece que llevan intención a formar una quimera o un monstruo que a hacer una figura proporcionada " ("I have not seen a book of chivalry that makes an entire body of fable with all its members, so that the middle corresponds to the beginning, and the end to the beginning and the middle, but that they compose them with so many members that it seems they intend to give shape to a chimera or a monster than to make a proportioned figure").[50] This aesthetics, which will become dominant for the following period, has at its core a gendered political element that can be seen within the genre of chivalry, in yet another mirror of the history of the political, as a transforming process from the invocation of Oriana in *Amadís* and the characterization of Andandona to the emplacement of female political activity at the center of *Primaleón*.

[50] Miguel de Cervantes, *Don Quijote de la Mancha*, Francisco Rico, ed. (Madrid: Crítica, 1998), Book II, p. 47.

Chapter 6
Experiments with Alchemy: Caterina Sforza in Early Modern Scientific Culture[1]

Meredith K. Ray

In the preface to a popular sixteenth-century collection of alchemical, medicinal, and cosmetic recipes entitled the *Secreti della Signora Isabella Cortese* (1561), the author admonishes a correspondent not to waste his time and money trying to uncover the secrets put forth by traditional alchemical authorities, who write in coded, intentionally obscure language.

> . . . se vuoi seguir l'arte delle Alchimia, et in quella operare, non bisogna che più seguiti l'opere di Geber, né di Raimondo, né di Arnaldo, né d'altri filosofi, perché non hanno detto verità alcuna i libri loro, se non con figure, et engimati, con sincopi . . . io ho letto e riletto e non trovo se non favole, e ciancie.
>
> (...If you wish to learn and practice the art of Alchemy, there is no need to follow the works of Geber, nor Ramon, nor Arnault, or any other philosopher, any longer, for they reveal no truths in their books, except through figures, and enigmas, with syncope . . . I have read and reread them, and found nothing but tall tales and rumors . . .)[2]

Better, she insists, to place one's faith in practice and experiment, as she has done herself, and as she now reveals to her audience. To be a successful alchemist, Cortese advises following a few simple rules: learn the properties of all metals and materials; use strong, well-made earthen or glass vessels for laboratory experiments; know how to regulate the flame; and keep a bellows at the ready.

---

[1] Research for this essay was supported by a 2008–2009 fellowship from the Penn Humanities Forum Mellon Research Seminar and a 2009 Research Grant from the Renaissance Society of America.

[2] Isabella Cortese, *I secreti della Signora Isabella Cortese*, Chicca Gagliardo, ed. (Milan: La Vita Felice, 1995), p. 31. First published in 1561 (not 1584 as incorrectly noted by Gagliardo), Cortese's work had seven editions by 1599 and was translated into German. On this work and its publishing history see William Eamon, *Science and the Secrets of Nature: Books of Secrets in Medieval and Early Modern Culture* (Princeton, NJ: Princeton University Press, 1994), pp. 136–7; see also Claire Lesage, "La litterature des 'secrets' e 'I secreti d'Isabella Cortese'" in *Chroniques italiennes* 36 (1993): 145–78.

Most importantly, find a trustworthy assistant and keep him always at your side; reveal the work to no one; and give thanks to God – and alms to the poor – when the work is complete.[3]

Replete with recipes not only for effecting the transmutation of metals, but also for treating a range of physical ailments and producing a host of cosmetics, soaps, and perfumes, Cortese's work raises important questions about the practice of alchemy in sixteenth-century Italy. First, her instructions suggest – and recent scholarship has demonstrated – that alchemy was not the arcane province of an élite few, those with the tools to access the hermetic works of ancient authorities. Rather, it was a vibrant arena of scientific investigation accessible to the layperson as well as the initiate, one based on observation and trial and applied broadly and profitably to a range of quotidian problems.[4] Indeed, Cortese's emphasis on the tested nature of her recipes situates her work – and others like it – solidly within an early modern culture of empiricism that increasingly privileged praxis over theory, as William Eamon has noted.[5]

Second, and of particular interest here, Cortese's book of "secrets" – the only such collection to be published under a woman's name in this period[6] – provides a useful starting point for thinking about the engagement of early modern women with alchemy, both as readers and producers of alchemical texts, and as practitioners

[3] Cortese, *Secreti*, p. 32.

[4] The literature on alchemy in early modern Europe is extensive. Among recent studies, see Lawrence M. Principe, ed., *Chymists and Chymistry: Studies in the History of Alchemy and Early Modern Chemistry* (Sagamore Beach, MA: Science History Publications, 2007); Tara Nummedal, *Alchemy and Authority in the Holy Roman Empire* (Chicago: University of Chicago Press, 2007); Kathleen Perry Long, *Hermaphrodites in Renaissance Europe* (Aldershot, UK: Ashgate, 2006), ch. 4; Allen Debus, *The Chemical Philosophy: Paracelsian Science and Medicine in the Sixteenth and Seventeenth Centuries* (revised edition, Mineola, NY: Dover Publications, 2002); William R. Newman and Anthony Grafton, ed., *Secrets of Nature: Astrology and Alchemy in Early Modern Europe* (Cambridge, MA: The MIT Press, 2001); Pamela O. Long, *Openness, Secrecy, Authorship: Technical Arts and the Culture of Knowledge From Antiquity to the Renaissance* (Baltimore: Johns Hopkins, 2001); Pamela H. Smith, *The Business of Alchemy: Science and Culture in the Holy Roman Empire* (Princeton, NJ: Princeton University Press, 1997); Piyo Rattansi and Antonio Clericuzio, ed., *Alchemy and Chemistry in the Sixteenth and Seventeenth Centuries* (Dodrecht: Kluwer, 1994); Gareth Roberts, *The Mirror of Alchemy: Alchemical Ideas and Images in Manuscripts and Books From Antiquity to the Seventeenth Century* (London: The British Library, 1994); Alison Coudert, *Alchemy: The Philosopher's Stone* (Boulder: Shambhala, 1980).

[5] Eamon, *Science and the Secrets of Nature*, p. 4. Many books of secrets privilege experiential knowledge in this way: see for example, the dedication to Timoteo Rossello, *Della summa de' secreti* (Venice: Bariletto, 1565, unnumbered), which shares similarities to Cortese's text (on this relationship, see Lesage, pp. 162–4); see also the well-known preface to the *Secreti del reverendo donno Alessio Piemontese* (Venice, 1555).

[6] There is some debate over Cortese's female identity, based primarily on a lack of biographical documentation about her; the debate is detailed in Lesage.

of the "great work" in their daily lives. Part of a wave of printed *libri di segreti*, or "books of secrets," that characterized much of sixteenth-century print production,[7] Cortese's volume is dedicated to a specifically female audience. Its recipes, which include rouges, waters, soaps, and perfumes along with others for calcinated mercury and potable gold, are deemed useful to "every noble lady" ("ogni gran signora") and meant to reflect the range of uses that Renaissance women made of alchemy.[8] While there is no dearth of printed sources against which to compare Cortese's recipes when considering their provenance (indeed, the intertextual web created between books of secrets, alchemical texts, medical treatises, herbals, and other such works was vast and complex), many of the recipes offered by Cortese also found their inspiration in women's incorporation of alchemical practice into aspects of their everyday activities.[9]

Recent scholarship has begun to stress the active role of women throughout early modern Europe in the "patronage, theory and practice of alchemy,"[10] pointing to examples such as Anna Maria Zieglerin, an alchemist in early modern Germany, or Marie Meurdrac of France, author of a seventeenth-century chemistry manual for women.[11] Not only did women engage in the quest to produce alchemical gold, but they also incorporated alchemical practice into their lives, most especially with regard to the management of the household and the care of their own bodies and their family members. As an examination of manuscripts and printed books – including Cortese's manual – reveals alchemical ingredients and processes commonly underlay instructions for the preparation of medicines and cosmetics and for the preservation of food and wine, areas closely associated with women's duties and activities. Women practiced science on a daily basis: as Lynette Hunter

[7] The most extensive study of early modern books of secrets is Eamon, *Science and the Secrets of Nature*; see also Allison Kavey, *Books of Secrets: Natural Philosophy in England 1550–1600* (Urbana: University of Illinois Press, 2007). Nancy Siraisi notes that, "From the early Middle Ages to the high Renaissance, medicinal recipes" – a major element of the content of books of secrets – "were the commonest form of medical writing," *Medieval and Early Renaissance Medicine. An Introduction to Knowledge and Practice* (Chicago: University of Chicago Press, 1990), p. 141.

[8] As Penny Bayer notes, "A published book of alchemical receipts for a female readership is evidence that women might wish to undertake or supervise alchemical work, a point reinforced when the author is named a woman" ("From Kitchen Hearth to Learned Paracelsianism: Women and Alchemy in the Renaissance," in *Mystical Metal of Gold: Essays on Alchemy and Renaissance Culture*, ed. Stanton J. Linden [Brooklyn, NY: AMS Press, Inc., 2007]), p. 369.

[9] On the possible printed sources for Cortese's work, see Lesage. Siraisi (speaking of medical writing in general) states that recipe collections, along with other related texts, "may be a better guide than more sophisticated medical literature to the kinds of medicines most frequently prescribed" (*Medieval and Early Renaissance Medicine*, p. 148).

[10] Tara Nummedal, "Alchemical Reproduction and the Career of Anna Maria Zieglerin," *Ambix* 49 (2001): 56–68 (57).

[11] On Zieglerin, see Nummedal, ibid.; on Meurdrac, see Lucia Tosi, "Marie Meurdrac: Paracelsian Chemist and Feminist," *Ambix* 48.2 (2001): 69–82.

notes, the "non-formal" nature of this practice and its location within the domestic sphere has traditionally led scholars to undervalue or ignore it, but the kinds of work carried out in the home – cooking, gardening, tending the ill – involve aspects of physical and organic chemistry, as well as "all aspects of preventive medicine and pharmacy."[12] Books of secrets increasingly reflected this activity as they began to target a growing audience of women.

This essay examines one manuscript, probably begun in the late fifteenth century but transcribed in the early sixteenth, that offers compelling evidence of the uses of alchemy by early modern women and presages in many respects the range of recipes described in the *Secreti di Isabella Cortese* as well as that work's pragmatic approach to alchemy. Compiled by Caterina Sforza (1463–1509), this rich collection of recipes entitled *Experimenti* (*Experiments*) is a vivid record of Sforza's engagement with scientific culture.[13] Most noted for her role as a political leader, Sforza also had a documented interest in medicine and alchemy, one that has received far less attention from scholars. Throughout her life, she sought out and circulated recipes and remedies, maintaining a close relationship with her own *speziale* (apothecary) in Forlì and sending to Mantua and other cities for ingredients and instructions regarding medicinal and alchemical preparations. This essay explores what Sforza's *Experimenti* can tell us about gender and alchemy in early modern Italy. What kinds of recipes did Sforza collect, and how did she obtain them? How did her efforts to compile and test these recipes establish her within a network of other alchemical adepts, and what role did gender play in the dynamics of this network? How did Sforza's interest in alchemy relate to her political position? Finally, how do the experiments described by Sforza relate to later, published representations of similar recipes in works such as that of Isabella Cortese?

To contextualize my discussion of Sforza's work, I will begin by considering the role of alchemy in the *libri di segreti* tradition in sixteenth-century Italy, along with the place of gender within such texts. Who was the audience for such works, and how did this condition their content and presentation? In the second part of the essay, I will move on to a discussion of Sforza's alchemical activity as reflected in her *Experimenti* as well as in her epistolary exchanges with male and female contacts who aided her in the staging of such experiments.

***

Over the course of the sixteenth century, Italy saw a proliferation of printed vernacular texts devoted to popular medicine, the production of cosmetics and perfumes, and the dissemination of "secret" recipes and remedies aimed at

---

12 Cf. Lynette Hunter and Sarah Hutton, eds, *Women, Science and Medicine, 1500–1700: Mothers and Sisters of the Royal Society* (Thrupp, Stroud, Gloucestershire, UK: Sutton, 1997), p. 2; and in the same volume, Hunter, "Women and Domestic Medicine: Lady Experimenters, 1570–1620," p. 95.

13 *Experimenti de la Ex[ellentissi]ma S]igno]ra Caterina da Furlj Matre de lo inllux[trissi]mo S[ignor] Giovanni de Medici*; see n. 40 below.

enhancing personal health, facilitating the management of the household, and effecting the transmutation of metals. As Deborah Harkness has argued, receipt books, with their exhaustive and sometimes contrasting remedies, may be seen as a product of a "culture of therapeutics" that derived from a broader curiosity about the self and the body characteristic of the early modern period.[14] Along with a focus on the physical body, books of secrets also display a great interest in uncovering and reproducing the workings of the natural world, together with an optimism that such knowledge might be manipulated to better the time spent in this life.[15] The earliest printed Italian work of this kind, Eustachio Celebrino's *Dificio delle ricette* (*New Work Entitled the House of Recipes*, 1525), for example – a kind of "general household recipe book"[16] – combines, in an accessible vernacular format, medical and chemical information of various kinds. In addition to sections devoted to health and personal hygiene, the *Dificio delle ricette* includes perfumes, culinary recipes, and even marvelous parlor tricks (such as making a candle burn under water, or writing on paper without ink).[17] Emphasizing the empirical nature of his information, Celebrino is careful to note that his are "tested recipes, which

---

[14] Cf. Deborah Harkness, "Nosce teipsum: Curiosity, the humoral body and the culture of therapeutics in late sixteenth- and early seventeenth-century England," p. 188: "Receipt books represent an important artefact of the culture of therapeutics in which many different accounts of illness, as well as many different therapeutic prescriptions and regimes, are often juxtaposed in a single text." In *Curiosity and Wonder From the Renaissance to the Enlightenment*, R.J.W. Evans and Alexander Marr, eds. (Aldershot, UK: Ashgate, 2006), pp. 171–92. Harkness' focus is on the context of early modern England, which she sees as distinct from that of Europe, but her comments here are applicable to books of secrets more widely.

[15] Cf. Lesage, p. 146, "... les auteurs des "Secreti" ont une vision positive de la réalité, univers mouvant plein de mystères, mais qu'on peut façonner et, peut-être, apprivoiser, afin de améliorer le passage de l'être humain sur terre" ("... the authors of the "Books of Secrets" have a positive vision of reality, a living universe full of mysteries, but one which can be shaped, and maybe tamed, in order the ease the passage of the human being on earth"). Much work has been done on nature and the marvelous in the early modern period: see for example Lorraine Daston and Katherine Park, *Wonders and the Order of Nature 1150–1750* (New York: Zone, 1998); *Wonders, Marvels, and Monsters in Early Modern Culture*, Peter G. Platt, ed. (Newark: University of Delaware Press, 1999).

[16] Eamon, *Science and the Secrets of Nature*, p. 127.

[17] Eustachio Celebrino, *Opera nova intitolata dificio de ricette*; I consulted the 1528 edition published in Venice by Giovanni Antonio e Fratelli da Sabbio. Eamon calls this work the "best known and most popular title in what eventually grew to be a large family of Italian all-purpose manuals for household use" (Eamon, ibid). On Celebrino see Giovanni Comelli, *Ricettario di bellezza di Eustachio Celebrino, medico e incisore del Cinquecento* (Florence: Sansoni, 1960) and Stanley Morison, *Eustachio Celebrino da Udene Calligrapher, Engraver, and Writer for the Venetian Printing Press* (Paris: Pegasus Press, 1929); see also Eamon, *Science*, pp. 127–30.

will teach you about many wonderful secrets."[18] Similarly, the influential *Secreti del reverendo donno Alessio Piemontese* (1555),[19] with more than 100 editions and numerous translations, offers treatments for ailments ranging from skin rashes and rotting teeth to impotence and infertility; recipes for face creams and rouges; and methods for preserving food and wine, removing stains from linens, and dyeing fabrics. While, as Eamon notes, Alessio's recipes are clearly aimed at an upper-class reader most likely to make use of his soaps and pomanders as well as his medicinal recipes, his *Secreti* constitute an "alternative pharmaceutical tradition" made accessible to a broad audience – a new approach to science and medicine gleaned from "surgeons, empirics, gentlemen, housewives, monks, and ordinary peasants . . . anyone but representatives of the medical establishment."[20]

The audience for early modern secrets-books included not only an élite, highly educated public, but also a wider bourgeois audience that was becoming increasingly literate in Italian.[21] This reading public included a growing number of women, a shift that did not escape the attention of authors and publishers. As an examination of sixteenth-century medical manuals and secrets books reveals, many of these works overtly targeted this public of female readers. In an effort to earn their attention, they honed in on issues such as feminine beauty, domestic management, and women's health; offering, among other things, numerous remedies for problems with menstruation, pregnancy, childbirth, and lactation.[22] Especially with regard to cosmetics, such collections offered a pragmatic and neutral alternative to the decidedly negative approaches to feminine adornment that abounded in prescriptive works such as Leon Battista Alberti's *I libri della famiglia* (*On the Family*) (where the use of cosmetics is linked to moral as well as

---

[18] "…varie sorte di ricette experimentate, le quale te insegnaranno di molti bellissimi secreti…" (Celebrino, *Dificio de ricette*, aii–r).

[19] Some critics speculate that the real author of Alessio's *Secrets* was Girolamo Ruscelli, author of his own such work, the *Secreti nuovi* (Venice, 1566). Others take a more circumspect position (see Eamon, *Science and the Secrets of Nature*, pp. 134–51; Eamon and Françoise Peheau, "The Accademia Segreta of Girolamo Ruscelli. A Sixteenth-Century Italian Scientific Society," in *Isis* 75 (1984): 327–42; see also Lesage, pp. 160–62).

[20] Eamon, *Science and the Secrets of Nature*, p. 144.

[21] Carlo Dionisotti has argued that the linguistic openness of the period between 1545–1563 engendered by the emerging primacy of the vernacular in Italy fostered the entry into the literary arena of marginalized groups with limited access to formal education, including women; but see Virginia Cox, *Women's Writing in Italy, 1400–1650* (Baltimore: Johns Hopkins University Press, 2008), pp. xx–xxi and 82-4, for a critique of Dionisotti's periodization. On literacy rates in this period see also Paul Grendler, *Schooling in Renaissance Italy: Literacy and Learning, 1300–1600* (Baltimore: Johns Hopkins University Press, 1989).

[22] Efforts to appeal to a female readership extended across genres, for example to letter collections, which sometimes incorporated aspects of the *libri di segreti*; see Ray, *Writing Gender in Women's Letter Collections of the Italian Renaissance* (Toronto: University of Toronto Press, 2009), pp. 10–11, 67–8.

physical decay) or in a well-known passage from Ariosto's *Cassaria* that similarly derides women's pursuit of beauty.[23] Many books of secrets overtly addressed this female audience in their titles or dedications as well as their content. In addition to Cortese's work, directed to "every great lady," Timoteo Rossello's *Summa de' Secreti* (1565) singled out "men and women of great intellect" ("huomini e donne, di alto ingegno"); while Celebrino's *Opera nuova ... per far bella ciaschuna donna* (*New Work ... For Making Every Woman Beautiful*, 1551), opens with a sonnet that addresses female readers directly, *Donne che desiate farve belle* ("Ladies, who wish to make yourselves beautiful"). Another sixteenth-century work, the *Notandissimi secreti dell'arte profumatoria* (1555), a collection of recipes devoted solely to perfumes and cosmetics, was introduced by a letter addressed to "those most virtuous ladies who enjoy the art of perfume" ("le virtuosissime donne le quali si dilettano de l'arte profumatoria").

Many of the medicinal recipes detailed in vernacular books of secrets rely on procedures and ingredients associated with alchemy, an area of scientific experimentation that was intricately intertwined with the practice of medicine in the early modern period and, increasingly, applied to cosmetic and "marvelous" secrets as well.[24] Celebrino's sonnet cited above, for example, interweaves alchemical practice with the feminine arena of cosmetic enhancement by evoking distillation – the "primary procedure" of alchemy[25] – in the preparation of rouges and face creams. Celebrino elaborates, "Here are colors white and red/ Diverse concoctions of waters distilled" ("Quivi beletti son blanche e vermigli/

23 Alberti, *The Family in Renaissance Florence*, ed. and trans. Renée Neu Watkins (Illinois: Waveland Press, 1994), Bk. III, pp. 84–5. Giannozzo's comments to his wife about the corrupting effects of cosmetics are based on the real dangers presented by arsenic, an ingredient commonly present in remedies for the complexion, but he explicitly links them to the moral character of the user. Ariosto's *Cassaria*, V, III (Venice: Zoppino, 1538), despairs of women: "Spendono queste femine pur assai tempo in adornarse, mai non vengono al fine . . . hor col bianco, hor col rosso, metteno, levano, acconciano, guastano . . ." ("Women spend so much time making themselves beautiful, they are never done . . . now with the white, now with the red: they apply, they remove, they prepare, they ruin . . ." [my translation]). Ariosto also composed a more general satire entitled the *Erbolario* that targets not women specifically, but rather the charlatans that hawked useless remedies, cosmetic and medicinal, to men and women alike (*Satire e rime, nuovamente ordinate e corredate di note con in fine: L'erbolario, Le lettere, Le poesie attribuite all'autore e I carmi latini*, Trieste: Sez. letterario-artistica del Lloyd austriaco, 1858).

24 Many scholars note the linked nature of alchemical and medical practice in the early modern period: see for example, Chiara Crisciani, "From the Laboratory to the Library: Alchemy According to Guglielmo Fabri," in *Natural Particulars: Nature and the Disciplines in Renaissance Europe*, A. Grafton and N. Siraisi, eds. (Cambridge, MA: MIT Press, 1999), pp. 295–319; and Katherine Park, "Natural Particulars: Medical Epistemology, Practice, and the Literature of the Healing Springs," in ibid. 347–67.

25 Cf. Bruce Moran, *Distilling Knowledge: Alchemy, Chemistry, and the Scientific Revolution* (Cambridge, MA: Harvard University Press, 2005), p. 11.

Varie composition d'acque stillate").[26] A 1563 work spuriously attributed to the physician Gabriele Falloppio, the *Secreti diversi et miracolosi* (*Diverse and Miraculous Secrets*) describes various "healthful waters" (*acque molto salutifere*) likewise produced through distillation.[27] A recipe for women's rouge ("rosso per la faccia") calls for mixing several ingredients in a clean glass alembic, a central component of the alchemical laboratory, and allowing them to rest for two days before boiling them until all the ingredients have dissolved, a kind of cosmetic transmutation. A recipe to enhance the beauty of women's hair (*a far belli li capelli*) also calls for the prolonged distillation of ingredients in an alembic.[28] The *Secreti* of Isabella Cortese, which professes itself a compilation of "things mineral, medicinal, alchemical, and artificial," applies alchemical procedures to the domestic economy that was so central to women's world (laundering clothing, manufacturing perfumes, preparing and preserving food and wine), as well as to turning base metal into gold. In addition, many of the recipes offered by books of secrets rely on the kinds of ingredients commonly present in alchemical experiments, for example minerals such as antimony, silver, and gold, or the Paracelsian *tria prima* of salt, sulphur, and mercury. Cortese's instructions for a soap capable of removing any kind of stain, calls for a mixture of calcinated alum and pulverized tartar pounded in a bronze mortar – ingredients, preparations, and vessels familiar to the alchemist.[29] Underscoring this link to alchemy, works including Cortese's *Secreti* and Celebrino's *Dificio delle ricette* are accompanied by illustrations depicting a series of interconnected vessels being heated at the hearth – images that explicitly evoke the alchemical laboratory.[30] Indeed, books of secrets often devoted entire sections to alchemy, as in Book II of Cortese's *Secreti*, or Alessio Piemontese's chapter on alchemy and metallurgy in his *Secreti* that contains detailed technical descriptions of working with alchemical materials.[31] Thus alchemy is seen to underlay a range of activities that encompass the medical and the cosmetic as well as the purely alchemical, thereby extending itself to the broader household economy in which women were central players.

---

[26] Celebrino, *Opera nuova...per far bella ciascuna donna*, unnumbered.

[27] The empiric Leonardo Fioravanti (author of his own book of secrets) was likely the real author behind this work (cf. Eamon, *Science*, p. 166).

[28] *Secreti diversi e miracolosi. Raccolti dal Falloppio...* (Venice, Zaltieri, 1588), pp. 315–6.

[29] Cortese, *Secreti*, p. 93.

[30] Celebrino, *Opera nova*, p. 16v.

[31] As Eamon points out, Alessio included some particularly valuable information here, including instructions for refining borax, which was imported to Europe via Venice, "thus violating an important trade secret" (*Science and the Secrets of Nature*, p. 146).

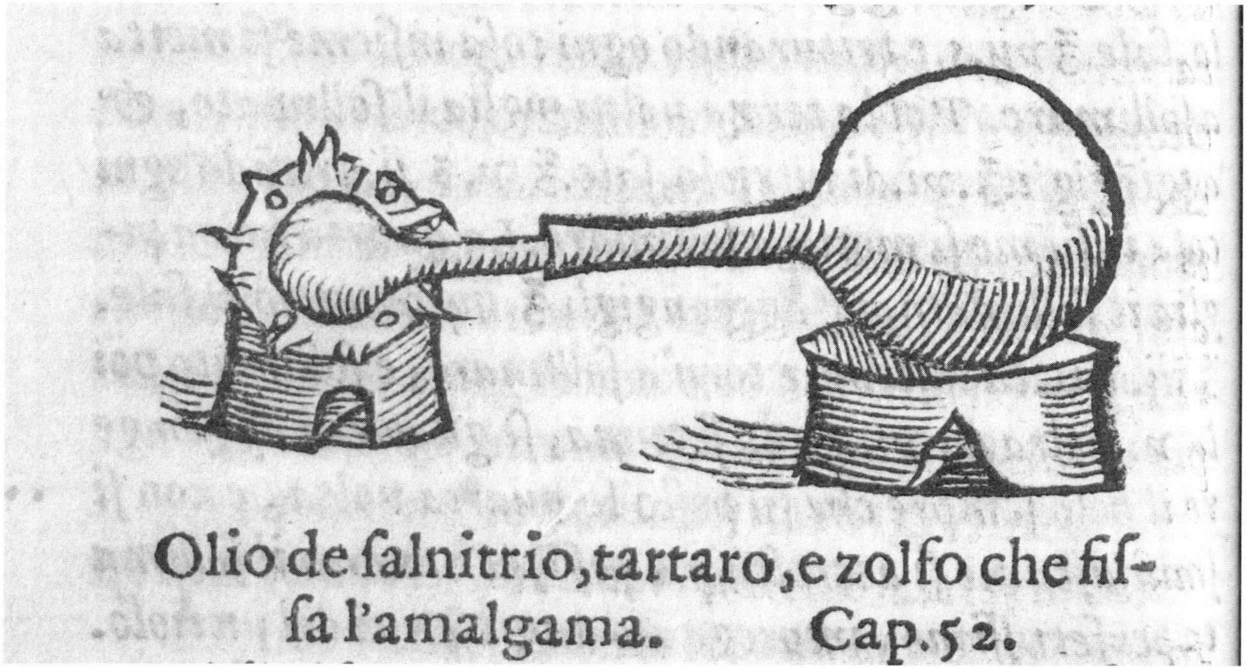

Fig. 6.1 Alchemical vessels, from *I secreti de la Signora Isabella Cortese, ne' quali si contengono cose minerali, medicinali, arteficiose, & alchimiche, & molte de l'arte profumatoria, appartenenti a ogni gran signora : con altri bellissimi secreti aggiunti*. (Venice, Bariletto, 1574). Courtesy of the Edgar Fahs Smith Collection, Rare Book and Manuscript Library, University of Pennsylvania.

***

If sixteenth-century books of secrets capitalized on a growing female audience for these kinds of recipes, women had long been collecting and experimenting with such information. When Caterina Sforza – the "Madonna of Forlì," as she was called by Machiavelli[32] – died in 1509, she left a record of her own pursuit of alchemical, medicinal, and cosmetic secrets in the form of a manuscript compilation of *Experimenti*, as well as in her correspondence. Sforza's example offers insight into the ways in which early modern women incorporated alchemical experiment into their daily lives – a frequent, if often unremarked, companion in the quest for physical health, beauty, and (in Sforza's case), the creation of wealth and the increased political stability to which such riches might contribute. Sforza's example also suggests that the pursuit of such knowledge resulted in the creation of a kind of alchemical network composed of both male and female practitioners who exchanged recipes with one another and kept each other informed of new discoveries, as attested to by her correspondence.[33]

The daughter of Duke Galeazzo Maria Sforza of Milan and his mistress Lucrezia Landriani, Sforza was raised and educated in her father's household. At age 14 she was married to Girolamo Riario, a nephew of Pope Sixtus IV whose fortunes were on the rise. Sforza followed Riario to Rome and then Romagna, where the couple was invested with the control of the towns of Imola and Forlì. Destined to become one of the most well-known women of the Renaissance, Sforza was regarded by her contemporaries with both admiration and trepidation for her fierce occupation of the Castel Sant'Angelo in Rome in 1484 following the death of Sixtus IV as well as for her tenacious governance of Imola and Forlì after Riario's assassination in 1488.[34] Especially legendary is the story of Sforza's defense of the Rocca di Ravaldino, the main fortress of Forlì, in the wake of the coup against Riario, wherein she successfully outwitted her enemies by overturning their expectations of her as a female ruler. Machiavelli, who had occasion to treat with Sforza on behalf of Florence, famously relates the story in his *Discorsi*, describing how Sforza, in response to her foes' threats to kill her hostage children, lifted her skirts,

---

32 See Niccolò Machiavelli, *Il principe* (ed. Luigi Firpo, Turin: Einaudi, 1984), chap. 20.

33 The exchange of recipes was common in many Renaissance courts, from that of Elizabeth I of England to those of the Empress Maria of Spain and Catherine de Medici of France. See Alisha Rankin, "The Practice of Pharmacology and Laywomen," in *Encyclopedia of Women in the Renaissance: Italy, France, and England*, Diana Robin, Anne R. Larsen, and Carole Levin, eds. (Santa Barbara, CA: ABC-CLIO Inc., 2007), p. 265.

34 The major biographies of Caterina Sforza remain Pier Desiderio Pasolini, *Caterina Sforza* (Rome: Loescher, 1893) and Ernst Breisach, *Caterina Sforza: A Renaissance Virago* (Chicago: University of Chicago Press, 1967). See also the essays collected in *Caterina Sforza: Una donna del Cinquecento* (Florence: La Mandragora, 2000).

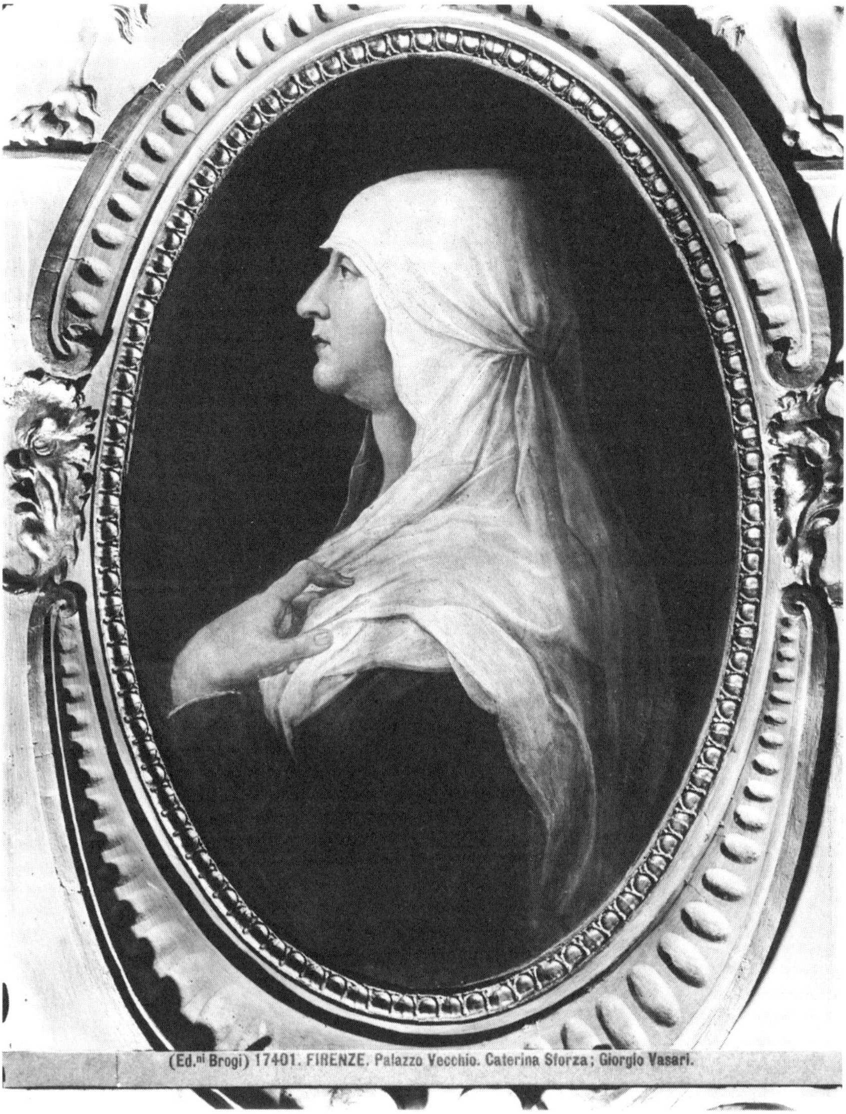

Fig. 6.2 Portrait of Caterina Sforza, Giorgio Vasari. Courtesy of Art Resource.

pointed to her genitalia, and retorted that she could make more.[35] While, as Julia Hairston has demonstrated, Machiavelli's account is rather more theatrical than contemporary chroniclers of the incident describe, his portrait of Sforza served to cement the enduring public image of her as a Renaissance virago who had defiantly preferred losing her children to losing her state.[36]

While serving as regent, Sforza continued to solidify her power through a combination of force, diplomacy, and the fostering of public works in the territories she controlled. She had relationships with (and probably secretly wed) Giacomo Feo and, after Feo's death (also by assassination), Giovanni de' Medici of Florence, with whom she had a son, the renowned condottiere Giovanni delle Bande Nere (father to Cosimo I, the first grand duke of Tuscany). Besieged by Cesare Borgia, who had his eye on the conquest of Imola and Forlì, Sforza was taken as a prisoner to Rome in 1500, where she was eventually charged with having attempted to poison Pope Alexander VI, Cesare's father. After a year of solitary confinement in the same Castel Sant'Angelo she had occupied so defiantly years earlier, Sforza was compelled to renounce her titles to Imola and Forlì. Released in 1501, she made her way to Florence. There she remained until her death in 1509, when she was buried in the convent of Le Murate, of which she had been a patron.[37]

While Sforza is well known for her importance as a political figure, her interest in alchemy and medicine has received less scrutiny.[38] However, Sforza's *Experimenti*, a repository of recipes for everything from dying dark hair blond and creating

---

35 Cf. Machiavelli, *Discorsi* III, 6, modified in *Istorie fiorentine* VIII, p. 34. Machiavelli, *The Prince*, chapter 20, cites Sforza as a (negative) example with reference to the usefulness of fortresses to rulers under seige.

36 Specifically, Caterina's lifting of her skirts would appear to have originated with Machiavelli. See Julia Hairston, "Skirting the Issue: Machiavelli's Caterina Sforza," *Renaissance Quarterly* 53.3 (2000): 687–712. On the incident at the Rocca di Ravaldino and Machiavelli's reworking of it, see also John Freccero, "Medusa and the Madonna of Forli: Political Sexuality in Machiavelli," in *Machiavelli and the Discourse of Literature*, ed. Albert Russell Ascoli and Victoria Kahn (Ithaca: Cornell University Press, 1993), pp. 161–78; and Francesco Bausi, "Machiavelli and Caterina Sforza," in *Archivio storico italiano* (1991), disp. IV: pp. 887–92.

37 On Sforza's patronage of this and other institutions see Joyce DeVries, "Casting Her Widowhood: The Contemporary and Posthumous Portraits of Caterina Sforza," in *Widowhood and Visual Culture in Early Modern Europe*, ed. Allison Levy (Aldershot, UK: Ashgate, 2003), pp. 77–92 (88).

38 With some exceptions: see, in addition to Pasolini, *Caterina Sforza*, v. III: Umberto Foschi, *Fantasia e superstizione delle ricette di Caterina Sforza…, Bollettino economico. Organo ufficile della C.C.I.A.A. di Ravenna*, 43.2 (1988): 31–6; Natale Graziani and Gabriella Venturini, *Caterina Sforza* (Milan: Dell'Oglio, 1988), pp. 141–9; Mario Tabanelli, "Ricette di medicina dal libro "Degli experimenti" di Caterina Sforza," *La piê* 39.4 (1970): 195–8; and *Ricettario di bellezza. Introduzione di Luigi Pescasio* (Castiglione delle Stiviere, 1971). See also the essays contained in the exhibition catalogue, *Caterina Sforza: Una donna del Cinquecento*. None of these works, however, deals in any great depth with Sforza's interest in alchemy.

beauty waters and creams to curing ailments such as asthma, cancer, and sciatica and turning base metal to gold, can indeed be interpreted as a "foundational text in the history of pharmacology," not to mention that of alchemy.[39] Sforza was not the only woman to experiment with remedies and recipes in this way, incorporating medical and alchemical knowledge to meet the needs of daily life. According to Monica Green, the "collecting of family remedies" was by the sixteenth century a common feminine pastime; certainly, Italian archives are filled with numerous such compilations. While many of these are anonymous and therefore their female authorship cannot be established with certainty, their attention to women's health and beauty suggests at the very least a female audience.[40] Sforza's own manuscript also presents some philological problems, for the original manuscript of the *Experimenti*, said to have been passed down by Sforza to her son Giovanni delle Bande Nere, has been lost. A contemporary transcription of the work by Lucantonio Cuppano, a colonel who served under Giovanni, survives in a private collection; it was published in the nineteenth century by Sforza's biographer Pier Desiderio Pasolini, who termed it the "most complete and important known document on medicine and perfume" of the early sixteenth century.[41] Cuppano's preface refers repeatedly to Sforza as the work's author, and to himself as the transcriber of her original, handwritten instructions. He takes care to underscore that he works from an autograph copy of Sforza's manuscript, thus emphasizing her direct engagement with the volume as both author and medical/alchemical practitioner:

---

39 Cf. Julia Hairston, "Out of the Archive: Four Newly-Identified Figures in Tullia d'Aragona's *Rime della Signora Tullia di Aragona et di diversi a lei* (1547)" in *MLN* 118 (2003): 257–63 (259).

40 Cf. Monica H. Green, *Women's Healthcare in the Medieval West* (Aldershot, UK: Ashgate, 2000), p. 20. See also T. Adolphus Trollope, *A Decade of Italian Women*, v. 1, 264: "The practice of forming and preserving such collections seems to have been a common one among the ladies of that time" (London: Chapman & Hall, 1859). A *Ricettario galante* dating to the sixteenth century contains alchemically derived cosmetic recipes attributed to Isabella D'Aragona, wife of Gian Galeazzo Sforza (Caterina's half-brother) and Elisabetta Gonzaga, wife of Guidobaldo da Montefeltro of Urbino (*Ricettario galante. Del principio del secolo XVI*, ed. Olindo Guerrini, Bologna: Gaetano Romagnoli, 1883, see below). Raffaele Ciasca, *L'arte dei medici e speziali nella storia e nel commercio fiorentino dal secolo XII al XV* (Florence: Olschki, 1927) cites several such manuscript compilations at the Biblioteca Nazionale di Firenze (pp. 350–53). Recent scholarship also shows that the nuns of Italy's many convents produced and dispensed pharmaceuticals and ran their own apothecaries; see Sharon Strocchia, *Nuns and Nunneries in Renaissance Florence* (Baltimore: Johns Hopkins University Press, 2009).

41 Pasolini, *Caterina Sforza*, v. 3, p. 601. The manuscript is now in a private archive (Archivio Pasolini) in Ravenna. Luca Antonio Cuppano appears as an interlocutor in the *Rime* of Tullia d'Aragona (see Hairston, "Out of the Archives," p. 259). On Cuppano, see Carlo Coppi da Gorzano, "Il Conte Lucantonio Coppi detto Cuppano, ultimo condottiero delle Bande Nere e dimenticato Governatore Generale di Piombino (1507–1557)," *Rivisita araldica* 3 (1960): 87–105.

> In nome de Dio in questo libro se noteranno alcuni experimenti cavati da lo originale de la illux.ma madonna Caterina da Furli Matre de lo illux.mo S.re joann de medici mio S.re et patrone et per essere lo originale scripto de man propria de dicta madonna . . . non me curarò durare fatiga a rescriverli . . . .
>
> (In the name of God in this book you will find some experiments taken from the original by the most illustrious madonna Caterina of Forli, mother of the most illustrious signor Giovanni de Medici my lord and patron; and since the original was written in said madonna's own hand . . . I will not mind the fatigue I undergo in copying them . . .)

Because the original manuscript is no longer extant, we cannot compare the hand in which it was composed to Sforza's own. We are forced to rely on Cuppano's testimony as to the work's authorship in his preface and at several points in the body of the text where the copyist again reiterates Sforza's ownership and mastery of these recipes: for example reminding the reader that a recipe for calcinated talc (a mineral used in many alchemical and cosmetic preparations) must be carefully followed, "just as Madame of Furlì used to do it."[42] As we will see below, however, letters attesting to the enduring business relationship between Sforza and her speziale in Forlì, along with others addressed to her that provide or request assistance with alchemical, medicinal, and cosmetic recipes, offer convincing evidence that she was actively involved in the collection of such recipes and support the proposition that she was compiling such a work before her death. A valuable cultural artifact, the *Experimenti* suggests that alchemy, in its many configurations (medical, chemical, cosmetic), was a central and continuing pursuit for Sforza, one that occupied her attention even amidst her most pressing political battles and up until the end of her life.[43]

Sforza's manuscript bears striking resemblances to the kinds of published collections of "secrets" discussed above, including that of Cortese, suggesting that, in some cases, such works may have found their models in quotidian practice. Certainly, the *Experimenti* shares with these later printed books of secrets an interest in experimental methodology. The brief foreword added to the *Experimenti* by Cuppano emphasizes that these are recipes that Sforza personally tried and tested; therefore "one must assume [all the recipes] to be effective, for they have been proven so by this great lady."[44] Like many printed books of secrets, Sforza's compilation is plain in style and devoid of narrative framework or flourish. Its

---

[42] Pasolini, *Caterina Sforza*, v. 3, p. 618, "il vero modo de calcinarlo sie questo, como usava madama da Furlì."

[43] Trollope's speculation that Caterina compiled the whole of her *Experimenti* only during her final years in Florence seems unlikely, although she was certainly collecting recipes until the year before her death. Pescasio surmises that the recipes were compiled over course of her life (*Ricettario di Bellezza di Caterina Sforza*, p. 5).

[44] Pasolini, *Caterina Sforza*, v. 3, p. 617, "se deve extimare tucti li altri essere veri per essere experimentati da cusi alta madonna."

recipes are often general in nature, assuming some prior knowledge or familiarity on the part of the user.[45] The recipes are presented as tools for navigating daily life and daily problems; some of the more overtly alchemical recipes seem to derive from Sforza's particular concerns as a ruler of two territories in need of financial backing (for example alchemical recipes for coloring or adding weight to metal so that it appears to be gold). Occasional asides inserted into the recipes underscore the collection's function as a practical manual. One such note, for example (whether Cuppano's or Sforza's own is unclear), explains that extra space has been left in the manuscript following a recipe for talc water so that anyone who discovers additional uses for the mixture can write them in for the benefit of future readers.[46] Indeed, the note elaborates, it would be "a mortal sin to keep such treasure [i.e., knowledge] hidden."[47] The tension revealed here between the secrecy and obscurity traditionally associated with alchemy, and the practical imperative to disclose and share information, especially (but not only) when it relates to health, is also characteristic of the printed books of secrets that Sforza's collection prefigures. Works such as the *Secreti di Isabella Cortese* must constantly negotiate the conflict between maintaining the privileged nature of the recipes even as they reveal them to the reader and ensure their still wider diffusion through print (seeking to maintain this aura of secrecy, Cortese, for example, cautions that to reveal a secret causes it to lose its power[48]). Further contributing to a veneer of secrecy is a handful of Sforza's recipes that are offered in Latin rather than Italian. These recipes are for the most part related to the transmutation of metals – the Latin intended to signal their particular gravity and importance, both

---

45 In her study of cookery and "household physick" books in early modern England, Elizabeth Tebeaux emphasizes the role of technical writing as a memory aid meant to supplement women's existing knowledge: "The fact that these books . . . gave less emphasis to exact quantities than to ingredients and placed little emphasis on precise instructions for the making and then using [of] foods and folk medicines implies that women readers had a basic knowledge of cooking which they learned through oral transmission and from demonstration" ("Women and Technical Writing, 1475–1700: Technology, Literacy, and Development of a Genre," in *Women, Science and Medicine*, p. 37).

46 Pasolini, *Caterina Sforza*, v. 3, p. 618. Regardless of how much blank space was available, readers were likely to make their own notes in the margin regarding the success of the recipe or any adjustments that should be made to it. A 1535 edition of the *Triumpho di ricette & secreti bellissimi composto per Giovanbattista Verini Fiorentini* at the Newberry Library, for example, is annotated throughout in this fashion.

47 Ibid., ". . . è mortale peccato tenere ascoso tanto tesoro." Highlighting both the secrecy and the utility of Sforza's secrets, Cuppano again adds that the recipes were "written down in [Sforza's] own hand, and so as not to keep these marvelous secrets hidden I now leave a record of them (Ibid., p. 617, "experimentati da cusi alta madonna e scripti de sua propria mano et perché questi mirabili secreti non siano ascosi per me se ne tira memoria . . .).

48 Cortese, p. 32, "il revelare de secreti fa perdere l'efficacia." On the traditions and strategies of secrecy associated with alchemical texts, see for example Long, *Openness, Secrecy, Authorship*.

in terms of their alchemical content and their possible significance as a political tool for the creation of currency (or perhaps simply to indicate their provenance from another source). Several of the alchemical recipes – particularly those that describe techniques rather than ingredients or uses – are partially presented in code, the key to which is provided on the manuscript's first page.[49]

Like Cortese's *Secreti*, Sforza's *Experimenti* encompass health, beauty, and alchemy. Of the 454 recipes she records, the majority are primarily medicinal in nature (358); while the others are divided among cosmetic and alchemical recipes.[50] However, it is difficult to draw real distinctions between the types of recipes, for here, as in the printed books of secrets discussed above, cosmetic and medical recipes rely heavily on alchemical ingredients and processes. Among Sforza's medicinal recipes, for example, are a number of distilled waters, unguents, and elixirs, produced through alchemical procedures such as multiplication, a kind of progressive distillation whereby a substance assumes greater and more diverse powers during the course of preparation. A "marvelous secret unguent" ("una untione mirabile segreta") for gout, sciatica, and nervous tension, for example, involves boiling meat and salad leaves in wine for eight hours, then draining the mixture and adding additional ingredients such as rosemary and other herbs over an additional period. To make a truly marvelous unguent, Sforza adds, leave the mixture outside for a month, so that it may gain force from the heat of the sun.[51] More general panaceas described by Sforza include an *elisir vitae*, an elixir capable of conferring perpetual health and youth – a principle goal of therapeutic alchemy: "… it causes a person to regain his youth and brings the dead back to life, and if someone were so ill as to have been abandoned by his physicians as an incurable case, it will restore him to health."[52] To create this elixir, Sforza advises mixing spices, flowers, herbs, fruit, and sugar in a pestle, then distilling the mixture with water in a tightly sealed glass alembic.[53] After two days the mixture is stirred over slow heat until the water changes color from clear to white. These stages recall the principle stages of the alchemical process as described in theoretical alchemical texts, in which the phases of transformation are marked by corresponding changes in color (rendering the use of a glass vessel of central importance to the alchemist).[54] Similarly, an "acqua mirabile et divina" ("a miraculous and divine

---

[49] The key reads b f h p x for A E I O U (cf. Pasolini, p. 615). It was not unusual to highlight the particular value of a recipe by providing it wholly or partially in code.

[50] Cf. Fabrizia Fiumi and Giovanna Tempesta, "Gli 'Experimenti' di Caterina Sforza," in *Caterina Sforza: Una donna del Cinquecento*, p. 140.

[51] Pasolini, *Caterina Sforza*, v. 3, p. 669.

[52] Ibid., p. 639, "… fa regiovenire la persona et de morto fa vivo ciò e si una persona fusse tanto gravata de infermitate che li medici labandonassino per incurabile et morta la reduce a sanità . . . ."

[53] Ibid.

[54] See for example William Newman, "The Homunculus and His Forbears: Wonders of Art and Nature," in *Natural Particulars*, p. 319–45.

water") produced from a mixture of spices, flowers, wine, and other ingredients improves memory, treats toothache, earache, and melancholy, and can even cure leprosy, paralysis, and other grave illnesses. Distilled over a period of several days, this recipe, like the elixir, also results in three separate stages of liquid, each more powerful than the last: here, the third stage produces the deep red color prized by alchemists and capable of bringing a patient back from the brink of death: ". . . the second [liquid] is better than the first but the third is the color of blood, and better than all the rest."[55] Sforza includes many other medicinal recipes to treat everything from lice and colic to wounds, poison, cancer, and plague, and even one for a powerful, opium-based surgical anesthetic that places the patient in a drug-induced sleep.[56] As befitting a ruler in a Renaissance court, Sforza also records recipes for poisons and their antidotes, along with others for invisible ink and the like.[57]

Sforza's recipes, like most medicinal preparations of the time, rely extensively on familiar herbs, spices, and foodstuffs, as well as on more exotic ingredients thought to contain magical and curative properties, such as heliotrope (a variety of quartz).[58] Many of them suggest that she subscribed to the law of similars, according to which a substance is thought to share a common characteristic with the disease it is used to treat (for example, using goat's spleen to treat the spleen) or, alternatively, to impart its characteristics to the patient (for example, egg whites to whiten the complexion).[59] A few of Sforza's recipes retain the mixture of pharmacy

---

55 Pasolini, *Caterina Sforza*, v. 3, p. 622, ". . . la seconda è meglio che la prima ma la terza è de color de sangue, e sopra tutte."

56 Ibid, p. 769, "A far dormire una persona per tal modo che porai operare in cirurgia quelche vorai e non sentirà est probatum." For Patrizia Catellani, this recipe is "… forse la più considerevole di tutto il libro" (http://chifar.unipv.it/museo/Catellani/catSforza/CaterinaSf.htm).

57 Cf. in Pasolini, *Caterina Sforza*, v. 3, several recipes for poisons and antidotes that take scorpion as a central ingredient; one of these is attributed to Pope Paul II (1464–1492) (pp. 679, 672, 673). Poison was certainly considered a real threat. Sforza herself was accused of having attempted to poison Pope Alexander IV (by sending him letters contaminated by plague), although it is widely agreed that this accusation was a mere pretext on Alexander's part for confining her to Castel Sant'Angelo. Also included in the *Experimenti* are recipes for concealing and protecting written documents in various ways (for example, an "Acqua da cancelare le lettere scritte" [p. 784] and another "Acqua da scrivere che non si veda" [p. 790], both offered in Latin). Similar recipes appear in Cortese's *Secreti;* see "Contra peste et veleno" (p. 17), "Olio di scorpione contra peste, et altri mali" (p. 19), "Inchiostro che in quaranta dì sparisce e non si vede" (p. 44), "Scancellar lettere senza guastar carta pergamena" (p. 45).

58 See Siraisi, *Medieval and Early Modern Medicine*, pp. 147–8; see also Anna Maria Guccini, "L'arte dei Semplici: Alchimie e medicina naturalistica tra conoscenza e credenza all'epoca di Caterina," in *Caterina Sforza: Una donna del Cinquecento*, pp. 131–8.

59 In some cases, the affinity is merely linguistic, as in "corallo" (coral) to treat the "core" (heart). Cf Pasolini, *Caterina Sforza*, v. 3, pp. 612–3.

and astrology that also characterizes some books of secrets, as in her instructions for a preparation of blessed thistle ("cardo Benedetto"), that cures headache when eaten in salad, body aches when taken with red wine, and, when distilled into a liquid during the months of May or August, rids the body of all "cattivi humori" ("bad humors").[60] Where did Sforza obtain the herbs and other ingredients for her medicinal recipes? Her correspondence indicates that she depended on her speziale, Lodovico Albertini, an apothecary based in Forlì, to supply her with what she required. When Sforza died in 1509 she owed Albertini more than 587 florins, a debt amassed during her years in that city. Sforza's third husband Giovanni de Medici also died owing Albertini money, suggesting that he probably participated in his wife's experiments as well.[61]

Like her medicinal remedies, Sforza's cosmetic recipes make similar use of herbs and plants distilled in alchemical vessels, as well as minerals, precious stones, and metals. Many recipes focus on smoothing and lightening the skin: a recipe to protect the complexion against unsightly spots ("A fare un acqua mirabile a conservare il viso contra ogni macula"), for example, suggests distilling a mixture of fennel, betony, endive, roses, and white wine. Over a period of days, the recipe will produce, in turn, "rose water," "silver water," and, finally, "golden water" or "balsam" – a precious panacea often named in books of secrets.[62] Her instructions recall similar recipes included in later, printed books of secrets, including a *Ricettario galante* dating to the early sixteenth century that likewise offers a recipe for a water distilled in three stages (here, the first water, a cosmetic remedy, removes freckles; the second cures fistulas; the third, the strongest, cuts iron).[63] Some of Sforza's cosmetic recipes are simple and straightforward, for example relying on egg whites or fava flowers distilled with water to whiten the skin.[64] More complex recipes, however, revolve around alchemical ingredients and procedures to produce multifaceted remedies akin to that described in the

[60] Ibid., p. 625.

[61] In a letter written by Albertini to Francesco Fortunato, Sforza's confessor, shortly after her death and suggesting their closeness during her life, he writes that he couldn't bring himself to mention her debt when he visited Sforza during her final illness: "non mi parse conveniente a notificarlo nequiquam parlarne, mi essere vero creditore dela prefata bona memoria di Madonna mia illustrissima de fiorini 587 et ultra in magiore somma per resto de robbe date a prefate sua llustrissima Signoria in Forli como appare uno clarissimo conto per li mei libri. Item de la bona memoria del magnifico Ziovann di Medici per robbe de la mia botega date a sua Magnificentia . . ." (ASF, Med. a Princ., unnumbered).

[62] Pasolini, *Caterina Sforza*, v. 3, p. 621, ". . . fa stilare ultra modo de acqua rosata la prima e quasi argento la seconda oro la terza e quasi balsino."

[63] *Ricettario galante*, p. 7: "La prima acqua manda vi lentiggine del volto . . . la seconda acqua . . . spegne le fistole. La terza, ch'e piu di tutte forte . . . rode il ferro . . . raunando insieme queste tre acque, fa bello et biondoil capo come fila d'oro da la mattina a la sera." When combined, the three waters cause the hair to turn a permanent golden color, a result also prized in Sforza's text, which offers more than a dozen recipes for dyeing the hair.

[64] Pasolini, *Caterina Sforza*, v. 3, p. 627, "Ad idem;" "Ad idem."

Ricettario galante. One such recipe for removing marks from the face is based on pulverized silver litharge dissolved in vinegar, a process that involves heating and distilling.[65] An "acqua perfettissima per far bella" ("perfect beauty water") requires mixing "argento vivo," or mercury – a central alchemical ingredient – in a rounded flask with sage and then pulverizing it in a stone mortar with a pestle made of walnut, followed by various stages of boiling.[66] Some of the most elaborate beauty recipes, such as one for "acqua di talcho" (talc water), demonstrate how tightly intertwined are cosmetics, medicine, and alchemy for Sforza. Calcinated and then slowly heated, this water can make a woman of 70 appear to be only 20 ("se una donna fuse de sesanta anni la fara parere de vinti"). Truly an alchemist's dream ("el disiderio de li alchimisti"), the substance not only confers youth and beauty, but in powder form and mixed with white wine it serves as an antidote to plague or poison, while the water itself can cause inferior pearls to increase their luster and even their size.[67] While this recipe describes the various cosmetic, medicinal, and alchemical uses of talc water, another recipe explaining how to actually produce the water is partially encoded, suggesting a deeper level of secrecy associated with the actual technique of alchemy, as noted above.[68] As Joyce DeVries notes, physical adornment and cosmetic enhancement functioned as part of Sforza's broader strategy of self-fashioning (an effort that also included actions from charitable works to the casting of portrait medals in her image). Just as the surviving inventories of Sforza's luxurious wardrobe suggest her concern to dress the part of power, so do her cosmetic recipes attest to a corresponding interest in achieving and maintaining the ideal of feminine beauty.[69]

If Sforza's medical and cosmetic recipes draw on elements of alchemical practice, the *Experimenti* also include 30 recipes that are overtly alchemical in nature: for example instructions for coloring metals, dissolving precious stones, calcifying mercury or converting it to water, and preparing various tinctures of gold. A recipe for a water that promises to "dissolve iron and any other metal and congeal mercury" as well as serve a medicinal use as a substitute for precious balsam is offered entirely in Latin, as are several others for turning tin to silver or silver to gold.[70] One particularly valuable recipe adds a reddish tint to any metal, giving it the appearance of 24-carat gold.[71] As Pasolini has noted, Sforza's is a

---

[65] Ibid., "A fare la faccia bianchissima et bella et lucente, et colorita."

[66] Ibid., pp. 630–31.

[67] Ibid., pp. 617–8.

[68] Ibid., p. 619, "A cavare l'acqua del talcho."

[69] Cf. Joyce DeVries, "Caterina Sforza's Portrait Medals: Power, Gender, and Representation in the Italian Renaissance Court,"*Women's Art Journal* 24.1 (2003): 23–8, 24.

[70] Ibid., p. 777, "Questa e una acqua mirabile che dessolve el ferro et tutti li altri metalli et congela el mercurio et si pone in loco de balsamo," see also recipes on pp. 781–2.

[71] Ibid., p. 782, "Aqua rubea fixa ad rubeum qua tingit omnia coloris auris sic fit 24 karatarum."

particularly practical sort of alchemical interest. Rather than seeking to create true alchemical gold, Sforza focuses largely on recipes for making metals and lesser coins appear to be more valuable than they are. A recipe for "adding greater weight to a scudo or golden ducat" ("A dare gran peso a uno scudo, o ducato de oro"), for example, calls for salt nitre distilled in water with "filings of Saturn" ("limatura de Saturno"), then calcinated and distilled again in an alembic. To add weight to the coin, it must merely be dipped in the mixture and weighed; and dipped again until it reaches the desired weight.[72] It is with a curious note of self-consciousness that this recipe is specified as one that allows the user to commit this fraud without pangs of conscience ("senza carigo de conscientia"). This is a seemingly important distinction, suggesting an awareness not only of any moral implications of such an action, but also the penalties that were associated with such fraud.[73] Other similar chemical recipes include instructions for "lending color to ducats" and coloring copper and pewter. All rely on the ingredients and processes of alchemy, demonstrating that Sforza saw the potential for the application of these theoretical practices to the realities of her own life, in which the need for money was presumably a constant burden.

Sforza's personal correspondence corroborates that she actively sought out and circulated recipes such as those included in her *Experimenti*. Indeed, surviving letters to and by Sforza show that the pursuit of alchemical, cosmetic, and medical secrets established her within a network of others, women and men, who called upon her for the same.[74] A letter written to Sforza in 1502 by Luigi Ciochi, for example, makes reference to a secret recipe, compounded from egg and saffron, that her correspondent has gleaned from the Mantuan court – one too precious to describe in a letter, but which Ciochi promises to reveal to Sforza in person. Ciochi's letter demonstrates not only that he was accustomed to seeking out such recipes for Sforza – often from the same source, for example the "Madona Costanza" named here, from whom he also obtains an unguent for the face and hands – but also that he had an established interest in performing experiments with Sforza. Insisting that he wishes to be present when Sforza tests the recipe, Ciochi

---

[72] Ibid., p. 620, "Quando voli dare peso alli scudi ponili drento et lassali stare un poco de poi cavali et vedi si è al peso se non mettili di novo et fa cusí finché serà al peso."

[73] Ibid. p. 620, "A dare gran peso a uno scudo, o Ducato de oro senza carigo de coscientia . . . ." This consideration was likely rendered more serious by the fact that alchemical fraud was punishable by law (on alchemical fraud, see Nummedal, *Alchemy and Authority*). As Trollope notes, Sforza's interest in fraudulently producing "gold" is the more curious given that Forlì was authorized by papal bull to coin money (p. 265).

[74] Caterina's correspondence, and hundreds of other letters and documents pertaining to her, are recorded, and many transcribed, in Pasolini's invaluable *Caterina Sforza*, vol. III. For an assessment of Pasolini's archival findings and suggestions for further work, see Cecil H. Clough's important critique in "The Sources for the Biography of Caterina Sforza and for the History of Her State During Her Rule, With Some Hitherto Unpublished Letters Illustrative of Her Chancery Archives," *Atti e Memorie, Deputazione di storia patria per le provincie di Romagna*, vv. 15–6 (1963): 57–143.

describes himself as an indispensable accomplice, possessed of all the requisite qualities of the alchemical adept:

> Ma zuro a Vostra. Exellentia di portarvela se ben dovesse venire aposta perchè io anchora mi voglio trovar presente a tanto experimento et a una tanta satisfactione . . et anche Vostra Exellentia non trovaria mai homo simile a mi perché c'é bisogna animosità, zoe non temere spiriti, fede, zoe credulo, secreto, zoe non se scoprire con homo del mondo et haver li istrumenti necessarii a tanta opera che né in el studio di Bologna né in Ferrara né in Parigi né a Roma non furono mai simili a li mei . . .
>
> (I assure your Excellency that I will bring you the recipe myself because I wish to be present for so great an experiment and so great a satisfaction . . . and besides, your Excellency would never find another man like me, because courage is required (that is, he can't fear spirits); faith (that is, he must believe); secrecy (that is, he can't disclose anything to anyone); and [he must] have the instruments necessary for such a great experiment and there are none in the laboratories of Bologna, nor Ferrara, nor Paris, nor Rome, similar to mine . . .)[75]

The qualities Ciochi praises in himself – courage, faith, discretion – are among those traditionally prescribed for the alchemist. Cortese's *Secreti*, for example, stresses these very attributes when describing the ideal alchemical assistant in the preface to Book II mentioned at the beginning of this essay: "a servant who is faithful, discreet, and courageous in spirit" ("un servitor fedele, e secreto, e buono d'anima").[76]

A second letter from Ciochi to Sforza similarly underscores his role as a procurer of recipes – this time a potent medical remedy – and a participant in the experiments performed by the Lady of Forlì. Like the other, this letter too reveals the links forged by Sforza with other noblewomen through her pursuit of marvelous secrets, as Ciochi passes on the same madonna Costanza's request for certain perfumes and "powder of cypress" ("polvere di cipri"). Ciochi urges Sforza to comply, so that Costanza may later have occasion to reciprocate (as, in fact, she does), and signs himself Caterina's "servant and faithful partner in undertaking all the experiments in the world."[77]

Sforza's other correspondents likewise provide her with a variety of cosmetic and medicinal remedies. A certain "Anna Hebrea" (Anna the Jewess), for example, sends, at Sforza's request, a black unguent for the complexion, capable of removing age spots and softening the skin – just the kind of cosmetic recipe that

---

75 Luigi Ciocha to Caterina Sforza, 23 March 1502 (ASF, Med. a. Pr., f. 77, n. 85; Pasolini, p. 606). I have modernized accents and punctuations here but have retained the original orthography.

76 Cortese, *Secreti*, p. 32.

77 Luigi Ciocha to Caterina Sforza, 5 May 1502 (ASF; Pasolini, p. 607), "io la prego a compiacerla perchè anchora le ha de le gentileze de recambiare Vostra Signoria;" "servitore et partigiano fidelissimo a farne tutti li esperimenti del mondo."

appears with great frequency in Sforza's own *Experimenti* as well as in virtually any printed book of secrets. Anna gives detailed instructions on how the cream is to be applied (at night, and rinsed off in the morning), along with a price list for her various products, of which she is certain Sforza will order more.[78] Frate Bernardino di Gariboldi sends Sforza another remedy that commonly appears, in various formulations, in printed books of secrets: three small flasks of "acqua celeste," a liquid capable of curing a range of maladies. As Bernardino explains, the first flask is for treating headache and stomachache; the second for the liver; and the third to protect against plague. Bernardino further promises to provide an oil, which he has not yet finished producing.[79] Remedies for all these complaints are included in Sforza's *Experimenti*, often in numerous forms, although which of these, if any, corresponds directly to the remedy furnished by Bernardino is impossible to tell.

Two final examples demonstrate still more clearly Sforza's real interests in the practice of alchemy, not only for the production of medicines and cosmetics, but for making alchemical gold. A letter from an unidentified correspondent who signs himself only "That faithful servant" ("Quel fidel servo") alludes to an exchange of secrets the two parties have agreed upon. For his part, Sforza's correspondent supplies a special cream for the face ("quel lustro del volto") that he has promised her, obtained through a lady of the Gonzaga family. In return, he fretfully awaits Sforza's recipe for making "eighteen- carat gold": "I beg Your Excellency to attend to that which you promised me; that is to send me that recipe for making eighteen-carat gold, and to send me the complete recipe and as soon as possible …" ("prego che la Vostra Exellentia me voglia attendere ad quel che la me promisse, cioè de mandarme quella ricetta da faro oro da xviii carati, et mandarmela intieramente et al più presto …"). His anxious tone and insistence that Sforza should immediately provide the recipe in its entirety, with no part left out, speaks both to the difficulty and the excitement of the experiment he seeks to undertake, and suggest that Sforza was known for performing such experiments herself. Indeed, as noted above, her *Experimenti* provide several recipes for tinctures of gold.

A second, more obscure letter is addressed to Sforza by a Lorenzo de Mantechitis, a correspondent who was imprisoned after playing a trick on one of Caterina's auditors in which he pretended to perform an alchemical operation:

---

[78] Anna Hebrea to Caterina Sforza, 15 March 1508 (ASF, Med. a Pr., f. 125, n. 228), "El quale unguento lo ponirete la sera et tenetelo fino ala matina e poi ve laverete con l'acqua pura di fiume . . . Lo unguento nero vale Carlini quattro l'oncia. . . Se Vostra Illustrissima Signoria ne adoperarà io mi rendo certo che continuo ce mandarete" (cf. Pasolini, p. 608).

[79] Frate Bernardino di Gariboldi to Caterina Sforza, 21 January 1504 (ASF, Med. a Pr., f. 125, n. 19; Pasolini, p. 607): ". . . mando a la vostra Signoria tre fiaschete de aqua celeste . . . de le quale fiaschete et ge ne una per il malle de testa e del stomaco. L'altra si è per el figato . . . L'altra si è contra peste pigliandone uno poceto la matina per quelo zorno non piara peste e cosí è scrito e ligato uno breve al collo per caduana fiasceta . . . De li oley non o potuto lavorare, ma di curto la vostra Signoria li haverà. . . ."

> . . . perchè non intendesse quello che se lavorasse, como da la Signoria Vostra hebbi in commissione; pure a l'ultimo li disse che non era nulla, immo non credeva fusse possibile ma che faceva per dare ad intendere al maestro, el quale era pertinace che non se potesse fare arzento né fusse possibile affarne per questa via alchimica, dove che monstrandoli questo argento calcinato et in sua presentia redurlo in corpo cum sapone negro, salnitrio overo borace, che in simile forma pare cenere, che lui remanerà stupefacto a vedere che quella polvere sia reducta in arzento.
>
> (. . . I was careful . . . that no one should know what we were doing, just as Your Ladyship advised me; even at the end I said it was nothing, and that I did not believe it was possible but that I was trying to show the master, who was certain that it is impossible to make silver or to make it by alchemical means, so that in showing him this calcinated silver and reducing it, in his presence, with black soap, salt nitre or rather borax, which in that form seems like ash, that he would be amazed at seeing that powder reduced to silver.)

Lorenzo pleads with Sforza to be freed and returned to her service, insisting he carried out the prank only to please her. Lorenzo seems to suggest that if indeed he were a successful alchemist, he would not find himself in these present straits ("... et non seria quasi in extrema necessità como sonno se havesse tale vertù"). At the same time, however, he also seems to refer to some prior success in this area, mentioning a little book that now constitutes the sum total of his activity in this area and promising to use his knowledge of alchemy only in Sforza's service.

> Quando ancora la Signoria Vostra o vero messer Jacomo [Feo] vorano che se faza alcuna prova de quelle cose che io ho, quale tengo per bone, se farà; et maxime circa quanto se contiene in quello libretto . . . perché ultra di quelle mai più intendo sopra ad ziò affaticarmi.[80]
>
> (If Your Ladyship or indeed messer Jacomo [Feo] should wish for some proof of those things I have, which I consider useful, I will provide it; and especially with regard to what is contained in that little book . . . because I have no intention of ever trying anything beyond that again.)

While difficult to interpret without further information about Lorenzo and his relationship to Sforza and her second husband Giacomo Feo, mentioned in the passage, the letter suggests that Sforza had a strong interest in experiments but also that she prized secrecy and discretion in their undertaking. As noted above, such experiments – especially the transmutation of base metal into gold or silver – would have held particular appeal for one in Sforza's position, as well as considerable risk. Indeed, the dangers of alchemy were not only legal or moral but also physical: a century later, for example, the Jewish writer Leone Modena would describe his son's death from the noxious fumes produced by his efforts in the

[80] Cf. Pasolini, p. 609, n. 2.

alchemical laboratory.[81] No longer practical or domestic alchemy, with this kind of experiment Sforza was undoubtedly seeking – no matter the risks – tools that would help to strengthen her rule. Thus she seeks recipes to create precious metals, or at least to simulate them, without succumbing (as specified in the *Experimenti*) to any pangs of conscience.

***

The example of Caterina Sforza offers important evidence regarding the use of alchemy by women in Renaissance Italy as well as its uses in a Renaissance court. Both her collection of *Experimenti* and her epistolary exchanges over the last decade of her life demonstrate that the pursuit of beauty, health, and wealth through alchemical means was an ongoing and central focus for Sforza even in the midst of political and personal turmoil. The recipes collected by Sforza offer valuable insight into the role of scientific inquiry in the lives of early modern women and provide important information regarding the specific ingredients and processes used in treating illness or performing experiments. They also shed light on the relationships and networks established while doing so, which in Sforza's case involved both men and women from her immediate circle and farther afield, for example Mantua; and from the highest echelons of society as well as from marginalized communities such as the Jews. The bonds of scientific community – not to mention the corresponding financial obligation – could run deep. When Sforza succumbed to quartan fever in 1509, not only did she leave behind a substantial debt to Lodovico Albertini for the materials she had used in her experiments, but she also left her apothecary with a great sense of sadness for the partner he had lost. In a letter dated 3 June, 1509, Albertini shared his grief with one of Sforza's Riario relatives, writing, ". . . never did I feel greater sorrow, along with Bastiano and my whole family, and never again will I be content for I have lost my sweet mistress and I grieve all the more because I was not there at the end . . . ."[82]

Sforza's example is also important in contextualizing the wave of printed books of secrets that flourished throughout the sixteenth century. Her *Experimenti* confirm that the therapeutic and cosmetic solutions offered in such works did in many cases

---

[81] In his *Life of Judah*, Leone Modena recounts his son Mordecai's death after experimenting with transforming lead into silver, speculating that the vapors and fumes of the "arsenics and salts" used in his efforts were to blame; see the *Autobiography of a Seventeenth-Century Venetian Rabbi: Leon Modena's Life of Judah*, ed. Mark R. Cohen (Princeton, NJ: Princeton University Press, 1988). See also Raphael Patai, *The Jewish Alchemists* (Princeton, NJ: Princeton University Press, 1995), pp. 399–401.

[82] Lodovico Albertini, 3 June 1509 (ASF, Med. a. Princ., f. 125, n. 258; cf. Pasolini, p. 549), ". . . mai non [ho] sentito el magior dollore insemo con Bastiano e tuta la famiglia mia et mai più non vivrò contento perch'io ho perso la mia dolce patrona e più me dolle ch'io non me so' ritrovato a la fine a li servitie . . . ." Breisach's view is that Albertini's grief stemmed mostly from the loss of Caterina's financial patronage (*Caterina Sforza*, p. 137).

find their models in quotidian practice, and that even some of the more strictly chemical recipes had roots in women's everyday lives and in the household economy (and Sforza's political position clearly lends still another facet of significance to her alchemical experiments). While the female authorship of a work such as Isabella Cortese's *Secreti* may make it an anomaly among sixteenth-century, male-authored *libri di segreti* (indeed, some have suggested that this was just a marketing ploy to draw increased attention[83]), its dedication to a readership of women deemed likely to find its recipes useful attests to the real effort it made to reach – and to reflect – a specifically female audience. The similarities between the types of recipes offered by Cortese and those recorded by Sforza further underscore the links between books of secrets and women practitioners of alchemy and medicine.

From Machiavelli's day to the present day, Caterina Sforza has served as a central character in efforts to understand the political contours of the Renaissance court and the role of women in relation to it.[84] From her military and diplomatic strategies to her strategies of self-fashioning as a female prince, Sforza's history has been profitably examined from many angles. Her alchemical activity, however, has remained largely in the background, a supporting actor in the larger story of her political significance. As this essay has shown, Sforza's experiments in the laboratory are not wholly separate from her political identity, but rather attest to the important and ongoing role of scientific culture in Sforza's life. Indeed, as Pasolini pointed out, even as Sforza was preparing for seige by Cesare Borgia – a pivotal moment in her political life – she was thinking of her next alchemical experiment. A letter addressed to her confessor, Francesco Fortunato, asks him to send her a series of glass vessels made to particular specifications, along with other ingredients known for their medicinal – and potentially poisonous – properties, as soon as possible. The letter is dated 2 November 1499 – only a few weeks before Borgia's conquest of Imola.[85]

To restore Sforza's activity as an alchemical practitioner and a collector of alchemical, medicinal, and cosmetic recipes to the broader picture of her historical importance allows us to see her in a more nuanced way. The resulting picture is one that integrates Sforza's political significance with her involvement with early modern scientific culture. It is also, as I have suggested here, one that can help to deepen our broader understanding of women and science in early modern Italy.

---

[83] See for example Rudolph Bell, *How to Do it: Guides to Good Living for Renaissance Italians* (Chicago: University of Chicago Press, 1999), p. 44.

[84] On the use made of Sforza by Machiavelli, see notes 31, 34, and 35 above. A more recent example is in Joan Kelly's influential essay, "Did Women Have a Renaissance?," in which Sforza serves as an exception to Kelly's argument (now problematized by many scholars) about women's diminished roles in the Renaissance period (in idem, *Women, History, and Theory: The Essays of Joan Kelly*, Chicago: University of Chicago Press, 1984, pp. 19–50).

[85] In a letter dated 2 November 1499, Sforza requested three glass balls with openings of a certain size, along with twelve sea onion bulbs (officinal squill): " "Mandatice palle tre de vetro tondo habiano il buco piccolo et che tengano doi bucali de mesura et xii cipolle marine che si chiamano schille . . ." (ASF, Med. a Pr., f. 70, n. 87, Pasolini, p. 606).

Chapter 7
Madame de la Martinville, Quercitan's Daughter and the Philosopher's Stone: Manuscript Representations of Women Alchemists

Penny Bayer

Introduction

This essay introduces a series of related alchemical manuscripts originating in France or the Swiss Cantons, with various active female subjects, named as Madame de la Martinville, Quercitan's Daughter, Mr de Chenis Quercitan's daughter, la docte damoiselle de France and Neptis (see Table 7.1). These manuscripts are rare in depicting woman as active alchemists, aware of Paracelsian and medieval literary sources, and working with allegories of sexual and spiritual generative power. They raise issues of the way in which female authorial identity and authority are expressed, concealed, established, supported or undermined. Authors are ascribed apparently real names (Madame de la Martinville), names that reference a male expert (Quercitan, the pseudonym of the Paracelsian chemist Joseph du Chesne (1544(?)–1609)), and vaguer descriptions (une docte damoiselle de France). It is conventional within the alchemical tradition for authorial identity to be obscured through use of pseudonym and alibi within a context of code, cipher, metaphor and paradox. Because there are so few references to possible women alchemists within the alchemical canon, the obscuring of their identity has greater significance than for male references in potentially removing all traces that real women were alchemists. In addition, symbolic interpretations of the concept of the philosopher's daughter, or soul, further detract from establishment of authorial identity.

These manuscripts suggest a father/teacher-daughter/student relationship for the passing on of alchemical secrets that has affinity with that of the traditional alchemist master-son. However, there is a fundamental difference for the woman who is situated in relation to a male expert figure rather than a mentor of her own sex (as is found in early alchemical history with the semi-historical Maria, Cleopatra and Theosebeia). Druidic references in these manuscripts introduce possible female role models with affinities to alchemical symbolism.

The texts use imagery of sexual generative power, pregnancy and birth which provide opportunities for reading women's involvement as spiritual midwifery (paralleling the reading of male alchemists as a form of lay priest). In diffusion the sexual metaphor is extended and developed into misogynist slurring in a later attempt to discredit the idea of female authorship or alchemical practise. This is a complication not found in master-son treatises or other alchemical texts.

The actuality of women alchemists in the circle around Joseph du Chesne, who was the most significant figure in the French Paracelsian movement, resonates comfortably with a tradition in which humanist Calvinist women were well educated and skilled in writing and translation. Evidence elsewhere supports the hypothesis that women in Paracelsian circles were more likely to engage in learned and technical alchemy. However by the mid-seventeenth century in diffusion of the texts into England, a different social climate with misogynist ideas sought to amend the historical record.

Alchemical Background

Frank Sherwood Taylor traces the history of alchemy back to Graeco-Roman Egypt, when, as Jack Lindsay's work indicates, women, both mythical and historical, are reported to have been active participants in alchemy.[1] Alchemy has technical craft aspects (including distillation, metal working and making and using specialised equipment such as the bain marie and furnaces) and a philosophical-magical-spiritual aspect. It was transmitted from Egypt to Europe through Islamic scholarship in 12th-century Spain. By the Renaissance there was a wide range of philosophical approaches, incorporating variously Christianity, natural magic, hermeticism, humanism and neoplatonism. The Paracelsian movement codified and developed the work of Paracelsus, the adopted name of Theophrastus Bombastus von Hohenheim, c.1493–1541. It had a wider social and education reform agenda, which involved opening up alchemical ideas and secrets to a wider cross section of society. Paracelsus valued the medical knowledge of ordinary people, including women, because it was tested against experience, not simply learned from books. Paracelsianism is important within the history of science for its experimental focus on learning from direct experience of the "book of Nature", and for the introduction of mineral-based medical preparations. The Paracelsian philosophy introduced a third element, salt, to the medieval idea of the coupling of mercury and sulphur.[2]

Alchemical texts describe a process that is said to transform a metallic or mineral prime material into gold or silver or a healing elixir of life through stages identified with death, purification and rebirth. Sometimes the process or material is

---

1 Sherwood Taylor, Frank, *The Alchemists, Founders of Modern Chemistry* (London: W. Heinemann, 1951); "The Origins of Greek Alchemy," *Ambix*, 1 (1937): 30–47. See also Jack Lindsay, *The Origins of Alchemy in Graeco-Roman Egypt* (London: Frederick Muller, 1970).

2 Walter Pagel, *Paracelsus: An Introduction to Philosophical Medicine in the Era of the Renaissance* (London: Karger, 1982).

named philosophic or refers to the making of the philosopher's stone. The chemical process is described in vivid metaphors. Various sequences are used. A four-colour sequence was described from Graeco-Roman times: initial chaos and blackness (known as nigredo), purification and washing of the matter into whiteness (albedo), a yellowing stage (citron) and the final stage of red or purple (rubedo). In the fifteenth century George Ripley (d.c. 1490) set out 12 stages in *The Book of Twelve Gates*: calcination, solution, separation, conjunction, putrefaction, congelation, cibation, sublimation, fermentation, exaltation, multiplication and projection. Variations to these stages occur in manuscripts, including those discussed in this essay, probably reflecting processes in specific experiments.[3]

The language of the alchemists, including the Paracelsians, is obscure. Metaphors are used widely in receipts and treatises. Modern scholarship is beginning to address the complex issues involved in identifying both chemical and philosophical meanings in these metaphors.[4] The case studies below illustrate the problems of identifying sources and interpreting symbols. For example, *Splendor Solis* by Solomon Trismosin [pseud.], teacher of Paracelsus, includes a summary of an alchemical process called the red lion.[5] A stellar lion is depicted in *Philosophia Reformata* (Frankfurt: 1622) by Johann Daniel Mylius, where it is described as the Universal Solvent, the Green Lion of Mercury of the Wise.[6] Both sources occur in adapted form in one of the manuscripts discussed below, t*he Epistola Nobilissime*. French manuscript translations under the name *La Toyson d'Or* were made in the sixteenth and seventeenth centuries which could have been known to Madame de la Martinville and Quercitan's Daughter.[7]

Where it is possible to interpret meanings of symbols this essay does so, elsewhere the metaphor or image is left to stand alone. However, for the discussion of alchemical female authorial identity it is not necessary to have fully solved these problems, only to have established that an alchemical process is being described.

Evidence for Historical Women

Historical evidence supports the feasibility that the daughter of Joseph du Chesne could have been an alchemist and that other named women in his circle also engaged in philosophical and practical alchemy. The evidence suggests there were probably at least two historical women in this circle – Jeanne du Port, the daughter of Joseph du Chesne and Madame de la Martinville.

---

3 For an introduction to alchemical language, colour sequences and stages see Gareth Roberts, *The Mirror of Alchemy* (London: The British Library, 1994), pp. 45–64.

4 See for example Betty Jo Teeter Dobbs, *The Founding of Newton's Alchemy or "The Hunting of the Green Lyon"* (Cambridge: Cambridge University Press, 1975).

5 London: K. Paul, Trench, Trubner and Co., 1921.

6 Reproduced in Stanislas Klossowski de Rola, *The Golden Game* (London: Thames and Hudson, 1988), pp. 176, 181.

7 See Oxford: Bodleian Library, Ashmole MS 1395.

The existence of Quercitan's daughter as an historical person with an interest in alchemical literature is tentatively backed up by the annotation "Mr de Chenis Quercitan's daughter" on a manuscript of English verses of some of the important alchemical text the *Rosarium Philosophorum*".[8] The association of her name with this manuscript is potentially significant. The *Rosarium Philosophorum* was first published in Latin, with German verses, at Frankfurt circa 1550.[9] No English translation of the *Rosarium* was published (the standard Latin text was published in a German translation) and there do not seem to have been many English manuscript translations. There is one English translation in manuscript in the Ashmole collection, in Edward Barlow's commonplace book dated 2 January 1579.[10] This translation has the full text but none of the poems.[11] For Elias Ashmole, in the mid-seventeenth century, the translated verses may have helped plug a gap in the English translation available to him. The verses in this text are those found after each illustration of the stages of the work, from calcination to perfection. The association of a woman with this translation of the *Rosarium*, suggests her knowledge of the esoteric symbolism and language of this key alchemical text, and, if she were the translator, fluency in German (High Dutch) and English, and high intellectual standards which cause her to provide two translations.

The inference of the annotated *Rosarium* manuscript, that the daughter of Joseph du Chesne had an educated interest in alchemy, is reinforced by the biography of the du Chesne family. This shows that Joseph du Chesne had a daughter whose upbringing could well have been conducive to development of alchemical, Paracelsian and hermetic interests and beliefs. Joseph du Chesne was the significant hermetic doctor and chemist who, after a period of exile in Germany, Basle and Geneva (caused by the persecution of Protestants in France) became court doctor and alchemist to Henry IV of France in 1593. Du Chesne reached the top of the French medical profession, became known for a literary output of drama and poetry, and also acted for a period as a secret agent for

---

8 Oxford: Bodleian Library, Ashmole MS 1459 Item III (1) ff. 464–5. *Rosarium Philosophorum* with marginal annotation at end, "Mr de Chenis Quercitan's daughter."

9 First published: *De Alchimia opuscula complura veterum philosophorum [...] Rosarium Philosophorum Secunda Pars* (Frankfurt: Cyriac Jacob, 1550).

10 In the large Ashmole collection of alchemical manuscripts there is only one attempt at a full English translation: Oxford: Ashmole MS 1487, item 23, Inc: "Here begynnethe the booke of the Rosarye of Philosophers" is annotated that it was the book of Edward Barlow, made 2 January 1579: its 20 illustrations were pasted on and have been removed. Otherwise there are only short extracts. An eighteenth-century English translation held at the University of Glasgow formed the basis of Adam McLean's recent edition, due to the lack of any suitable earlier version.

11 The text is very close to that transcribed and edited by Adam McLean from the eighteenth-century Glasgow: Ferguson MS 210 with the major omission of the poems. See *The Rosary of the Philosophers*, ed. by Adam McLean (Edinburgh: Magnum Opus Sourceworks, 1980).

Henry IV.[12] Allen Debus regards him as one of the important French Paracelsians, and has traced du Chesne's influence on English Paracelsians.[13]

Du Chesne married Anne Trye, grand-daughter of the humanist Guillaume Budé, during the period (circa 1570s) when du Chesne practised medicine at Lyons, as 'docteur ordinaire' to Francois-Hercule, Duke of Anjou. His medical practice is presumed a success since his bride, Anne Trye, came from a wealthy background with a rich inheritance. Their daughter Jeanne probably received a good education, given her status as only child and the humanist tradition in her female line of descent. Anne Trye's cultural family inheritance, which brought intellectual vigour in a blend of humanism and Calvinism, was exactly the sort to produce an educated daughter. Since Erasmus' famous wish that women should read the Bible in the vernacular, humanists had favoured some education for women.[14] Jeanne's grandfather Guillaume Budé was internationally known and respected among fellow humanists and himself acted as a principal conduit for the reception of humanist thinking in France. Nancy L. Roelker, who identifies the significant role of French noblewomen in the vanguard of the Huguenot movement, describes Jeanne's grandmother Roberte le Lyeur, Madame Budé (d. 1550) as a correspondent of Calvin who was active in evangelical reform.[15] Anne may have influenced du Chesne towards a particular blend of humanism and Calvinism.[16] The inclusion of Paracelsian alchemy in Jeanne's area of interest is supported not only by her father's expertise in this subject, but also by the trend away from Erasmus' negative view of alchemy as deceitful, to the alignment in the late sixteenth century of Paracelsianism with French Calvinism.[17]

The use of the name Madame de la Martinville name in different sorts of manuscript and textual sources provides the strong suggestion that she was a real woman in the circle of Joseph du Chesne. There is no known biographical evidence of a woman with this name but the manuscripts show an expert learned alchemist scholar who has worked with alchemical experiments over some 20

[12] *Dictionnaire de Biographie Française*, ed. by Roman d'Amat et R. Limouzin-Lamothe, 11th vol. (Paris: Librairie Letouzey et Ane, 1967), pp. 1239–240.

[13] Allen Debus, *The French Paracelsians* (Cambridge: Cambridge University Press, 1991), p. 33.

[14] Norman Davies, *Europe: A History* (Oxford; New York: Oxford University Press, 1996), p. 478. On the complex inter-relationship of Calvinism, humanism and women see John Lee Thompson, *John Calvin and the Daughters of Sarah: Women in Regular and Exceptional Roles in the Exegesis of Calvin, his Predecessors, and his Contemporaries* (Geneva: Droz, 1992), particularly pp. 4–6.

[15] "The Appeal of Calvinism to French Noblewomen in the Sixteenth Century," *Journal of Interdisciplinary History*, 2 (1972): 391–418.

[16] D'Amat and Limouzin-Lamothe, *Dictionnaire de Biographie Francaise*, pp. 1239–40.

[17] Will Ogrinc, "Western Society and Alchemy from 1200 to 1500," *Journal of Medieval History*, 6, (1980): 103–32 (114). Hugh Trevor-Roper, "Paracelsianism made Political 1600–1650," in *Paracelsus,* ed. by Ole Peter Grell (Leiden; Boston; Koln: Brill, 1998), pp. 119–33.

years. In addition to her philosophical alchemical discourses which reference Joseph du Chesne, there is a record of her expertise in making a medicine for high fever, removal of vermin, blemishes on the face, languid and heavy limbs, gout and smallpox. A mixture of mercury of *sol* is dissolved, fixed, coral added and boiled in an athanor until a white snow-like substance forms. The mixture is distilled repeatedly to wash the essence. Children of 5 to 6 years are recommended a dose of six grains dissolved in white wine, or if they refuse it, in food or syrup. The dose increases with age: adults can take eight grains in thistle water, or 12 grains in a pill of theriac.[18]

Real Women and Purposeful Obscurity

Whilst Madame de la Martinville and Jeanne du Port appear to be real women, there is lack of clarity over the names Quercitan's daughter, la docte demoiselle de France and Neptis. Some of the confusion arising from the variety of names may be a consequence of purposeful obscurity through the use of pseudonyms and alibis. This veiling of identity reflects the tradition of anonymity and secrecy in alchemical literature: the large number of alchemical texts and manuscripts of anonymous authorship, including the most famous, such as the *Rosarium Philosophorum* and the *Turba Philosophorum*, as well as probably thousands of uncredited manuscripts on alchemical themes.[19] Even when not anonymous, male and female alchemists sometimes take pseudonyms or use initials. Anonymity or semi-anonymity may be linked to the tradition of secrecy by which from antiquity alchemists used code, cipher, riddle, paradox and enigma with intentional obscurity. [20] From the start of alchemical mythology texts are attributed to "great names" of the alchemical tradition when Hermes, Isis and Democritus became authorial identifiers of texts. By the Renaissance a large *corpus* of work had spurious names. Once a "name" entered the tradition it might be attached to other similar works. The use of "authorities" indicated the place of a text in a revealed tradition: the antiquity of alchemy was an important part of its mythology. There are, no doubt, many other alchemical manuscripts whose authorship has not yet been established, and await careful study: the lack of knowledge about minor alchemists, scribes and writers probably makes the literature appear more obscure than it might otherwise be.

The tradition by which the secrets of alchemy were passed orally from master to son is also significant.[21] The "Filius Sendivogii" was known under the monogram "J.H.F.S." and has been identified by Joachim Telle as Johann Harprecht (Fortitudio) Starcke.[22] Sendivogius and Joseph du Chesne were contemporaries in the circle of

---

18 ff. 194v–196v.

19 Gareth Roberts, *The Mirror of Alchemy*, p. 66.

20 Roberts, p. 66.

21 Roberts, p. 18.

22 Joachim Telle, "Zum 'Filius Sendivogii' Johann Harprecht," in *Die Alchemie in der europäischen Kultut- und Wissenschaftsgeschichte*, ed. by Christopher Meinel (Weisbanden: Harrassowitz, Wolfbütteler Forschungen Band 32, 1986), pp. 119–36. I am grateful to Jan Bäcklund for this reference.

Oswald Croll: the son of Sendivogius is contemporary with Quercitan's daughter. In both cases the reduction in identity of the "son" or "daughter" reinforces the significance of the "master". In this context it is of note that, even though she and Croll were about the same age, the poetess Elizabeth Jane Weston used the vocabulary of admiring daughter to father figure in her prefatory poem to Oswald Croll's *Basilica Chymica*, a classic work of hermeticism and alchemical medicine. In this poem she claims special status by expressing her great admiration for Croll: "aeternum Phoebus Apollo mihi est".[23] It seems that in a few instances alchemical "masters" taught or included in their circle women who took on the mantle of a special sort of "daughter".

The resonance of the alchemical daughter differs significantly from that of the alchemical son. The authority of the female pupil is lessened by her deference to a male teacher. Quercitan's daughter is an identity comprised of a male authority and female dependant. On the other hand where Madame de la Martinville is cited as author without reference to du Chesne, for example in some receipts, she is acknowledged as expert.

The question of whether it was Quercitan's biological, spiritual or symbolic daughter who wrote the *Quercitan's Daughter's Letters* is prompted by the image of the philosopher's daughter found in the alchemical tradition. The translated epigram from the *Rosarium Philosophorum*, *Revivicato*, which is annotated with the name of Mr de Chenis Quercitan's daughter, uses the image of the philosopher's daughter:

> Heere cometh the Soule from heaven faire & cleere,
> And raiseth the Philosophers daughter deare./[24]

Whether she read, translated or copied these words, a reinforcement of her own image as daughter of a philosopher can be imagined, as she wrote "the Philosophers daughter deare". A later translation places a slightly different, and less human, emphasis:

> Here the Soul descendeth gloriously from heaven
> And raiseth up the Daughter of Philosophy.[25]

The philosopher's daughter provides an analogy for the revived androgynous body of the philosophers' stone, which is now raised to the spiritual realm.[26] Lyndy

---

23 Apollo's daughters were the muses.

24 The German text printed in *De alchimia opuscula*, p. 259, reads "hye compt die Seele vom himel schon und clar/ Und macht ausserstehen der philosophi dochter fur (war)". Ruland, p. 357, gives Daughter of the Grand Secret as a synonym for the Philosophers' stone.

25 *The Rosary of the Philosophers*, ed. by McLean, p. 94.

26 The female gender may refer to the philosophic body created from the merging of *Sol* and *Luna*, who perhaps represent father and mother.

Abraham discusses the widespread use of the symbol of the philosophical child as the new-born philosopher's stone. She suggests that in some cases, for example by Johann Valentin Andreae (1586–1654) and Johann Mylius (c.1585–post 1630), the infant Stone is personified as a female child representing Sophia or wisdom.[27] In this sense, letters from the philosopher's daughter might be read literally as the words of wisdom.

The question of whether the representations of women are real or symbolic is further complicated by the widespread use by alchemical texts of serious and playful language, pseudonyms and purposeful obscurity. In the *Epistola Neptis, Operation de Neptis au Druide communiquée par M. Landrivier Calend.* Madame de la Martinville's name is substituted with the pseudonym *Neptis*, and the name Quercitanus is playfully substituted with the Druid, an obvious identification of Quercitanus based on Druid reverence for the oak tree. In the frequent mentions in the Theodore de Mayerne papers of Neptis as an alchemical authority Neptis is clearly associated with Quercitanus and his circle: the reference to Neptis, the Druid and Don Philippon mirrors the trio in *Quercitan's Daughter's Letters* of the author, Quercitanus and Monsieur Philippon.[28] Several hands write mainly in French with some English and Latin. These papers suggest a circle of people in France/Geneva who took on pseudonyms as part of their mutual endeavours in alchemy, and a mingling and merging of identities and names and perhaps a playful enjoyment of mythology in the tradition of what Michael Maier calls the alchemical serious game.[29]

The Theodore de Mayerne papers suggest a larger network around "the Druid" and Neptis, some of whom made use of pseudonyms. A reminder of Jeanne du Port's Swiss upbringing is The Old Genevan: other male participants are Bathodius, Maurice, Bea[r?]ardeau, Purpurmantel-Basilu and Basilius (f. 134v.). The apparently feminine name forms of Druida, and Haligraphia suggest additional women participants (f. 134v). Also mentioned in relation to Neptis or the Druid are "Monsieur \Q/uané D.M. a Paris", Trogny, M de la Vallée, M. Landrivier and Camilles.[30]

It is probable that some of these names were pseudonyms with resonances with the *opus*. A footnote to a French version of the *Epistola Nobilissime* in the Theodore de Mayerne papers mentions "au manuscript du Druide, je trouve Le Livre J +alibi

[27] *A Dictionary of Alchemical Imagery* (Cambridge: Cambridge University Press, 1998), pp. 148–9.

[28] London: British Library, Sloane MS 693, f. 156r, 134v, 156r.

[29] London: British Library, Sloane MS 693, ff. 134v–137v. Hugh Trevor-Roper ("Paracelsianism made Political," in Grell, *Paracelsus*, pp. 119–33 (p. 130)) states that Théodore de Mayerne, du Chesne and Guillaume de Trogny formed a secret group in Paris to perform alchemical work, but does not discuss any female participants. On the serious game see Michael Maier, *Lusus serius* (Oppenheim: Lucas Jennis, 1616). Elias Ashmole displays the same tendencies in using an anagram of his name, James Hasolle, in the subtitle of his edition of Arthur Dee's *Fasciculus Chemicus*.

[30] ff. 130, 152,139r–144r, 145r–146r.

93" (ff. 139r–144r). The two implied pseudonyms or alibis for du Chesne, "the Druid" and *Quercitanus* or oak tree, are etymologically related: "druid" may mean "oak knower" and refer to secret tree lore.[31] It is also relevant that the *Discours Philosophical* draws on Bernard Trevisan's allegory of the fountain, in which the old oak tree from which the fountain flows has central significance. These images of a spirituality of rebirth associated with the earth hark back to pagan antiquity, and the idea of a purer wisdom in the Celtic Druid tradition, as well as other pre-Christian traditions, which in sixteenth-century France found a popular focus in the claim on a Gaulish Druidic past.[32] Guy le Fèvre de la Broderie in *La Galliàde* represents the Gaulish Druid priesthood as the font of the wisdom traditions.[33]

Gallic tradition preserved legends of druidesses and other women closely associated with druidism.[34] Although accounts by Caesar and other classical sources speak of the priesthood as if exclusively male, it is not impossible that literary references to women druids were known to Christian humanists in sixteenth- and seventeenth-century France. Both druids and druidesses were closely associated with prophecy and divination, and there is an account of a Druid prophetess in Gaul. The acceptability of the theme of the woman alchemist as prophetess is demonstrated by the development of the legend of another woman from antiquity, Maria the Jewess, into Maria the Prophetess during the seventeenth century.[35] Celtic representations of the Roman God Mercury holding a caduceus accompanied by his consort the Celtic Rosmerta, who carries her own caduceus, also indicate a female role model for the hermetic tradition with resonance to the images of the alchemical king and queen in medieval and Renaissance alchemy.[36]

The Manuscripts

A series of nine manuscripts now in libraries in Copenhagen, Glasgow, London and Oxford comprise alchemical letters, discourses or poems, written between 1609 and the mid-seventeenth century, with references to active female subjects. These fall into two sets of attributions which situate these female authors in ways that give them different degrees of authority, both as authors and alchemists. One refers to Madame de la Martinville, Matrone de Martinvilla and Madame Martin Viel; another to Quercitan's daughter, Mr de Chenis Quercitan's daughter and Neptis (meaning female descendant or grand-daughter). The manuscript descent

[31] Geoffrey Ashe, *Mythology of the British Isles* (London: Methuen, 1990), p. 122. Druids have been associated with oak trees since Pliny.

[32] Desirée Hirst, *Hidden Riches: Traditional Symbolism from the Renaissance to Blake* (London: Eyre and Spottiswoode, 1964), p. 20.

[33] Hirst, p. 73.

[34] Miranda Green, *Celtic Goddesses, Warriors, Virgins and Mothers* (London: British Museum, 1995), pp. 138–42.

[35] Raphael Patai, *The Jewish Alchemists: A History and Source Book* (Princeton, NJ: Princeton University Press, 1994), p. 14.

[36] Miranda Green, *The Gods of the Celts* (Gloucester: Alan Sutton, 1986), p. 97.

is confused by the way these names are used in different versions of similar texts, including an additional attribution to a learned woman of France. All the references include or infer a relationship to the Paracelsian chemist Joseph du Chesne (c.1544–1609), whose published pseudonym was Quercitanus.[37]

Within the first sequence of manuscripts, the earliest document is probably a 12-page letter in Latin with the title *Epistola Nobilissime Matrone de Martinvilla ad Dom Quercitanum +1609*,[38] which, according to annotations by Isaac Harbrecht, was translated from French into Latin in 1615 in Stuttgart.[39] This text situates Madame de la Martinville as author and expert alchemist, with over 20 years of alchemical-Paracelsian experience. Madame de la Martinville recalls that in 1589 Quercitanus gave her several alchemical remedies. Twenty years later, in 1609, the year of du Chesne's death, she writes to him, recounting her experiments. In 1610, the year after Joseph du Chesne's death, Madame de la Martinville writes a 4-page *Discours philosophical*, the second manuscript in the sequence.[40] Like the *Epistola Nobilissime*, the *Discours philosophical* is written in the mixture of chemistry and symbolic language that characterises Paracelsian alchemical writings. Additional evidence for an expert woman alchemist in the Paracelsian tradition called Madame de la Martinville is presented by papers belonging to Theodore Turquet de Mayerne (1573–1655), the young doctor, friend and colleague of Joseph du Chesne, which refer to methods from and approved by "M. Mlle" and "Observatione de M de Mlle" on a "Methode por faire l'operation du Δ de vie [Sole]ea", a method for making a water of life from gold.[41] Since Theodore de Mayerne knew du Chesne and his French circle well, the evidence of his papers carries weight.

Within the second sequence of letters are four copies of a document titled *Quercitan's Daughter's letters*, three of which appear to date from the seventeenth century.[42] *Quercitan's Daughters Letters: An Alchemical Treatise* has two parts, the

[37] See Table One. I refer to him as Joseph du Chesne except when referring to manuscripts using the name Quercitanus.

[38] Copenhagen: The Royal Library, MS 1776, ff. 1–12. The author is referred to as Matrone de Martinvilla in the title of this Latin document: I refer to her in her native French form throughout: Madame de la Martinville.

[39] Isaac Habrecht (1589–1633) owned or wrote a number of manuscripts in the Royal Library, Copenhagen.

[40] Paris: Bibliothèque Mazarine MS 3681 (2679), no 22, ff. 77–81.

[41] London: British Library, Sloane MS 693, ff. 148r, 145r–146r, 194v–196r, and Allen Debus, *The French Paracelsians*, pp. 15, 48.

[42] In addition to Oxford: Bodleian Library, Ashmole MS 1440, and Glasgow: University of Glasgow, Ferguson MS 163, which have been used in this study, there are at least two others which have not been viewed. From the seventeenth century is London: British Library Sloane MS 3729, ff. 19–38 Quersitan's Da[f]ters letter: an alchemical tract translated from the Latin, with the second part titled "Quersitan's Da[f]ters letter". Apparently from the early nineteenth century is *The Theory and Practice of the Philosophers Stone described by Quercitan's Daughter. Copied from an antient manuscript* (Philadelphia: the Manly Palmer Hall collection, MS 199, ca. 1805, Source: Alchemy CD rom). I have inserted an apostrophe into *Daughter's* throughout this study for ease of understanding.

first theoretical, the second practical, as do many other alchemical writings.[43] The first is a letter signed by "your most humble affectionate handmayd"; the second contains technical information which provides practical details of her alchemical practices. The basic text presents Quercitan's Daughter (who is not given her own name) as a deferential diligent practising alchemist whose experiment has failed through her tiredness. Later versions include insertions which seek to denigrate any idea of female identity or authority.

A similar text titled *Copie d'une lettre escripte a Monsieur du Chesne d'une Docte damoiselle de france*[44] dates probably from the first half of the seventeenth century. This text situates the author as a wise woman even though her experiment failed. By the mid-seventeenth century, an English translation of this text (with a large additional passage) had been renamed *The Copie of a Letter sent me by ye late Madam Martin Viel, wch was found after her death.*[45] Madam Martin[e] Viel is most likely an English phonetic translation of Madame de la Martinville. This aspect of the manuscript descent raises the question of whether Madame de la Martinville and Quercitan's daughter were the same person, or whether their identities or representations become confused over time as a copyist sought to identify an authorial identity, with Madame de la Martinville being regarded at some point as Quercitan's biological or spiritual daughter.

Another example of the situation of a female alchemist in relation to a male expert is through references to a woman known as Neptis, apparently an alchemist granddaughter or female descendant of Quercitanus. The Theodore de Mayerne papers include *Epistola Neptis, Operation de Neptis au Druide communiquée par M. Landrivier Calend. i68.*[46] These papers are problematic to date: Theodore de Mayerne died in 1655, and the whole manuscript includes dates from 1580 to 1625.[47] In this French version of the *Epistola Nobilissime*, the pseudonym Neptis is substituted for Madame de la Martinville's name. The same substitution has taken place in *The work of Neptis communicated to Quercitanus*, a later English version of the *Epistola Nobilis,* copied into a notebook dating from the mid-seventeenth century.[48]

A manuscript in the University of Oxford Ashmole collection. "The English of the Dutch also in Rosarium Philosophorum" is annotated "Mr de Chenis

43 See Gareth Roberts, *The Mirror of Alchemy*, p. 65–6.

44 Denmark: Copenhagen, Royal Library MS. 1792.

45 Scotland: University of Glasgow, Ferguson MS 163, ff. 1–34.

46 London: The British Library, MS. Sloane 693 particularly ff. 139r–144r Epistola Neptis. Operation de Neptis au Druide communiquée par M. Landrivier Calend. 16[0?]8.

47 1580, 1593 (ff. 116v, 116r); 1625 (f. 122v); 1621 (f. 133v); i68 (possibly 1608) and 1610 (f. 159r). London: British Library, Sloane MS 693, ff. 116v, 226r, 122v, 133v, 159r.

48 Glasgow: University of, Ferguson MS. 163, ff. 35–56, *The worke of Neptis communicated to Quercitanus.*

Quercitan's daughter".[49] This suggests that the daughter of Joseph du Chesne either translated the two verses of the *Rosarium Philosophorum* in this manuscript, as indicated by William Black, Ashmole manuscript cataloguer, or that she transcribed or owned it.[50]

Representations of Women as Active Alchemists

The main writings of these French women alchemists are finely focused on alchemy as the making of gold, medicine and spiritual-philosophical work. There is no association with related household management activities such as the distillation of perfumes, waters, the making of art pigments or metalwork, as is the case in other examples of women's involvement with alchemy, such as Isabella Cortese's book of secrets for noblewomen, which includes a section on alchemy.[51] The main texts discussed indicate intellectual Paracelsian alchemy using the imagination and text-based learning, as well as practical equipment, a wide range of costly materials and sensual testing of experimental results, for example by watching colour changes.

The Writings of Madame de la Martinville

In the *Discours Philosophical* Madame de la Martinville outlines alchemical practice as the philosopher's craft, in which the key to the work takes place as matter passes through the philosopher's hands: a quasi-priestly quality is involved in preparing the philosophic holy tincture which cannot be separated from physical alchemical activity (f. 77r). She writes as an expert alchemist, drawing on the authority of her own practise and learning. She outlines three ways of obtaining philosophical mercury. A first method aims to separate mercury from gold and silver through digestion in a *bain marie* for 30 to 40 days, until the matter becomes black, when the mercury can be cooled off in quantity (f. 77r). This is based on the concept that to augment gold (or silver), the seed, sperm or mercury of gold (or silver) is required. This concept is one manifestation of the alchemists' belief that mercury was the transforming agent, and its seed the potent active principle. A second method extracts mercury from resuscitating salts found in sublimated water. Sublimation is the conversion of solid to vapour, followed by condensation

---

49 Oxford: Bodleian Library, Ashmole MS 1459 Item III (1) ff. 464–5. Rosarium Philosophorum with marginal annotation at end, "Mr de Chenis Quercitan's daughter".

50 Black, 1265.

51 Isabella Cortese, *I Secreti de la Signora Isabella Cortese: Ne'quali si contengo cose minerali, medicinali, artificiose, e Alchimique, & molte de l'arte profumatoria, appartenenti e ogni gran Signora* (Venice: Giovanni Bariletto, 1574). For a general overview see, Penny Bayer, "From Kitchen Hearth to Learned Paracelsianism: Women and Alchemy in the Renaissance", in *"Mystical Metal of Gold": Essays on Alchemy and Renaissance Culture*, Stanton J. Linden, ed. (Brooklyn, NY: AMS Press, 2006).

of the vapour in solid form on a cool surface. A second method extracts mercury from resuscitating salts found in sublimated water. These salts are metaphorically reduced to death through sublimation, revived with distilled vinegar, oil of tartar and *sal ammoniac*, when mercury is then extracted through sublimation and mixed with crude tartar for further digestion (f. 77r). Thirdly antimony is used, praised as the premier metallic substance, the lead of the philosophers, made of a sulphur and a living silver (i.e. mercury; f. 77v). Madame de la Martinville then describes how to sublime a reduction of antimony with *sal ammoniac*, adding red *luna* (silver), and putting the mixture into what she calls philosophical distilled vinegar and sulphur until the *luna* stops reacting and is cemented. The prefaced word "philosophical" here is obscure but probably means that the distilled vinegar has been through a process that the alchemists considered part of their art. She describes the result of fermenting mercury from the pure sulphur of antimony, with *sol*, as the fountain, perhaps a visual image of the chemical reaction taking place. A powder of "cinnabar of antimony" is mixed with saltpetre and salt, sublimated and revived over a low heat with black tartar, lime, a half-burnt crust of bread and *sal ammoniac*, which mixture, she claims, provides mercury for the "bel oevre" (f. 79r). Finally she gives a method to obtain mercury from the flowers of antimony in order to then multiply gold. Ten ounces of mercury are amalgamated with calcined gold, put in an athanor for 10 to 20 days, until the blackness is removed, the substance becomes white, then red, and the substance proceeds to multiply to the same weight as the mercury (ff. 80r–v). Throughout she provides specific weights, guidelines on the amount of heat and visual clues to measure the success of the experiment.

Madame de la Martinville's writings are explicit examples of immersion in the learned Paracelsian tradition. In the *Discours Philosophical*, her careful referencing to the works of Paracelsus, whom she regards as the best interpreter of the wisdom of antiquity, to Arnold de Villanova and Bernard Trevisan not only suggests that it may have been intended for circulation, but also displays her own expertise.[52] She draws her authority from the ancients, stating that in antiquity the "mercury of saturn" was used for its ability to coagulate and dissolve all others in the separation of the good from the earthy (f. 77r). Whilst unspecified philosophers believed Saturn to be their hidden sun, because it purged and dissolved the body of common gold, she prefers Paracelsus' approach using antimony, asserting that this is also the choice of most true philosophers who have attained the perfection of the [philosophers'] stone (f. 77v). She refers to Paracelsus' book on antimony, to his *Archidoxes*, *De Vita Longa,* and his writing on the *ens* of gold, in relation to the nature of antimony and its parts, sulphur, mercury and salt, concluding that nothing is more prized than the mercury of antimony.[53] Antimony is the dissolved

---

52 See *The Discours Philosophical,* f. 77v, re. *Archidoxes* and *De Vita Longa*; f. 78r on Paracelsus, Arnald de Villanova; f. 78v for Trevisan.

53 Paracelsus, *Archidoxae* (Kracow: 1569), *Archidoxa. De tinctura physicorum; de occulta philosophia* (Strasburg: 1570); and versions published at Munich in 1570, Basel in 1570, 1572, 1582, and Strasburg 1574. An English translation of *Paracelsus his Archidoxis:*

stone which in turn dissolves the body and fixes the spirits, which is why, she states, Paracelsus, in his chapter on Saturn, describes mercury as the medium of antimony, which in congelation by a certain sympathy receives an invisible sulphur or spirit of Saturn. This invisible sulphur runs to the centre of the mercury to stop and retain there the part of the mercury which is of the same substance as gold; it is also the mediator between the two extremes of gold and mercury by means of its two qualities, heat and coldness.[54] Implicit in her argument is the Paracelsian idea of the trinity of salt, mercury and sulphur, or body, soul and spirit, with the body of gold, the mercury of antimony and the invisible sulphur.

Whilst this is based on alchemical recipes, clearly there is a metaphorical level at which this work operates. As she describes the alchemical process which unfolds, Madame de la Martinville makes extensive use of allegorical images which display her knowledge of the alchemical literary canon. The devouring lion, the fountain, the white eagle and the blood of the red lion are mixed with chemical references in classic alchemical symbolism. Her sources are textual and based on received alchemical authority, with authority for these symbols drawn from Paracelsus' interpretation of earlier alchemical philosophers, or directly from those authors. Paracelsus, she asserts, found that the allegories of the ancients refer to antimony, the lead of the philosophers, as the devouring lion, because it digests all other metallic substances except gold, and its sperm contains the living mercury which it digests at the bottom of its stomach in the red stone.[55] She argues that, according to Arnold de Villanova's *Specule Oculto*, this symbol has a relationship to the sign of the mercury of the philosophers.[56] The image of the fountain is introduced at the point when mercury from the pure sulphur of antimony is fermented with *Sol* (f. 78v). By specifically mentioning that this is the fountain in which Trevisan praised his King,

---

disclosing the genuine way of making quintessences [...] tincture of the philosophers [...] the philosophical medicinal stone was made by James Howell (Oxfordshire: 1660) with further versions in 1661, 1663. *De Vita Longa* was included in *Archidoxorum* (Basel: 1570). *Ens* is Latin for "entity". Paracelsus gave an account of five entities: *ens veneni* (poison); *ens naturale* (natural); *ens astrale* (the astral entity); *ens spirituale* (spiritual entity); and *ens deale* (the divine or God-given entity). See Mark Haeffner, *The Dictionary of Alchemy* (London: Aquarian Press, 1991), p. 203.

[54] f. 78r. Martin Ruland, *A Lexicon of Alchemy*, A.E. Waite, trans. (Lond.on: Watkins, 1964), p. 306, explains that sulphur is the seed of the stone and is of two kinds: one is external, the other internal, born in mercury. The internal sulphur is the power which makes and prepares the body and cannot be separated from it, being in its very heart and substance. It is the soul and ferment of the stone, the husband, the bridegroom, king and husband.

[55] f. 78r. Newman, *Gehennical Fire*, pp. 184–5, associates raw antimony ore drawing in celestial influences with the green lion devouring the sun, and emitting a vivified mercury symbolised by blood. Newton describes "spiritual semen" received by the philosophic gold or star regulus of antimony.

[56] f. 78r. This complex image may refer partly to the properties of antimony in the purification of gold. The more well-known association is of the green lion devouring the sun in the *Rosarium Philosophorum*, often attributed to Arnald de Villanova, where the green lion symbolises mercury: see *The Rosary of the Philosophers*, ed. by McLean, p. 104.

Madame de la Martinville signals that at least part of the work is operating on the visionary or meditative level which is the basis of Bernard Trevisan's *The Allegory of the Fountain*.[57] The white eagle is introduced as an image in the extraction of the *regulle* or *rebis* (double thing, or hermaphrodite) from antimony.[58] The *rebis* contains a sulphur and a mercury which by the hands of the artist are made one matter, and this process of *conjunctio* is described by quoting Paracelsus' enigmatic statement that the *rebis* is transformed into a white eagle, by the aid of nature and the skill of the artist himself, so that, paradoxically, two are produced out of one.[59] A later reference in the same sentence links the white eagle to sublimed mercury.[60] Whilst the imagery has a transcendental quality, practical instructions follow which appear close to practical chemistry. The transformation in the white eagle is made with the *regulle* or cinnabar of antimony in a powder, mixed with saltpetre from Hungary and a salt (f. 79r). A substance is made described as a beautiful flying eagle in the mode of sublimed mercury. This is sublimed and revivified with black tartar, lime, a half burnt crust of bread, *sal ammoniac* and low heat. The mercury is captured in a receiver half full of cold water. This makes an excellent eagle (i.e. prepared mercury) for fermentation with the lime of whichever metal chosen, to make decoctions of the *bel oevre* (f. 79r). Later, even more inscrutably, she argues that God has graced Paracelsus with a path shorter and easier than that of those who made long imbibitions in the pelican which feed the *rebis* or lily by its own blood.[61] A transfer is indicated between the red lion, its red blood and the flying white eagle.[62] The blood of the red lion (possibly an extract from antimony) is

---

[57] f. 78v. This allegory is given in full in Martin Ruland, p. 450.

[58] f. 79r. Haeffner, p. 140.

[59] f. 79r. " Hoc id est rebis per auxilium natureas nec non per arte artistae ipsius spiritus in aquilam albam transmutari sic ut ex duo fiant."

[60] Ruland, p. 32, gives the eagle as symbol for *sal ammoniac* because of its lightness in sublimation, but he notes that in many places Paracelsus uses it for precipitated mercury. Stanton Linden, *Darke Hierogliphicks: Alchemy in English Literature from Chaucer to the Restoration* (Lexington: University Press of Kentucky, 1996), p. 176, provides a diverse iconography for the eagle, including the mercurial spirit. The various meanings of the word sublime (from which sublimation is derived) are suggestive within an alchemical context: it can mean to subject a substance to the action of heat to convert it into a vapour which on cooling is deposited in solid form; to exalt a person; to raise or refine to a high degree of purity or excellence and make spiritually or morally sublime; to transmute a thing into something nobler, higher or more excellent. *Oxford English Dictionary*, p. 3119. Here the implication is that mercury becomes volatile and rises in a white vapour, to which the metaphor of the white eagle is applied.

[61] f. 80r. Imbibing is the term favoured by alchemists for soaking, steeping or infusing in a liquid.

[62] f. 80r. Ruland, p. 112, explains the conjunction of male and female in various ways. One is what Paracelsus described as the joining of the congealed spirit within the dissolved body: when the blood of the Red Lion and the blood of the White Eagle are united, the Red Lion can become the White Eagle, and be one with it. The Red Lion becomes white in order that the white may become red.

added to sublimated mercury, creating a sublimation of the flowers of antimony (f. 80v). Again, this derives from the authority of Paracelsus, whom she quotes. The rose-coloured blood is extracted from the lion and the gluten from the eagle, taking much trouble to ensure that the blood is separated out and no flesh taken (f. 80r).

This double level of working, simultaneously symbolic and chemical, is also shown in Madame de la Martinville's earlier work, the *Epistola Nobilissime*, which is less structured than the *Discours Philosophical*, and leads the reader into a labyrinth of mysterious secrets and often inscrutable symbolic imagery, suggesting that this was a private letter intended for Quercitanus alone. Nonetheless, the text situates her as an expert alchemist, and named author. In the *Epistola Nobilissime* she first accounts for the materials she puts into her vessel, and then appears to describe an interior process reflecting her understanding of the Paracelsian cosmos (f. 1seq.). She describes methods to animate mercury, to marry animated mercury with the vitriol of copper and to transmute unrefined antimony (which is associated by analogy with the symbol of the black lion) into various stages of purification (symbolised by images of the red lion, the stellar lion and the azure lion) and the use of sublimated mercury (symbolised as a flying eagle). The dragon is associated with the sulphurous earth, and the blood of the red lion is used to make Azoth, another name for the mercury of the philosophers (ff. 9 and 10). Within these processes she writes about the tinting of mercury and *luna* to a golden colour, which she associates with the creation of 24 carat gold, and the elixir of medicinal alchemy (ff. 1, 5, 6, 7, 8, 11, 12). The images of lions and eagles are not disembodied symbols, nor can the practical work be understood without reference to the soul and spirit of the matter. Many of the symbols she uses appear in later published texts as spiritual emblems although I am not aware of a sequence mirroring exactly the series of images described here.[63]

Quercitan's Daughter's Letters

Quercitan's Daughter's Letters tell the story of a woman with considerable time and money to spend on alchemical experiments, providing a striking image of a woman in her laboratory. Although the way she is named, in relation to Quercitan, gives her less authorial identity than Madame de la Martinville, this text gives a vivid account of a woman alchemist carrying out experiments, seeking to give birth to transformed matter, and evaluating her own work. She has manuscripts of receipts (from her teacher-mentor, and from the *Book of Morienus* and the *Turba Philosophorum*).[64] She records her experiments and results to share with

---

63 The starry lion, which is mentioned at f. 1, is shown in Mylius' *Philosophia Reformata*, 1622.

64 p. 62, The *Turba*; p. 65 Morienus, and p. 66: "I have in these few words S[ir] described openly (according to my Instructions receaved from your owne selfe)".

her mentor, takings a critical view of her mistakes. [65] Her vessels are made of earth, glass and brass, and, in response to the failure of an experiment, she has a window made in her athanor to watch the colours change: black, white, citron, carnation to purple.[66] After 3 months preparing the initial ingredients, she watches the experiment herself, only leaving a servant to watch when she develops a severe headache (pp. 79, 91). Her accounts of measurements and amounts are very specific and, despite the Paracelsian alchemical language, in modern terminology she can be regarded as an experimental chemist.[67] She watches what happens, records it carefully, analyses what she believes to have happened in accordance with the theories she has been taught and amends her approach as she sees fit. She does not mention that she is making medicine, the most documented alchemical activity for women.[68] Her account describes a focused alchemist or mystical chemist, who believes that not only is it possible to multiply silver and gold but also that she has performed the operation, claiming, for example, that 1 ounce of her powder would convert 25 ounces of silver into gold (p. 70). Her language, however, is not that of the alchemical "puffer", making a lot of noise about gold-making for profit. She is engaged in the activity of the alchemical-priest, involving preparation of the "Liquor of Life" and the Paracelsian triad of body (calx of gold), soul (the "blessed liquor of the soule") and spirit (mercury; p. 79). Animation of antimony and quicksilver requires that they "have passed through the hands of the philosophers", who know how to give them their true temperature, the temperature of gold (p. 78).

The author of *Quercitan's Daughter's Letters* presents herself as a learned alchemist-scholar.[69] She displays some contemporary Paracelsian themes but also shows her Christian humanist background by drawing more strongly on older sources: Aristotle's theory of the four elements, the *Turba Philosophorum* and the *Book of Morienus*. She uses imagery of sexual generative power, pregnancy and birth, beginning with a conventional alchemical discourse of the recreation of the four elements into the form of metals, arguing that everything should be

---

65 For example, p. 70: "I was not perfectly skilled in the poynt of fermentacion"; p. 71: "I hand not as yett learned the art of animating […] mercury"; p. 75: "I perceived yt there ws one Errour committed in the very beginning, in that we did not put in Δ enough for ye better Augmentacion"; p. 88: "I had fayled in mistakeinge the Figure 7 for 3"; p. 91: "whether through my servants negligence in attending of the Fire, or whether I had putt too much matter into my Glasse; itt breake in 1000 peeces".

66 See p. 89 (mislabelled 79) "I passed through all the Colours untill I arrived att y[e] pure purpurine w[ch] I took great Joy to see for I had made a Window in my Athanor".

67 See for example, pp. 70, 74, where she cites one ounce of the "red worke" to convert 25 ounces of silver into gold; the use of 9 ounces of powder; 50 ounces silver; and 22 carats.

68 See for example Linda Pollock, *With Faith and Physic: The Life of a Tudor Gentlewoman Lady Grace Mildmay 1552–1620* (London: Collins and Brown, 1993) on Lady Grace's medicinal practice which included alchemical receipts.

69 Page 69, "beying your unworthy Scholler".

sought and found in its own kind (p. 49). Each metal is "engendered, formed and produced" by its own sperm or seed, properly called mercury (p. 49). This sperm, mercury, "in which we ought to travaile and buisy our selves", contains the matter of the stone, and has special sympathy with silver and gold (p. 49).

Although the theory is medieval, it is provocative to read the text in relationship to a female alchemist. Several twentieth century authors have argued that male alchemists sought to appropriate the powers of the feminine and recreate women's biological and psychic secrets. In 1980, Sally G. Allen and Joanna Hubbs argued that the masculinist bias in Michael Maier's *Atalanta Fugiens* indicates that the alchemist sought the magic of maternity to be conferred on men with a vehement absorption and denial of the feminine by the masculine, which they saw as the precursor of the test-tube baby.[70] David Noble argued in 1992 that the alchemists aimed at an arrogation of the powers of the feminine, especially those of procreation.[71] However in this text, the reverse is true. Quercitan's daughter works just as explicitly with the symbolic powers of the biological masculine in this magical transformative sperm. She seeks to create the resurrected body, drawing on the *Turba* to explain that through conjunction, the imperfect and dead body receives and is clothed in perfect brightness by the ferment of his soul (p. 62). The resurrected actor is gendered male, in the tradition of Christianity and of the *Turba Philosophorum*, which she cites as a source for creation of a king from the perfect infant, a metaphor used to explain the colour changes taking place in the vessel, from white to "orientall purpurean red". [72] This red substance embodies and symbolises the ultimate patriarch: "our king which cometh out of the Fire tryumphing and crowned" has "all power and Authority given him over his subjects" (p. 66). Joining of body (common gold) and spirit (mercury) by the vegetative soul; creating the resurrected body in a birth process.

The interpretation of the secrets of nature as a pregnancy process has a long tradition in alchemy. Although its first proponent may have been the semi-mythical Alexandrian woman alchemist Cleopatra, it has most often been promulgated by men.[73] When the narrator is a woman the female alchemist takes on the mantle of the midwife-philosopher who is helping give birth to new life through the material

---

70 'Outrunning Atalanta: Feminine Destiny in Alchemical Transmutation', *Signs*, 6 (1980): 210–29 (213, 221).

71 *A World Without Women: The Christian Clerical Culture of Western Science* (New York: Alfred A Knopf, 1992), pp. xvi, 178.

72 See 66. *The Turba Philosophorum or Assembly of the sages* has been translated and edited by A.E. Waite (London: George Redway, 1896).

73 "The Book of Comarius, Philosopher and High Priest who was Teaching Cleopatra the Divine the Sacred Art of the Philosophers' Stone," in Marcelin Berthelot, *Collection des Alchemistes Grecs*, 3 volumes (Paris: Steinheil, 1887–8), vol. 2, pp. 278–87 and vol. 3, pp. 289–99. See also Jack Lindsay, *The Origins of Alchemy in Graeco-Roman Egypt*, 253–61. In an unpublished note F. Sherwood Taylour asks whether the text from Comarius to Cleopatra is particularly significant because of its great similarities with the *Rosarium Philosophorum* (Oxford: Museum of the History of Science, MS Taylour, p. 122).

and spiritual changes taking place in the alchemical vessel. There is an affinity between women's presence at human births in early modern Europe, and the birthing role within the alchemical process. Certainly Lady Margaret, Countess of Cumberland, who is a well-documented alchemist, is also recorded as helping at births.[74] In *Quercitan's Daughter's Letters* this birth process takes place between body and spirit. To follow nature's steps is to introduce form into matter (mercury): to make silver the form is silver, for gold the form is gold. To join matter and form, or body and spirit, something called the vegetative soul is needed "without which nothing is done" (p. 56). In the joining of spirit, body and soul a purification takes place. The process becomes a spiritual one, and the three parts become one through conjunction. The vegetative soul is significant for its ability to quicken the body with vigour and virtue, and to alter common silver and gold into the *luna* and *sol* of the philosophers. The female philosopher acts as a cross between a priest and a midwife in this extraordinary birth process: the change into *luna* and *sol* happens as the material passes through her philosopher's hands. She acts also as an empiricist, who seeks to learn by experience and recorded experimental work, including work within the soul. She is a student of philosophy whose mystical chemistry is presented within the context of a consistent natural philosophy.

Distinguishing the Representations of Women Alchemists

A comparison of the text of *Une docte damoiselle* and *Quercitan's Daughter's Letters* with the earlier works of Madame de la Martinville shows some similarities between the texts. All the manuscripts describe an alchemical process both philosophical and chemical, separating spirit from bodily dross. They are both Paracelsian, and include textual references. They agree that the work requires philosophical animated mercury and all include specific time frames for the experiments. A reference to "Philiponnus" in the *Epistola Nobilis* is mirrored by one to "Philiponny" at Monsieur de la Fin's in *Quercitan's Daughter's Letters*.

However, there are significant differences in tone, style and content. *Quercitan's Daughter's Letters* is considerably longer, with a more detailed experimental and theoretical explanation, and a clear narrative. Madame de la Martinville's texts lack a story-line, but describe chemical processes using a wide range of materials and images. The key thought process in *Quercitan's Daughter's Letters* is that body (common gold) and spirit (mercury) can be joined by means of a vegetative soul. Madame de la Martinville seeks what she calls interior fusion of *sol* and *mercurius*. In the *Epistola Nobilis* she describes the fusion in the interior of the *sol* of antimony with mercurius; in the *Discours Philosophical* she discusses interior gold and interior mercury. Although both processes may refer to the standard alchemical idea of conjunction, traditionally of mercury and sulphur, there is

[74] Penny Bayer, 'Women's Alchemical Literature 1560–1616 in Italy, France, the Swiss Cantons and England, and its Diffusion to 1660' (unpublished PhD thesis, University of Warwick, 2003), chapter 5.

a clear difference between the language of interior fusion or mediation of the vegetative soul between body and soul.

Whilst *Quercitan's Daughter's Letters* emphasises recording and understanding the experiment, using only one symbolic animal, a double flying eagle, Madame de la Martinville makes extensive use of emblematic symbolism. In the *Epistola Nobilis* she uses a stellar lion, flying eagle, white stone, marriage of *mercurius* with his love, eternal *sol*, dragon and heavenly *menstruum*; in the *Discours Philosophical* she uses the metaphor of the stone, lily, devouring lion, *rebis* and fountain.

Madame de la Martinville uses a wider range of experimental materials. In the *Epistola Nobilis* she works with mercury, *sol*, *luna*, *aqua fortis*, Cyprian vitriol, the spirit of sulphur, vinegar, distilled *aqua vitae*, tincture of the sun and spirit of wine. In the *Discours Philosophical* her ingredients include mercury, mercury of saturn, resuscitating salts, distilled vinegar, oil of tartar, *sal ammoniac*, antimony, the magnesium of the philosophers, a sulphur and living silver, the invisible sulphur, sulphur and cinnabar of antimony and distilled philosophical vinegar. *Quercitan's Daughter's Letters*, on the other hand, uses only philosophic mercury, *sol*, vegetative soul, lead ore, coppelled silver, oyle of tartar, gold and cinnabar. Very specific equipment is used in *Quercitan's Daughter's Letters* – an egg-shaped vessel, a perpetual lamp, and a copper vessel with windows specially made for the author. These do not appear in Madame de la Martinville's treatises though she refers to a pelican, and various crucibles, receivers and collectors. Finally, both the *Discours Philosophical* and *Quercitan's Daughter's Letters* are referenced but with different sources. The *Discours Philosophical* is emphatically Paracelsian whilst *Quercitan's Daughter's Letters* does not cite Paracelsus at all, drawing authority from the *Turba Philosophorum*. The works of Madame de la Martinville are clearly dated at 1609 and 1610, and the earliest also refers to a specific date in 1589 when, she says, du Chesne gave her some remedies. *Quercitan's Daughter's Letters* includes no dates at all and can be dated only on the evidence of the handwriting. Madame de la Martinville is therefore not likely to have been the author of *Une docte damoiselle/Quercitan's Daughter's Letters*, and there appear to be two different women, Madame de la Martinville and Quercitan's daughter.

Diffusion

The diffusion of these manuscripts shows ambivalence to the stories of active women alchemists. On the one hand they are perceived to have been experts. For example the reputation of Madame de la Martinville as a fine experimenter in the contemporary French alchemical tradition is suggested from the Theodore de Mayerne papers where she is associated with words to do with testing and observation. A "belle experience et concordance chymique" is said to have been received by Paracelsus from his father, but is also valued as "un tres bon secret" because it is similar to one tested by "M. Mlle"(ff. 145r–146r). Another receipt is included "de la dite M Mlle qu'elle a esprouvé" (f. 148r). Her "methode por faire l'operation du Δ de vie [Sol]ea" is headed "Observatione de M. de Mlle" (ff. 194v–196r).

On the other hand their stories are considered unbelievable and slurs cast upon them. Even whilst contemporaries kept alive the writings of Quercitan's daughter and Madame de la Martinville, under different but still female names, these papers show that some seventeenth-century collectors or copyists questioned or actively sought to undermine women's contribution. One avenue for attack was the use of sexual status.[75] At the of end of *une Docte damoiselle de France* an additional note, in the same handwriting as the rest of the manuscript, indicates a powerful dislike of the idea of a woman working in tandem with a man on alchemy. The failed experiment (the vessel exploded) is explained as a tragic outcome which is God's punishment for the adulteress with the adulterer.[76] The strong language of this sexual insult conveys the message that it is adulterous for a woman other than a man's wife to correspond with him and to be party to a relationship of some intimacy based on alchemical experimentation.

In the case of *Quercitan's Daughter's Letters* textual insertions significantly alter the tone and obscure the woman authorship.[77] A new voice in parts of *Quercitan's Daughter's Letters* not present in *une Docte damoiselle* has strong opinions and a penchant for defensive criticism. An attack on false alchemists is introduced for the first time in any of these documents: the recipient of the letter is advised to "not willfully wander from the beaten path of truth, in following ye fancies, and follies of Ignorant and false pretenders to ye Arte whoe knowe, now intend nothinge but to deceave the covetous and Credulous" (p. 51). A reference to the parts of the alchemical work referred to traditionally as "Child's Play and Women's Work" is introduced, along with a slur on women for defiling men with their sin (p. 57). Within this sequence the traditional colour sequence which alchemists sought with wonder and delight is inappropriately (in the context of alchemical tradition) referred to as "gaudy colours" (p. 57). Intensely sexual imagery is also introduced with references to conjunction in the *Cubili Nuptiali*, the *Thoro Hymento* and the *vase semanario* with "ye Male or Masculine nature operating actually upon the female and ye Female sweetly clasping and embraceing ye Masculine" (p. 58). Finally, without the vegetable work the whole operation is regarded as "senseles & vain" and the body is stated to be "grosse and solid" (p. 60). This voice carries undertones of self-aggrandisement and veiled aggression, and may belong to a copyist or translator.

---

[75] Laura Gowing, in *Domestic Dangers: Women, Words, and Sex in Early Modern London* (Oxford: Clarendon Press, 1996) explores the prominent use of the sexual insult in disputes between men and women, and the perceived significance of female chastity for notions of obedience and household order.

[76] f. 21: "Eximum est huius historiae bis tragice, speculum, Aliene periculo sapiens sapit, […] Adultoram cum Adultero punivit Deus".

[77] The insertions are on page 50 from "but wth Gold Especially" to p. 51 "[…] of all things"; again p. 51 "& not willfully wander […] deceave the Covetous and Creduous"; and pp. 56–7 "All is ready to bee done […] For itt is they t. first defiled us with syn,"; pp. 58–61 "such as Union […] convert them into their owne nature".

A second new voice, expressed through an annotating hand, cannot believe the author to be a woman. When Quercitan's daughter ends her first letter as "your unworthy Scholler", and "humbly/beg/your Acceptance from her … Your most humble Affectionate Handmayd", the annotating hand writes "who is?", which might be taken as a straightforward enquiry into the identity of Quercitan's daughter if it did not follow an attack on the idea of the authorship of the text by a woman (p. 69). The text has a major insertion, an uncredited enlarged extract from the *Turba Philosophorum*:

> "Opus Mulierum Weomens Work which is to roast, and Boyle & Cooke, or dyett, & wash, and wringe us, to keep us Cleane. And well they owe itt to our Sex. For itt is they y^{t} first defiled us with syn". (p. 57)

The annotating hand uses this insertion to claim that the text is not written by a woman, underlining "And well they owe itt to our Sex" and adding in the margin "Ergo this was not written by Quercitan's daughter nor in ye person of a woman, but of a man else shee should forget her selfe" (p. 57). The original phrase about women's work in the *Turba* is " Now, therefore, I have demonstrated the disposition of the white lead, all which follows being no more than women's work and child's play,"[78] followed with a statement of the value of male and female in the alchemical work, in which "the female rejoices in receiving the strength of the male, because she is assisted by the male. But the male receives a tingeing spirit".[79] The comments that women defiled men with their sin, and consequently owed men and were to be punished by keeping men clean, among a host of other jobs, do not originate from the *Turba*. This biblical generalised gloss is not alchemical philosophy. The voice provides no explanation of why a man would label his work as Quercitan's daughter and sign himself "your most humble Affectionate Handmayd". Even in a world of secret agents and pseudonyms the use of the name of the daughter of a famous court alchemist would hardly have been uncontroversial. The strong misogynist tone of this paragraph stands out from the rest of the text in which rather than concern for sin and defilement, the tone is one of wonder at witnessing what is considered to be a philosophical process at work plus technical specificity over experimental details. It appears that the English versions of *Quercitan's Daughter's Letters* were amended from the earlier French one to include more contentious material that set up dissonance with the attribution of female authorship. The addition of more sexually explicit material took the text further from the type of literature that women were expected to write, and the piece on women's sin and defilement clearly placed women into the category of "other" by the use of the third person plural. The annotator of the Ashmole manuscript then used these amendments to conclude that the text could not have been written by a woman at all.

---

78 *The Turba Philosophorum*, p. 57.

79 Waite, p. 57.

Conclusion

This series of manuscripts provides evidence for at least two women alchemists, Madame de la Martinville and Quercitan's daughter, who may be Jeanne du Port, the biological daughter of Joseph du Chesne. Female identity and authority as author and alchemist is presented variously. In both cases the relationship with the alchemical master is an avenue to female authority. The texts associated with Madame de la Martinville situate her as named author, expert in the learned Paracelsian alchemical tradition. The texts associated with Quercitan's daughter show a woman alchemist at work within the Paracelsian tradition, but with lessened authorial identity. The reading of these texts present particular problems over and above those required for a text by a male alchemical author. The use of pseudonyms and alibis to veil alchemists' identity is common to both genders but the idea of the philosopher's daughter (whether biological, spiritual or symbolic) resonates differently from that of master-son same gender alchemical apprenticeships. The author's use of deference, and the failure of her reported experiment situate Quercitan's daughter as an apprentice alchemist learning from a male mentor.

Both Madame de la Martinville and Quercitan's daughter can be read as midwife-philosophers giving birth to the philosopher's stone, working with the masculine principle via the alchemists' transformative sperm. This is a reading that complements twentieth-century scholarly arguments that male alchemists sought to arrogate the powers of the feminine.

The manuscript diffusion of Quercitan's Daughters letters indicates that some seventeenth-century copyists and annotators had difficulty accepting that there had been more alchemical authors or practitioners and actively sought to discredit the concept. Their amendments sought to remove the identity of "Quercitan's daughter", and to remove any authority she might have through what we might interpret as a form of character assassination. The actuality of women alchemists around Joseph du Chesne, who lived in France and the Swiss Cantons, is supported by what is known of the Calvinist-Paracelsian circle he lived in, which included educated women.

Table 7.1 Manuscripts referring to women in the circle of Joseph du Chesne (Quercitanus)

Name	**Possible dating**	Abbreviated name
Copenhagen: The Royal Library, MS. 1776, assumed ff.1–12 (from photocopies), *Epistola Nobilissime Matrone de Martinvilla ad Dom Quercitanum +1609*	Original 1609 (?), this translation dated 1615	*Epistola Nobilissime*
Paris: Bibliotheque Mazarine, MS. 3681, ff.77–81, (from photocopies) *Discours philosophical de Mademoiselle de la Martinville*	Dated 1610	*Discours philosophical*
Copenhagen: The Royal Library, MS.1792, ff.1–24, (from photocopies) *Copie d'une lettre escripte a Monsieur du Chesne d'une Docte damoiselle de france*	Undated, handwriting consistent with 1600–1650	*Une docte damoiselle*
Oxford: The Bodleian Library, Ashmole MS. 1440 item 6, ff. 48–98, *Quercitan's Daughter's Letters: An Alchemical Treatise*	Undated, handwriting and other information consistent with mid-seventeenth century	*Quercitan's Daughter's Letters*
Glasgow: University of, Ferguson MS. 163, ff. 1–34, (from photocopies) *The Copie of a letter sent to me by ye late Madam Martin Viel wch was found after her death*	Undated: handwriting and other information consistent with mid-seventeenth century	*Madame Martin Viel's copy*
Glasgow: University of, Ferguson MS. 163, ff. 57–90, (from photocopies) *Quercitan's Daughter's Letters*	Undated: handwriting and other information consistent with mid-seventeenth century	
Glasgow: University of, Ferguson MS. 163, ff. 35–56, (from photocopies) *The worke of Neptis communicated to Quercitanus*	Undated: handwriting and other information consistent with mid-seventeenth century	*The worke of Neptis*
Oxford: The Bodlean Library, Ashmole MS. 1459, Item III (1), ff. 464–5. *Rosarium Philosophorum*	Copied and annotated mid-seventeenth century	

Name	**Possible dating**	Abbreviated name
London: The British Library, MS. Sloane 693 particularly ff.139r–144r *Epistola Neptis. Operation de Neptis au Druide communiquée par M. Landrivier Calend. 16[0?]8*	Textual references to dates from 1580–1625	*The Theodore de Mayerne papers*
also references through MS., eg.: ff. 22v-24v, Operatio Analoga Processus Neptis. Tinctura Vitriolo f.127v, Neptis in Epistola ita fecit Oleum ff. 131–7, Medulla operation […] Druidae, Neptis, Hermetis ff. 145r-146r Oeuvre excellente […] Ex per M. Mlle f. 148r Advertisement sur le fait de miniere tiré du L.X de la Dite M. Mlle ff. 194v-6r, Observatione de M. de Mlle		*Epistola Neptis*

Chapter 8
Women and Chymistry in Early Modern England: The Manuscript Receipt Book (*c.* 1616) of Sarah Wigges[1]

Jayne Elisabeth Archer

Introduction

In the Wellcome Library of the Royal College of Physicians there is a seventeenth-century manuscript receipt book, a stout quarto of just over 400 pages.[2] The owner/compiler of this book is identified on the ninth leaf: "Sarah Wigges 1616." In many ways, Sarah Wigges's book is entirely characteristic of other manuscript receipt books owned by early modern Englishwomen. It is heterogeneous, bringing together receipts for medicines, confectionary, perfumes, washing powders, rat powder, ink, cosmetics, perfumes, and household accounts. Like other books compiled by and for women shortly before or after marriage, it has been separated into two sections, with medical recipes entered at the beginning of the book and recipes for sweetmeats and sugar-craft at the end. There is a list of contents at the back, and tables for weights and measures at the front. Corrections and annotations to existing recipes are entered in a different hand, providing evidence of continuing use and experimentation. And as with other examples of this genre, this book was compiled over a long period of time, with at least three hands contributing: the earliest apparently dating back to 1616; another, working between the period 1616 into the 1620s, possibly a little later; and a final hand writing during the second half of the seventeenth century. From internal evidence that I will detail later in this essay, there seem to have been two main periods of compilation: in and around 1616, which may correspond to Sarah's marriage; and the period 1650–1670, when

---

[1] Early versions of this essay were presented at the Perdita Project Colloquium on women's manuscript receipt books (University of Warwick, September 2001), and at the Centre for Health, Medicine and Society Research Seminar at Oxford Brookes University (March 2004). I am grateful to Dr Elizabeth Clarke, Dr Jonathan Andrews, Professor Steven King, and to those present at the Colloquium and Seminar for their helpful comments and suggestions.

[2] London, Royal College of Physicians, MS 654.

the book may have been passed on to one of Sarah's children or grandchildren, or another close relative.

But there is something extraordinary about this book. For it is also filled with recipes for manufacturing the Philosopher's Stone, and for concocting the Star Regulus of Antimony (a crystal believed by many chymists to be an important stage in attaining the Stone). There are extracts from works on spiritual – or esoteric – chymistry, in which the chymist who works to refine metals in his or her crucible is also required to undergo a parallel process of spiritual refinement. On the final leaves of this book, written in the same neat italic hand, are recipes for sugar-craft and for counterfeiting precious stones. And on the final binding leaf, which distils or, perhaps, forms the quintessence, of this little book, there is a recipe for puff pastry and a recipe for making diamonds.

In this essay I will argue that this coming together of everyday household work and chymistry is, in fact, quite natural, even inevitable. For the early modern housewife was an important producer and consumer of chymical literature, knowledge, and practices.[3] In the first part of this essay I will briefly explore the relationship between chymistry and housewifery in early modern England. In the second part, I will provide an overview of women's receipt books, and, in particular, manuscript receipt books. Considering these books as material artefacts, with distinct methods of compilation and transmission, I will survey and evaluate the evidence they afford for women's knowledge of chymical theory and practice. In the final part I will outline two important ways in which chymistry informed the work of Englishwomen in their roles as housewives, and, in particular, healthcare providers: distilled waters and oils; and operations on metals and minerals.

Before proceeding, a brief word on terminology is necessary. For the purposes of this essay, I will follow the example of Lawrence M. Principe, who has written of "the inadequacy of the common practice of juxtaposing a monolithic 'alchemy' as a foil to early modern science," and suggests that we use the label "chymistry" to denote this field of inquiry, meaning "*the sum of total of alchemical/chemical topics as understood in the seventeenth century*."[4] This entails a range of pursuits not commonly regarded as alchemy/chymistry in existing histories of science. For to open the field of inquiry to take in the various definitions of alchemy/chymistry as outlined, for example, by Elias Ashmole in the Prolegomena to his *Theatrum Chemicum Britannicum* (1652), means that chymistry ceases to be purely about the transmutation of base metals into gold and the search for an Elixir of Life, but expands, to take in the manufacture of precious stones; distilled oils and quintessences; dyes and tinctures; aids to gardening; and communication with astral intelligences.[5]

---

[3] See Jayne Archer, "Women and Alchemy in Early Modern England," unpublished PhD dissertation, University of Cambridge, 2000.

[4] Lawrence M. Principe, *The Aspiring Adept: Robert Boyle and his Alchemical Quest* (Princeton, NJ: Princeton University Press, 1998), pp. 215, 9.

[5] Elias Ashmole, *Theatrum Chemicum Britannicum* (London, 1652), sig. A4^{v}–B2^{r}. Ashmole identifies four main types of Stone: the "*Minerall Stone,*" which will transmute "any *Imperfect Earthly Matter* into its utmost degree of *Perfection*"; the "*Vegitable*"

The Opus Mulierum: The Housewife as Alchemist

Arguing in 1673 for the need for thrift in prospective wives, Richard Allestree draws upon the popular notion that women are "more apt to waste, than to make Gold." Confirming the assumption that there exists a specific relationship between gender, gold, and the transmutation of matter into spirit, Allestree warns that the "vanity" of women will "infect" the "very walls" of the limbeck that is the material home, until it is "consumed" in the "variety and excess" of a never-ending *multiplicatio* of material goods:

> Women are now skillfull Chymists, and can quickly turn their husbands earth into Gold: but they pursue the experiment too far, make that Gold too volatile, and let it all vapor away in insignificant (tho gaudy) trifles.[6]

For Allestree, women are eager, but ultimately unsuccessful chymists: like chymists, women are forever trying to convert materials such as land, goods, and foodstuffs into superior forms, such as medicines, gold plate, silks, and jewellery. But they lack the ability to "fix" the gold that they project – a familiar complaint of many unsuccessful chymists – and it is over-refined, spiritualised away into "vapour." Although Allestree uses this metaphor in order to reinforce the stereotype of women as wasteful and vain, destined to sublimate their husbands' lands away into airy nothingness, he was only able to do so because of a long-standing correspondence between housewives and chymists.[7]

Writing from a very different perspective, Thomas Vaughan (1621–1666) remarks upon women's aptitude for chymical operations, and in particular for "the work," the chymical opus, the end product of which is the Philosopher's Stone:

> As for the work itself, it is no way troublesome *a Lady* may reade the *Arcadia*, and at the same time attend this *Philosophie* without disturbing her *fansie*. For my part I think *women* are fitter for it than men, for in such things they are more *neat* and *patient*, being used to a small *Chimistrie* of *Sack-possets*, and other finicall *Sugar-sops*.[8]

Stone, which will encourage plants to "*Grow, Flourish & beare Fruit*"; the "*Magicall* or *Prospective Stone*," by which "it is possible to discover any *Person* in what part of the *World* soever"; and "the *Angelicall Stone*," which "affords the *Apparition of Angells*, and gives a power of conversing with them".

[6] Richard Allestree, *The Ladies Calling* (London, 1673), p. 173. I am grateful to Dr Juliet Fleming for alerting me to this passage.

[7] Elsewhere in *The Ladies Calling*, Allestree sanctions women's medical work in the stillroom, commending those gentlewomen who open up their "dispensatories … providing medicines for such as either by disease, or casualty want that sort of relief" (p. 56).

[8] Thomas Vaughan, *Magia adamica or the antiquitie of magic* (London, 1650), p. 118. Margaret Cavendish argues that the feminine, creative faculty "fancy" is essential to an understanding of natural forms and processes: see Sylvia Bowerbank, "The Spider's Delight: Margaret Cavendish and the 'Female' Imagination," *English Literary Renaissance* 14.3 (Autumn 1984): 392–408.

Vaughan draws upon the idea, a commonplace in chymical literature, that 'the work', or latter stages of "the work," are deceptively simple, so simple that an uneducated child might accomplish it where a learned man might fail.[9] Vaughan's remark might seem to demean women's abilities, but this instinctual wisdom, attributed to women both by virtue of their sex and their work in the household – a skill that is simultaneously innate and acquired – could potentially put women in a privileged position with respect to chymical knowledge. Indeed, Thomas Vaughan's chymical workbook, *Aqua Vitae, Non Vitis*, was composed alongside his wife, Rebecca (d. 1658), whose ideas and insights into chymical theory and practice are accorded a privileged significance.[10]

Margaret Cavendish (1623?–1673) develops this perceived privilege to enable her own critique of the role of empiricism and experimentation in the study of natural philosophy. In the prefatory material to her *Philosophical and Physical Opinions* (1663), Cavendish draws a playful but telling distinction between her endeavours as a published writer of natural philosophy and her work as a housewife: "*I cannot for my Life be so good a Huswife, as to quit Writing*," she laments, "*the truth is, I have somewhat Err'd from good Huswifry, to write Nature's Philosophy, where, had I been prudent, I should have translated Natural Philosophy into good Huswifry*."[11] Cavendish, in exile and on the move for much of her adult life, probably did little, if any, actual housework. But her notion of the translatability of natural philosophy into housewifery and back again is striking, and legitimates her discussion of a range of topics, including chymistry, astrology, meteorology, and experimental science. Cavendish expands on this motif in her *Observations upon Experimental Philosophy* (1666), in which she compares Nature, "a wise and provident Lady," to a good housewife.[12] Nature, Cavendish asserts, successfully

[9] See, for example, the fourteenth-century "Opus Mulierum et Ludas Puerorum," in which the stages of the chymical opus are compared to "women's work" and "child's play." The "Opus Mulierum" was first published in *De Alchimia Opuscula Complura Veterum Philosophorum* (Frankfurt, 1550), and was reprinted in *Artis Auriferae*, vol. 2 (Basle, 1572), pp. 184–219.

[10] The manuscript is London, British Library, Sloane MS 1741. It has been edited and translated by Donald R. Dickson as *Aqua Vitæ: Non Vitis: Or, The radical Humiditie of Nature: Mechanically, and Magically dissected By the Conduct of Fire, and Ferment* (Tempe, AZ: Arizona Center for Medieval and Renaissance Studies, 2001). On Rebecca Vaughan see Donald R. Dickson, "The Alchemistical Wife: The Identity of Thomas Vaughan's 'Rebecca,'" *The Seventeenth Century* 13 (1998): 34–46, and Jennifer Speake, 'Vaughan, Thomas (1621–1666)', *Oxford Dictionary of National Biography*, Oxford University Press, 2004 <http://www.oxforddnb.com/view/article/28148> [accessed 18 April 2009].

[11] Margaret Cavendish, *Philosophical and Physical Opinions* (London, 1663), "To his Excellencie the Lord Marquis of Newcastle." On this point, see Kate Lilley, "Blazing Worlds: Seventeenth Century Women's Utopian Writing," in *Women, Texts & Histories*, ed. Clare Brant and Diane Purkiss (London: Routledge, 1992), pp. 101–32 (pp. 126–7).

[12] Margaret Cavendish, *Observations upon Experimental Philosophy* (London, 1666), p. 101.

manages her household, examining the goods at her disposal, and treats each according to its needs in an endless cycle of preserving, distilling, washing, and cooking. In contrast, Cavendish ridicules the authority of male scientists who claim sole right to 'inform the world' with their experiments and theories.[13] This playful juxtaposing of masculine and feminine modes of knowing culminates with a consideration of chymistry:

> I am confident, Women would labour as much with Fire and Furnace, as Men, for they'l make good Cordials and Spirits; but whether they would find out the Philosophers-stone, I doubt; for our Sex is more apt to waste, then to make Gold: however, I would have them try, especially those that have means to spend; for, who knows but Women might be more happy in finding it out, than Men (p. 102–3)

Of all the branches of natural philosophy, it is chymistry that, Cavendish believes, is most easily translatable into housewifery, and it is the diligent, careful, and meticulous housewife who makes the best chymist.

Writing from very different perspectives, Cavendish, Allestree, and Vaughan all write within a culture in which the chymical work, the *magnum opus*, was frequently called the *opus mulierum*, or "women's work."[14] In chymical literature would-be chymists are urged to meditate upon and imitate various aspects of women's work in the household, including washing (corresponding to the chymical process of distillation) and cooking (which is variously identified with fermentation, digestion, and putrefaction). Of the many examples of this motif, two emblems from Michael Maier's *Atalanta Fugiens* (Oppenheim, 1617) are representative.[15] Emblem 3 depicts a housewife pouring water from a bucket into a cauldron of boiling water. In the motto to this emblem, "Go to the woman

---

[13] On this point see, for example, Eve Keller, "Producing Petty Gods: Margaret Cavendish's Critique of Experimental Science," *English Literary History*, 64.2 (Summer 1997): 447–71.

[14] In his *A Lexicon of Alchemy* (Frankfurt,1612), Martin Ruland identifies the "Work of the Woman" as a synonym for "The Great Work" (i.e. the alchemical opus), on account of "the facility with which the Stone may be composed by those who are instructed in the proper method of operation" (Ruland, *A Lexicon of Alchemy or Alchemical Dictionary*, trans. A.E. Waite (London: John M. Watkins, 1964), p. 462).

[15] All quotations from *Atalanta Fugiens* are taken from *Michael Maier's Atalanta Fugiens: Sources of an Alchemical Book of Emblems*, ed. and trans. H.M.E. de Jong (Leiden: E.J. Brill, 1969). On the representation of housewifery in *Atalanta Fugiens* and other alchemical texts, see Gillian Beer, "*Square Rounds* and Other Awkward Fits: Chemistry as Theatre," *Ambix* 41.1 (March 1994): 33–44, and M.E. Warlick, "The Domestic Alchemist: Women as Housewives in Alchemical Emblems," *Emblems and Alchemy*, ed. Alison Adams and Stanton J. Linden (Glasgow: Glasgow Emblem Studies, 1998), pp. 25–47. For a very different reading of gender in this work, see Sally G. Allen and Joanna Hubbs, "Outrunning Atalanta: Feminine Destiny in Alchemical Transmutation," *Signs: Journal of Women in Culture and Society*, 6.2 (Winter 1980): 210–21.

who washes the sheets and do as she does," Maier directs the chymist to observe and learn from women's daily, domestic routines. Maier elaborates upon this instruction in an epigram:

> Don't you see how a woman is accustomed to cleaning dirty laundry
> By pouring hot water over it?
> Follow her example, so that you will not fail in your art,
> For the water washes the precipitation of the black body away.

The thorough washing of sheets corresponds to the chymist's initial washing of the *prima materia*, in readiness for the stages in the *opus*, and anticipates a later stage, the *solutio*, when, having been subjected to intense, dry heat, the charred *materia* is revivified by the introduction of healing waters.

The lessons of this emblem are developed in Emblem 22 of *Atalanta Fugiens*, in which a pregnant woman stands before a large open hearth. In the motto for this emblem Maier writes: "When you have obtained the white lead, then do women's work, that is to say: COOK." The accompanying epigram reads:

> Whosoever wants to achieve much with little trouble,
> Should throw snow in Saturn's black face:
> And the whitest material of lead will fall to you,
> After which only women's work remains.
> Then you should cook, like a woman, who puts her pans on the fire,
> But take care that the Truta dissolves in its own fluid.

Like a housewife cooking trout, the chymist must ensure that the lid is well sealed at all times. If there are any leaks, the vessel could easily break – a common complaint in chymical narratives – and the resulting loss of heat or vapour would prove disastrous to the final results. The housewife is visibly pregnant in this emblem – an image that again reinforces the need for the integrity of the womb-like vessel, and perhaps suggests that this knowledge and practice is something innate to women, held within their bodies and reinforced by social roles. As if to remind the chymist that this knowledge and practice is gendered, the vessel shown in the emblem is a *bain marie* – Mary's bath, one of the first chymical instruments, popularly attributed to a third-century CE Alexandrian chymist, "Mary the Jewess," and routinely used during the early modern period.[16] What I want to emphasise here is the popular notion that the housewife did indeed make an ideal chymist: that she possessed by virtue (and not in spite) of her sex, a unique

[16] Whether or not she can be identified with a single historical figure, "Mary the Jewess" (also known as Mary the Copt or Mary the Egyptian) is frequently cited as an authority in early modern chymical books, and the works attributed to her are collected in manuscript and printed miscellanies. See, for example, "The Practice of Mary the Prophetess in the Alchymicall Art" (London, British Library, Sloane MS 3461, fols. 1–8), which was printed in a number of publications, including Arnald de Villanova, *Opus Aureum* (Frankfurt, 1604). See also Raphael Patai, "Maria the Jewess – Founding Mother of Alchemy," *Ambix*, 29 (1982): 177–97.

and privileged knowledge of the secrets of the natural world, and that each day, as part of her routine housework, she could be perceived to be – and could perceive herself to be – performing aspects of "the work" and achieving tangible, profitable results. When Cavendish "apologised" for having failed to translate "Natural Philosophy into good Huswifry," therefore, she reasserted the fact that in early modern England natural philosophy and housewifery were believed to be related at a fundamental level.

Of course, we cannot assume that iconographic representations such as Maier's emblems translated into lived reality. But there is evidence to suggest that early modern Englishwomen did indeed engage in chymical work.[17] Queen Elizabeth I (1533–1603) and Mary Sidney Countess of Pembroke (1561–1621) were both reputed to have practiced chymistry in their own private laboratories – the latter is attributed authorship of medicinal recipes in contemporary manuscripts.[18] Anne Clifford recalls that her mother, Margaret Russell Countess of Cumberland (1560–1616), "was a lover of the study and practice of alchimy, by which she found out excellent medicines, that did much good to many," and a receipt book, possibly owned by Margaret, has recently been discovered.[19] Women also served as patrons of chymical literature. George's Baker's *A Newe Jewell of Health* (1576), a book of chymical medicine based on a work by Conrad Gesner, was dedicated to Anne de Vere Countess of Oxford (1556–1588). John Thornborough's "A Letter of Chemistry" (1614), a work of esoteric chymistry, including a chymical interpretation of the Pythagorean tetractys (or decad), was dedicated to Elizabeth,

---

[17] For examples drawn from England and Continental Europe, see Archer, "Women and Alchemy in Early Modern England," and Penny Bayer, "Women's Alchemical Literature 1560–1616 in Italy, France, the Swiss Cantons and England, and its Diffusion to 1660," PhD thesis, University of Warwick, 2003.

[18] On Queen Elizabeth I, see Archer, "Women and Alchemy in Early Modern England," chapter 1, and '"Rudenesse it Selfe She Doth Refine": Queen Elizabeth I as Lady Alchymia', in *Goddesses and Queens: The Iconography of Elizabeth I*, ed. Annaliese Connolly and Lisa Hopkins (Manchester: Manchester University Press, 2007), pp. 45–66. On Mary Sidney, see Margaret P. Hannay, "'How I These Studies Prize': The Countess of Pembroke and Elizabethan Science," in *Women, Science and Medicine, 1500–1700*, ed. Lynette Hunter and Sarah Hutton (Stroud: Sutton Publishing, 1997), pp. 108–21, and Archer, "Women and Alchemy in Early Modern England," chapter 2.

[19] Anne Clifford, *Lives of Lady Anne Clifford Countess of Dorset, Pembroke, and Montgomery (1590–1676) and of her parents summarized by herself*, ed. J.P. Gilson (London: Roxburghe Club, 1916) p. 20. The MS receipt book, "Alkumiste extraction of distillations and excellent medicines," is portrayed in Anne Clifford's triptych at Appleby Castle. It is discussed by Daniel Scott, "Recent Discoveries in the Muniment Rooms of Appleby Castle and Skipton Castle," *Transactions of the Cumberland and Westmoreland Antiquarian and Archaeological Society* 18 (1918): 189–210 (p. 200), and has been identified by Penny Bayer, "Lady Margaret Clifford's Alchemical Receipt Book and the John Dee Circle," *Ambix* (November 2005): 274–81.

Lady Knowles (1586–1658).[20] Perhaps the best evidence for the perceived correspondence between chymistry and housewifery is the appearance of chymical recipes and procedures in receipt books targeted at a female audience. Book 3 of Hugh Platt's *Jewell House of Art and Nature* (1594), for example, features a step-by-step guide to stillroom practice, and *The Ladies Cabinet Enlarged and Opened* (1654), which draws on the work of the Scottish-born chymist Patrick Ruthven, and the Italian chymical physician, Leonardo Fioravanti, includes sophisticated recipes for extracting quintessences, balms, and oils from metals and minerals.[21] Indeed, on a couple of occasions, women were ascribed authorship of printed receipt books with chymical recipes: *A Choice Manuall* (1653), attributed to Elizabeth Grey, Countess of Kent (1582–1651), contains recipes for mineral-based medicines, including the Countess's famous "Powder"; while *Natura Exenterata* (1655), attributed to Grey's sister, Aletheia Howard, Countess of Arundel (d. 1654), boasts a whole section, "*Chymicall Extractions*," devoted to operations on metals, including recipes for "*The quintessence of all manner of Herbs, flowers, roots, flesh, blood, or Eggs*" and "*Aurum Potabile.*"[22]

Early Modern Women and Their Books of Chymical Receipts

From Queen Elizabeth, Queen Anna, and Queen Henrietta Maria downwards, early modern Englishwomen were required to be – and, perhaps most importantly, show themselves to be – good housewives.[23] Being a good housewife involved a range of intellectual and practical skills that were intimately linked to a set of moral, specifically Christian and "feminine" qualities. To help women become good housewives, printed receipt books targeted at a female readership began to appear from the 1570s onward. In publications such as Gervase Markham's *The English Huswife* (1615) provision of medical care is shown to be an important part

---

20 London, British Library, Sloane MS 1799. Thornborough alludes to Lady Knowles's interest in chymistry in the opening paragraph: "Good madame, vnderstanding that yow haue a desier to spend yor howers freed from greater occasions in distilling waters & extracting tincktures, I thought good to write to your Ladishippe" (fol. 75^{r}).

21 Hugh Platt, *Jewell House of Art and Nature* (London, 1594), Book 3 ("Divers Chimicall Conclusions concerning the Art of Distillation"), pp. 3–7; *The Ladies Cabinet Enlarged and Opened* (London, 1654), pp. 154–68.

22 *A choice manuall, or rare and select secrets in physick and chyrurgery collected, and practised by the Right Honourable, the Countesse of Kent, late deceased* (London, 1653); *Natura exenterata: or Nature unbowelled by the most exquisite anatomizers of her* (London, 1655), pp. 375–6. On these publications, see Hunter, "Women and Domestic Medicine: Lady Experimenters 1570–1620," in *Women, Science and Medicine, 1500–1700*, pp.89–107, and *Seventeenth-Century English Recipe Books: Cooking, Physic and Chirurgery in the Works of Elizabeth Talbot Grey and Aletheia Talbot Howard*, ed. Elizabeth Spiller (Aldershot: Ashgate, 2008).

23 On the significance of housewifery to queenship, see Jayne Archer, "The Queens' Arcanum: Authority and Authorship in *The Queens Closet Opened* (1655)," *Renaissance Journal* 1.6 (June 2002), pp. 14–26.

of the household economy.[24] Charles Estienne, who acknowledged the scarcity of licensed practitioners in rural areas, stipulated that the "huswife" should run her own "Countrie Dispensatorie," and that she should be "skilfull in naturall Physicke, for the benefite of her own folke and others."[25] For Markham and Estienne, who situate their comments within the context of the larger domestic economy, allowing the housewife this much scope makes sound economic sense: a housewife who is "skilfull in naturall Physicke" is, Estienne maintains, good for "the profit of the house" (pp. 38–9).

At about the same time, from the latter half of the sixteenth century, women began to compile their own manuscript receipt books.[26] Ranging from four-page booklets, loosely bound with string, to large, leather-bound folios with gilt stamps, tooling and metal clasps, these books were one of the most important ways in which women accomplished Cavendish's ideal, translating domestic work – housewifery – into natural philosophy, and translating both into writing.[27] Early modern women were encouraged to collect, compose, and distribute recipes. Such activities were seen to be essential to their ability to fulfil their roles as healthcare providers in the home and neighbourhood. In his memoir of his late wife, Elizabeth (1623–1690), Anthony Walker offers an account of the compilation of such a book:

> She caused her daughters to transcribe her best recipes for things which were curious, but especially for Medicines, with directions how to use them … Her first and main stock she acquired from a Brother-in-Law, a very able Doctor of the *London* College, who Married her Sister, and was very freely communicative, who wrote her many Receipts, and directed her what methods to proceed in for most common Diseases … and she was very inquisitive of other Doctors, and had many English Books, *Riverius*, *Culpeper*, *Bonettus*, &c. which she read, not to say studied.[28]

---

24 Gervase Markham, *The English Huswife*, in Markham, *Countrey Contentments* (London, 1615), pp. 4–5.

25 Charles Estienne, *Maison Rustique*, trans. Richard Surflet (London, 1600), pp. 38–9.

26 On this phenomenon, see Sara Pennell, "Perfecting Practice?: Women, Manuscript Recipes and Knowledge in Early Modern England," in *Early Modern Women's Manuscript Writing: Selected Papers from the Trinity/Trent Colloquium*, ed. Victoria Burke and Jonathan Gibson (Aldershot, UK: Ashgate, 2004), pp. 237–58, and Elaine Leong and Sara Pennell, "Recipe Collections and the Currency of Medical Knowledge in the Early Modern 'Medical Marketplace'", in *Medicine and the Marketplace in England and Its Colonies c. 1450-c. 1850,* ed. Mark Jenner and Patrick Wallis (Basingstoke: Palgrave Macmillian, 2007), pp. 133–52.

27 The Wellcome Library for the History and Understanding of Medicine in London holds a particularly large and diverse collection of early modern women's manuscript receipt books. Some of these manuscripts can now be viewed online: http://library.wellcome.ac.uk/etexts.html.

28 Anthony Walker, *The Vertuous Wife: or, the Holy Life of Mrs Elizabeth Walker* (London, 1694), pp. 177–8. Walker observes that one of Elizabeth's principal duties was to care for the health of her neighbours, and that she imparted to their daughters "whatever required more Art or Curiosity, for the Closet or the Parlour, as Preserving, drawing Spirits in an Alembick, or cold Still" (p. 89).

Elizabeth Walker actively sought out recipes, drawing upon the knowledge and experience of her brother-in-law, who was a licensed physician, but also rifling through printed receipt books, and employing her daughters to transcribe her recipes.[29]

Women's manuscript receipt books have principally been used as evidence for women as healthcare providers.[30] But these books also testify to the wide range of skills required of the housewife, including distillation, preservation, cookery, accounting, gardening, and basic astrological lore. Although medical and culinary recipes predominate, it is important to emphasise the heterogeneous nature of these books. The manuscript receipt book of Lady Ann Fanshawe (1625–1680), for example, contains an eclectic, often dizzying range of material.[31] Begun in 1651, 7 years after Ann's marriage to Sir Richard Fanshawe, this elegant folio, entitled "Mrs Fanshawes Booke of Receipts of Physickes, Salves, Waters, Cordialls, Preserves and Cookery" (fol. 3^r), includes medical, culinary, and other household recipes, including prescriptions for perfumes, cleaning agents, costume jewellery, and a wide range of other literature, such as letters, printed advertisements for medicines, menu plans, and shopping lists. The recipes and other texts are written in English, Latin, and Spanish. Loose leaves and scraps written in a variety of hands have been sewn or pasted onto the pages of the volume to produce a text that works, quite literally, on many different levels.

In the case of Ann Fanshawe, we are lucky: Ann left several literary remains, including a memoir of her husband.[32] Her life is well documented, and it is possible to trace her movements and her milieu; we can, for example, identify a number of the named donors of Ann's receipts. But with Sarah Wigges, we are not so fortunate, and her life appears to be undocumented. There are a few clues to Sarah's identity within the volume. "Wigges" would appear to be Sarah's married

---

29 A "Mrs. Elizabeth Walker" is named as the source for a "Receipt for the Eyes" in a manuscript receipt formerly owned by the Duke of Norfolk: Worthing County Museum, MS 3574, p. 56. Elizabeth Walker, *née* Sadler, the daughter of a pharmacist, was the wife of Anthony Walker, chaplain to Mary Rich, Countess of Warwick, and afterwards Rector of Fyfield. Elizabeth may have collaborated with Mary and her sister, Katherine Lady Ranelagh, in the stillroom at the Warwicks' residence, Leighs Priory in Essex. A MS receipt book (Wellcome Western MS 1340), associated with Mary and Katherine, may incorporate receipts contributed or "approved" by Elizabeth.

30 See, for example, Lucinda McCray Beier, "The Character of a Good Woman: Women and Illness," in Beier, *Sufferers and Healers: The Experience of Illness in Seventeenth-Century England* (London: Routledge and Kegan Paul, 1987), pp. 211–41; John B. Blake, "The Complete Housewife," *Bulletin of the History of Medicine* 49.1 (1975): 30–42; Doreen F. Nagy, "Women's Role in Stuart Medicine," in Nagy, *Popular Medicine in Seventeenth-Century England* (Bowling Green, OH: Bowling Green State University Press, 1988), pp. 54–78.

31 Wellcome Western MS 7113.

32 London, British Library, Add. MS 41161. Ann's memoir has been edited by John Loftis in *The Memoirs of Anne, Lady Halkett and Ann, Lady Fanshawe* (Oxford: Clarendon Press, 1979).

name, for the name of her husband, "Richard Wigges" (pp. 283–4), features in one of the recipes, a charm to cure toothache.[33] Sarah's maiden name may have been "Speght," for "my one Mo Speght" (p. 106) is mentioned in connection with one medicine. "My Mother" is identified as the source for two other recipes: "A Sweete Water" and a method "To distill an excellent damaske rose water" (pp. 538–9). There is only one reference to place in the manuscript: a recipe "To plant Licoras" is attributed to "one that hath hadd much experience Mrs Nevell in Yorkeshere" (fol. 3^r). In the absence of other evidence, it is tempting to conjecture that Sarah Wigges may have been born into the Speght family of Yorkshire. The Speght family included Rachel Speght (*b.* 1597?, *d.* in or before 1661?), the author of two published books, *A Mouzell for Melastomus* (1617) and *Mortalities Memorandum* (1621) – the former publication a defence of the nature of women, the latter a defence of female education.[34] Rachel's father, James Speght (*c.* 1564–1637) from Horbury near Wakefield in Yorkshire, was a member of the London Society of Goldsmiths. Thomas Moundford, Rachel's godfather, was six times president of the Royal College of Physicians and personal physician to Arbella Stuart; his reputation among women at court is suggested by the appearance of a recipe for "Doctor Monford's Cordiall water" in the Countess of Arundel's *Natura Exenterata* (1655).[35] Boasting educated women, goldsmiths, and physicians, the Speght family would have provided an ideal environment for the compilation of a book such as that owned by Sarah Wigges.

Suppositions apart, what can this book tell us about Sarah's circumstances, her social milieu, and intellectual world? The first mention of Sarah Wigges herself comes on the recto of the ninth leaf of the volume, which also serves for a title page. At the top of this page is the inscription "Sarah Wigges hir Booke," the date "1616," and the motto "Live wel, dye neuer: Dye wel, liue euer." There follows a brief note on the "Climactera," which is defined as "The perilous time of ones life att every 7 or 9 yeres end, or at the end of 63 yeres when 7s and 9s meete." Perhaps, then, in 1616, when she set about the task of putting together this manuscript, Sarah was at such a point in her life – perhaps a newlywed of 18 or 21 years. On the verso of this title page is a table explaining the symbols for weights and measures used in the recipes. This leaf, dated and named, would seem to constitute the "start" of the book proper. When Sarah Wigges began to compile this book, therefore, she left eight blank leaves, possibly for further tables, directions, or other "keys" to using the rest of the book. Five of these blank leaves have been filled with general household recipes and a partial list of contents, written in a rapid, rather messy mid-seventeenth-century italic hand. These recipes, including one "To make sope" (fol. 2^r) and another "To catch Fowles without a nett" (fol. 1^r),

---

33 No one of the name "Richard Wigges" is recorded as having entered the universities of Oxford and Cambridge during the sixteenth and seventeenth centuries.

34 For Rachel Speght's life and works, see Barbara Kiefer Lewalski, ed., *The Polemics and Poems of Rachel Speght* (Oxford, Oxford University Press, 1996), pp. xi–xix.

35 *Natura Exenterata*, p. 336. On Moundford's connection to Arbella Stuart, see *The Polemics and Poems of Rachel Speght*, p. xiv.

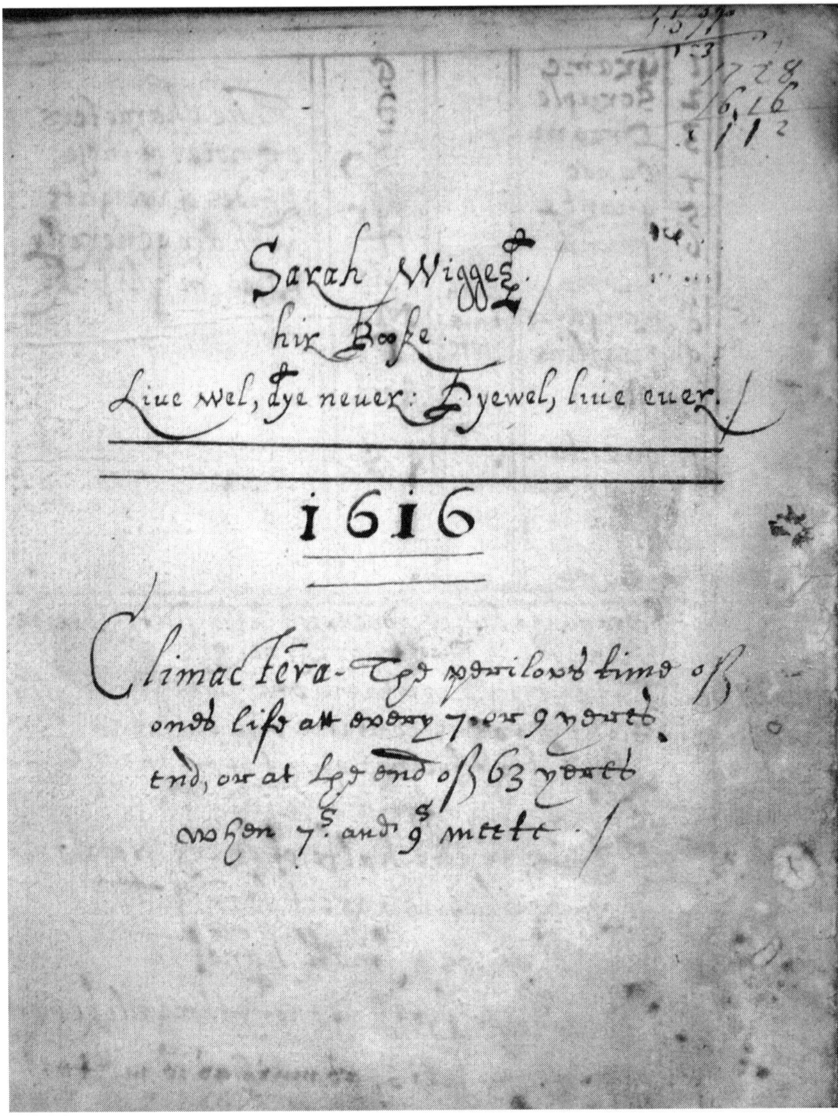

Fig. 8.1 The title page of Sarah Wigges's Receipt Book. London, Royal College of Physicians, MS 654. Courtesy of the Royal College of Physicians.

are short and simple. As with the following prescription, "To fetch staynes from Lynen," they serve not so much to instruct the reader in new knowledge, but as a memorial aid, confirming something that the reader already knows, perhaps from oral instruction: "Before the cloth hath beene put in any liquor after the stayning of it; you must wash the staynes place in new mead and urine probatum" (fol. 1^{r}).

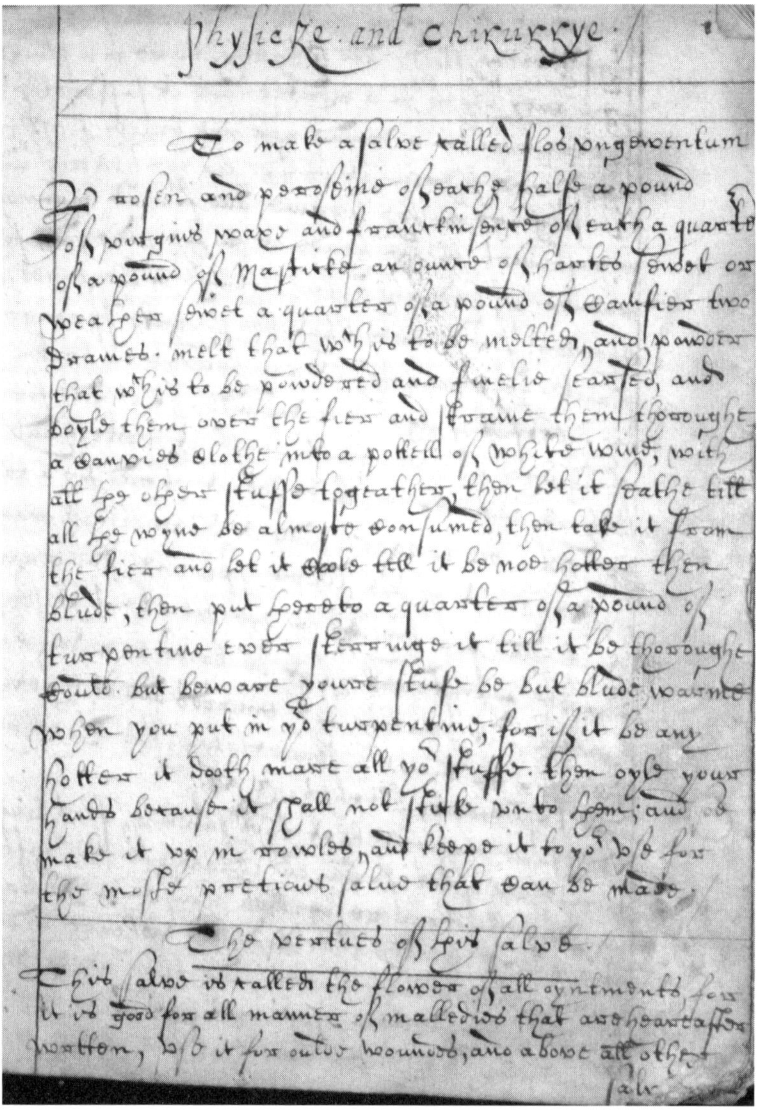
Physicke and chirurrye

To make a salve called flos unguentum

Take rosen and perrosine of each halfe a pound of virgins waxe and frankinsence of each a quarter of a pound of Mastike an ounce of harts suet or weathers suet a quarter of a pound of camphire two drames. melt that wch is to be melted, and powder that wch is to be powdered and finelie sarsed, and boyle them over the fire and straine them thorought a canvies clothe into a pottell of white wine, with all the other stuffe togeather, then let it seathe till all the wyne be almost consumed, then take it from the fire and let it coole till it be noe hotter then bloud, then put hereto a quarter of a pound of turpentine ever stirringe it till it be thorought coole. but beware your stuff be but bloud warme when you put in ye turpentine, for if it be any hotter it dooth marre all ye stuffe. then oyle your hands because it shall not stick unto them; and make it up in rowles, and keepe it to yor use for the moste pretious salve that can be made.

The vertues of this salve.

This salve is called the flower of all oyntments for it is good for all manner of malladies that are hearafter written, use it for outer woundes, and above all other salve.

Fig. 8.2 The first page of Sarah Wigges's Receipt Book. London, Royal College of Physicians, MS 654. Courtesy of the Royal College of Physicians.

Following the ninth leaf, and Sarah's mark of ownership, the leaves are paginated and the recipes begin under the title "Physicke and chirurrye" (p. 1). The bulk of the recipes are written in a clear, upright italic hand, with headings and margins clearly lined. It would seem that an amanuensis was used to transcribe these recipes, for Sarah's own hand, a neat italic script written in a lighter ink, annotates them, occasionally giving additional information, as when she notes against a recipe "to preserve apricots," "this way is nought," or personal endorsement, as in the case of a recipe "For the green-sickness," which, she notes, "hath helped myself" (pp. 71, 73). This phase of work on the book continued until at least 1625, as one recipe, entered in the same neat italic hand, is dated, and bears testimony in Wigges's annotating hand: "This was taught by a Jew w[hi]ich came from Jurey 80 yeares a goe. it will helpe if the party be 10. myle from you having his nam and how many teeth aketh." An earlier, aborted attempt to transcribe this complicated charm is also annotated by Wigges, who notes that it "hath helped all th[a]t have used it," and that it was "taught 1625" (pp. 283–4)

"Human knowledge," Londa Schiebinger has written, "develops through conversations, observations and exchanges."[36] A receipt, as the name suggests, was something given and received. Wigges intercedes to acknowledge the sources of her information on many occasions, and this testifies to the circulation of manuscript materials between early modern women. Such networks, Margaret Ezell has argued, provided an informal means to education for early modern women, providing them "with opportunities for intellectual engagements and insights which their circumstances, excluded from universities and learned societies, might not immediately suggest."[37] The attribution of certain recipes to specific individuals is a characteristic of receipt books, and women's receipt books in particular. Robert Boyle conceded that "In all Actions, the Autority of the Person giues Autority to the Example."[38] The appearance of named donors serves both to give authority to a recipe, and, perhaps, to locate the compiler within a specific network of acquaintances, a particular intellectual and social world. William Eamon has noted that in the latter half of the seventeenth century all kinds of secrets and receipts retained their value as commodities and articles in gift exchanges: secrets were tokens of exclusiveness and privilege, distinguishing those who could be entrusted from those who could not, creating bonds of mutual obligation and trust between like-minded individuals.[39] To refine Boyle's comment, therefore, "authority" was constituted not in the individual, but in ongoing transactions between individuals.

Wigges's "authority" as a housewife and practitioner was principally constituted through her interactions with female donors and printed books. Female donors – particularly female relatives – often predominate in women's manuscripts. In fact women's manuscript receipt books, which were frequently passed down from mother to daughter, testify to the strength of the mother-daughter bond in early

---

36 Londa Schiebinger, *Nature's Body: Sexual Politics and the Making of Modern Science* (London: Pandora, 1994), p. 211.

37 Margaret J.M. Ezell, *The Patriarch's Wife: Literary Evidence and the History of the Family* (London: The University of North Carolina Press, 1987), p. 73.

38 Cited in Steven Shapin, *A Social History of Truth: Civility and Science in Seventeenth-Century England* (Chicago, IL: University of Chicago Press, 1994), p. 126.

39 William Eamon, *Science and the Secrets of Nature: Books of Secrets in Medieval and Early Modern Culture* (Princeton, NJ: Princeton University Press, 1994), pp. 319–50.

modern England. On preparing to leave the parental house to set up a home with their new husband, young women often had their mother's or prospective mother-in-law's recipes copied down for them into a new manuscript book, as a guide to being a housewife and mother in their own right. Sarah's book follows this pattern, with her possible mother-in-law, "Mo Wigges," the most significant source, being credited with over 50 recipes. A couple of licensed physicians are identified as sources, including "Dr Pratt" (p. 339) and "Dr Allott" (p. 103) who has supplied a remedy for an ague.

As in the case of Elizabeth Walker cited earlier, women also gleaned recipes from printed books. Often, the source is not credited, and the recipe is altered in the act of copying so that it becomes difficult to trace specific printed sources. Wigges's manuscript is unusual in the number of recipes and extracts identified as coming from particular authors and publications. Towards the centre of the book, following the first batch of medical recipes entered by the amanuensis, there are passages and notes transcribed from other sources, apparently printed books, including John Gerard's *Herball* (1597; rev. ed. 1633);[40] Rembert Dodoens's *Herball* (4 edns 1578–1619),[41] Andreas Libavius's *Alchymia* (1606);[42] Andrew Borde's *The Breviarie of Health* (1575);[43] Giambattista della Porta's *Natural Magick*, which was first published in an English translation in 1658;[44] and, somewhat curiously, Boethius's *Consolation of Philosophie* (English translations were published in 1536, 1556, and 1609). Recipes are also attributed to Nicholas Culpeper (p. 356), Paracelsus (pp. 116–8, 355), and Galen (p. 246), although the particular works are not specified. The latter two authorities could have been gleaned from intermediary sources – indeed, Culpeper was a translator of Paracelsian literature.[45] Of these sources, only Nicholas Culpeper wrote works specifically targeted at a female readership; as we have seen, Alexander Walker identified Culpeper as one of the authors from whom his wife, Elizabeth, took down her recipes. Although there

[40] "Jarruts earball" (p. 307), i.e. John Gerard's *The Herball or Generall Historie of Plantes* (London, 1597) was published in a revised edition by Thomas Johnson in 1633.

[41] "Dodoneus" (p. 246), i.e. Rembert Dodoens's *A Niewe Herball: Or, Historie of Plantes*, trans. Henry Lyte, appeared in four editions between 1578 and 1619.

[42] "History of Andreas Libavius" (p. 606). Libavius's *Alchymia* is commonly credited as the first chemistry textbook. Featuring illustrations of chymical equipment and utensils, *Alchymia* appeared in several Latin editions, published on the Continent during the first decade of the seventeenth century. I have not been able to trace an early modern printed edition in English, but material by Libavius was available in Joannes Jonstonus's *An History of the Wonderful Things of Nature* (London, 1657).

[43] "the breviary of health Compiled by Andrew Boord, doctor in Phisick: an Englishman" (p. 340).

[44] "*magia*" of "Baptist Porta," (p. 606).

[45] Culpeper translated Simeon Partlicius's *A new method of physick: or, A short view of Paracelsus and Galen's practice* (London, 1654).

are testimonials to women reading herbals in early modern England,[46] this list of sources – particularly in a non-aristocratic woman, and especially in the field of natural philosophy – suggests that women's reading matter could be wider and more eclectic than has often been supposed.

The recipes at the beginning of Wigges's MS cover most of the typical medical complaints dealt with in such books, beginning with a method for making the "salve called flos vngewentum" (p.1) and a description of its "vertues." Some rudimentary attempt has been made to group the recipes according to disease, with sections devoted to the canker, gout, bruises, consumption, toothache, and backache. Recipes for women's illnesses are well represented, with several remedies for sore breasts, painful periods and other menstrual irregularities, the green sickness (for which "A purgatorie" (p. 19) is recommended), and for all stages in pregnancy and childbirth, including breast-feeding. More frequently, however, recipes are grouped according to type of medicine: vomits, plasters, unguents, syrups, waters, oils, and purges. The remedies betray the strong influence of Galenic medicine. The chief ingredients are herbs, flowers, seeds, and nuts – all items that a thrifty housewife could collect from her own garden or from her neighbours. Animal parts also appear among the ingredients: the water of a distilled pig is endorsed as a restorative (p. 9), while swallows' oil (p. 13) and "Powder of vipers" (p. 379) are recommended for their general health-giving powers. Following on from this general overview, I now want to turn to consider two specific medical interests as reflected in Wigges's manuscript, and to investigate the influence of chymical theory and practice on both.

Chymical Medicine in the Receipt Book of Sarah Wigges

Roger Bacon (*c.*1214–1292?) defined "*Alchimy*" as "a science teaching how to make and compound a certaine medicine, which is called *Elixir*, the which when it is cast upon mettals or imperfect bodies, doth fully perfect them in their verie projection."[47] During the sixteenth century, European chymistry underwent an important transition, as chymists increasingly turned away from the transmutation of base metals and the never-ending search for a single Elixir of Life, and redirected their efforts towards the manufacture of medicines that could bring specific and tangible results. Central to this transition were the revolutionary ideas of Paracelsus (1493/4–1541), who identified chymistry as the "third part, or pillar of true medicine."[48] For Paracelsus, anyone who wishes to practice

---

[46] See, for example, Margaret Hoby, *Diary of Lady Margaret Hoby, 1599–1605*, ed. Dorothy M. Meads (London: George Routledge & Sons, 1930), p. 71.

[47] Roger Bacon, *et al.*, *The Mirror of Alchimy* (London, 1599), sig. A3ʳ.

[48] Paracelsus, *The Hermetic and Alchemical Writings*, ed. and trans. A.E. Waite, vol. 2 of 2 (London: J. Elliott, 1894), p. 148. On the assimilation of Paracelsian medicine in England, see Charles Webster, "Alchemical and Paracelsian Medicine," in Webster, *Health, Medicine and Mortality in the Sixteenth Century* (Cambridge: Cambridge University Press, 1979), pp. 301–33.

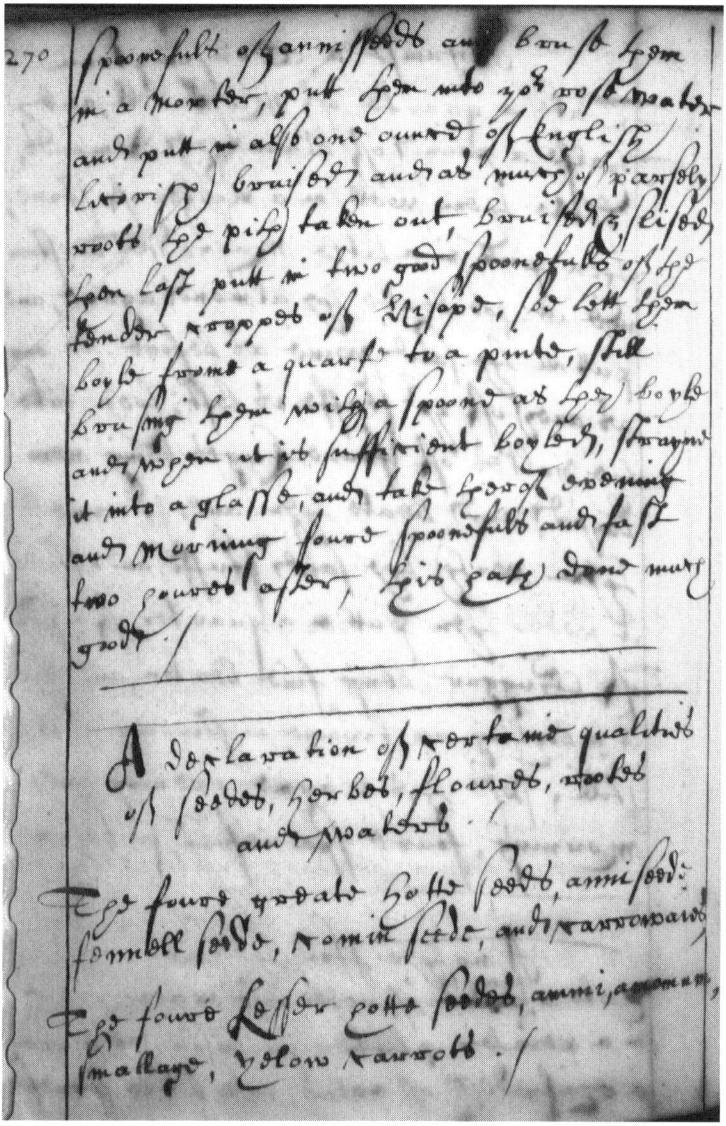

270 spoonfulls of annisseedes and bruse them
in a morter, put them into the rose water
and putt in also one ounce of English
licorice bruised and as much of parsley
roots the pith taken out, bruised, slised
then last putt in two good spoonfulls of the
tender croppes of Hisope, so lett them
boyle from a quart to a pinte, still
brusing them with a spoone as they boyle
and when it is sufficient boyled, strayne
it into a glasse, and take thereof evening
and morning foure spoonfulls and fast
two houres after, this hath done much
good. /

A declaration of certaine qualities
of seedes, herbes, flowers, rootes
and waters. /

The foure greate hotte seedes, annisseede:
fennell seede, comin seede, and carroway

The foure lesser hotte seedes, ammi, amomum,
smallage, yelow carrots. /

Fig. 8.3 Page 270 of Sarah Wigges's Receipt Book. London, Royal College of Physicians, MS 654. Courtesy of the Royal College of Physicians.

"true medicine" is also, by definition, "an Alchemist": a physician or healer participates in that general desire – which underlies the chymical enterprise – to bring (or, rather, to return) all created things to the state of prelapsarian perfection which God had intended. As Robert Multhauf has argued, the assimilation of distilled waters and oils into the work of chymists created a new category of chymical products, "a group of intermediary distillation products between the raw material and the elixir."[49]

In early modern medicine, distillation was the single most important chymical process. "Distillation," however, was a rather fluid term. For some writers, distillation became synonymous with chymistry itself; for others, it was simply an important stage within the opus. Konrad Gesner belonged to the former group, and pointed to "Phisicke" as one of the principle beneficiaries: "The Art of destillation (whiche they call *Chymia* …) hath inuented many profitable things for mans life, and in Phisicke also certain meruelous thinges."[50] As late as 1651 John French called his chymical receipt book *The Art of Distillation*, arguing that the difference between chymistry and distillation is one of emphasis rather than kind: "there are degrees" in "this spagyrical art," French writes, "there is the accomplishing of the Elixir it self, and there is the discovering of many excellent essences, magisteries, and spirits, +c … which abundantly recompence the discoverers thereof with profit, health and delight" (sig. a1^{v}).

As healthcare providers for the household and wider neighbourhood, this change had important consequences for women. Reflecting women's particular skill, distillation is typically gendered feminine in early modern narratives. Addressing Lady Knowles in 1614, John Thornborough writes:

> This Ladye [i.e. Lady Alcumy] speaketh out of a window to your Ladishipp (for yet she dareth not open her chamber dores) that she hath onelie two children: Th'one a faire daughter named *Distillation*, on whom do waite many handmayds, as *Extrac[t]ions* of *Tinctures* & *Saltes*, drawing oyles by Serpentines, forcing of Sperites by retortes with many other of that kinde:[51]

Women, who had long excelled in producing substances of intermediate status, such as waters of life – based on wine and alcohol – but also simple distilled waters, such as rosewater and cinnamon water, thus became not just participants, but potential experts in an enlarged chymical field. Between the Philosopher's Stone and rosewater, the chymist and the amateur healer, there ranged a continuum of beliefs, from which individual healers and/or chymists could draw according to each specific situation.

Like many of her female contemporaries, Wigges's medicines, and several of her other recipes, including perfumes, cosmetics, and foodstuffs, were largely based on distilled waters and oils – either the distilled extractions of single substances

---

[49] Robert Multhauf, "The Significance of Distillation in Renaissance Medical Chemistry," *Bulletin of the History of Medicine* 30 (1956): 329–46 (pp. 330–31). In an unpublished paper, Anne Stobart has identified a gradual decrease in the use of distillation and in the number of ingredients used in Englishwomen's medicine waters during the seventeenth century: "'A uery good Cordiall water without the trouble of a Still': Changing practise in early modern domestic medicine in South West England" (Medicinal Receipts Conference, Oxford Wellcome History of Medicine Unit, February 2004). I am grateful to Ms. Stobart for allowing me to read her paper.

[50] Konrad Gesner, *The Treasure of Euonymus* (London, 1559), sig. A1^{r}.

[51] London, British Library Sloane MS 1799, fol. 75^{v}.

("simples"), or compound waters, using as many as twenty ingredients. Among the simple distilled waters are recipes for rosewater, cinnamon water, and swallows' oil, each having quite specific and limited virtues. Among the compound waters are versions of a number of popular polychrests, with more general, often miraculous, restorative powers, including "Aqua Mirabilis" (p. 329), "Doctor Stevens Water" (pp. 544–5), "A Excellent restorative called the Electuary of life" (p. 129), and a water "For all Evill in the bodies" (p. 83).

Distilled waters formed the basis of almost all aspects of housewifery, and the stillroom (or "distillatorie") was the centre of the housewife's activities. But what did women such as Sarah Wigges think they were doing when they distilled a substance? How did they understand the transformation of, say, rose petals into rosewater? We can gain some insight into these questions from the definitions provided in printed receipt books aimed at a female readership. John Shirley opens his printed book of household receipts, *The Accomplished Ladies Rich Closet of Rarities* (London, 1687), with the following definition of "*Distilling*":

> Alimbecking and Distilling are held by many to be Learned, or taken by the Ancients from the Operation of the Sun in its effectually Exhaling the Sublunar moisture, and Rarifying the gross and indigested Vapours in a more subtil Region; and indeed Distillations participate of a Solar vertue, as being by their penetrating Qualities, and insensible Operations, more quick, subtil and enlivening. (p. 1)

Distillation perfects a substance. The gentle application of heat (Shirley's "Solar vertue") releases the spirit – or "Quintessence" (p. 2) – of a substance, briefly releasing it from its material shell, before refining it further and then reincorporating it within matter, which has in turn undergone a physical metamorphosis. The various products of the stillroom – whether they were used to concoct perfumes, cosmetics, medicines, or in cookery – were fashioned in the belief that the powers (or "virtues") of a substance were more powerful ("more quick, subtil and enlivening") after having been submitted to the appropriate method of distillation, which separated the poisonous or gross part of the substance from its more spiritual and beneficial essence. Usually, this separation was brought about by immersing the substance in a liquid and applying heat; the vaporized essence would then rise to the top of the alembic, where it condensed and was channelled into a separate vessel (the "receiver"), leaving the impure residue (the "filtrate") at the bottom of the limbeck.

Guides to distillation, combining theoretical and practical knowledge, appeared in numerous printed books, including John Fitzherbert's *Fitzharberts Booke of Husbandrie* (1598); Charles Estienne's *Maison Rustique* (1600); John Partridge's *The Treasurie of Hidden Secrets* (1633); and John French's *The Art of Distillation* (1651).[52] The books by Estienne and French include illustrations of stills, and such

[52] John Fitzherbert, *Fitzharberts Booke of Husbandrie* (London, 1598), pp. 104–5; Charles Estienne, *Maison Rustique* (1600), Book 3, chapters 58–61; John Partridge, *The Treasurie of Hidden Secrets* (London, 1633), sigs. D1^r–D1^v; John French *The Art of*

an illustration, of a furnace equipped for basic distillation, appears in the central section of Wigges's manuscript.[53] In such guides, the reader is required to tailor their equipment, method, timing, and source of heat (fire, dung, or sun) to the ingredients. Again, these concerns are reflected in Wigges's recipes, in which a range of stills is specified – earthen, glass, copper, and silver-lined. Wigges is also careful to acknowledge that different ingredients (or "simples"), require precise handling and treatment, certain times of harvesting, and the use of specific solvents. Her book thus features a guide to distilling oils, "To make certaine Oyles" (p. 39), and to the virtues of various simples, "A declaration of certaine qualities of seedes, herbes, flowers, rootes and waters" (pp. 270–72).[54]

Despite the Galenic emphasis in these herb-based waters, metals and minerals also feature in Wigges's book. Two methods "To kill quicke-silver," appear at the beginning of the book, and describe the ways in which mercury can be prepared for use in other recipes. The first method requires the following operation on an unspecified quantity of "quicke-silver": "mingle with it your fasting spittell in a peece of a broken glasse or in an oyster shell stirring them too geather with your finger until it looke blacke, and then it is killed" (p. 18). The equipment specified in this recipe – broken glass or an oyster shell – demonstrates the improvisatory skills of the housewife. The second method, again quite simple, requires the addition of wine vinegar to the mercury, and their mingling in "a vial glasse" (p. 17).

The introduction of metals and minerals into medicine was another of the legacies of Paracelsus and his followers. Although apparently controversial, this trend was picked up by some female healers.[55] Medicinal recipes involving mercury, gold, and other metals appear in printed receipt books directed towards a female readership, such as *A Closet for Ladies and Gentlewomen* (1608), and *The Ladies Cabinet Opened* (1639), but they also appear in women's manuscript receipt books.[56] *A Poore Mans Talent* (*c.* 1623), a manuscript receipt book written

---

Distillation (London, 1651), pp.1–2, 12–6. See also Platt, *Jewell House of Art and Nature*, Book III, Figure 1 (note 23, above).

53 The manuscript receipt book compiled by Lady Frances Catchmay (*c.* 1625) features a similar hand-drawn diagram, alongside a recipe "For to draw Chymicall Oyles out of anny hott herbe": Wellcome Western MS 184a, fol. 60^{v}.

54 A similar guide, "How to order each Herbe or Flower before it is distilled," appears in the manuscript receipt book of Ann Fanshawe: Wellcome Western MS 7113, fols. 263^{v}–64^{r}.

55 Margaret Pelling has argued that "the female irregulars in London were … fully involved in applying the drastic, novel remedies based on metals which were being used against unpleasant new diseases": "Thoroughly Resented? Older Women and the Medical Role in Early Modern London," in *Women, Science and Medicine, 1500–1700*, pp. 63–78 (p. 76). See also Pelling, "Defensive Tactics: Networking by Female Medical Practitioners in Early Modern London," in *Communities in Early Modern England: Networks, Places, Rhetoric*, ed. Alexandra Shepherd and Phil Withington (Manchester: Manchester University Press, 2000), pp. 38–53.

56 *A Closet for Ladies and Gentlewomen* (London, 1608), p. 89; *The Ladies Cabinet Opened* (London, 1639), p. 57.

by Thomas Lodge for Anne Howard, Dowager Countess of Arundel (1557–1630), features a number of recipes based on silver and mercury.[57] Lady Torrington's recipe for "orange water," which appears in the manuscript receipt book of Diana Astry Orlebar (*bap.* 1671, *d.* 1716), requires the addition of "2 leaves of gold," and Lady Grace Mildmay (*c.*1552–1620) collected a number of recipes based on gold, mercury, and antimony, the most ambitious of which is her "tincture of gold."[58]

Some of the printed sources cited in Sarah Wigges's book – Paracelsus and Libavius, for example – suggest a particular interest in iatrochymistry, the medicinal use of metals and minerals. Indeed, the central portion of Wigges's book is taken up with a set of longer extracts from printed books, directly alluding to chymical theory and procedures. The first extract, written in the hand of Wigges's original amanuensis, is a set of "Annotations and practicall Receipts and Processes" (p. 332), taken from *The Triumphant Chariot of Antimony* by the mythical chymist and Benedictine monk, Basil Valentine, complete with chapter and page references. In *The Triumphant Chariot* – or "Twelve Keys," as it was popularly known – Valentine tells how, after years of trying to use plants and herbs as medicines, he discovered the superior powers of metals and minerals, specifically antimony. *The Triumphant Chariot* was published in three English editions, between 1660 and 1678. The medicinal uses of antimony were debated throughout the first half of the seventeenth century, but the presence of these notes from Valentine suggests a particular interest in the use of antimony in the preparation of the Philosopher's Stone.[59] Although changes have been made in the process of copying, and errors introduced, it appears that the scribe was using the 1660 edition – or, perhaps, a manuscript copy of this edition. Either way, this pushes back the date of composition of this part of Wigges's book to at least 44

---

[57] Lodge endorses "*Lac virginis*" ("Virgin's Milk"), a mixture of "Litharg of silver," "white wine vineger," salt, and "raine or fountaine water," as a facial wash that will help "to cleare the countenance, drie up virulent pimples, and to destroy the frecknes [*sic*]": *The Complete Works of Thomas Lodge*, ed. Edmund Gosse, vol. 4 of 4 (Glasgow: Hunterian Club, 1883), p. 12. "Lac virginis", or "Virgin's Milk," was an alternative name for the Philosopher's Stone: see, for example, Ben Jonson, *The Alchemist*, ed. Elizabeth Cook, 2nd edn (London: A & C Black, 1995), 2.3.62, 184.

[58] "Diana Astry's Recipe Book," ed. Bette Stitt, *The Publications of the Bedfordshire Historical Record Society* 37 (1957): 83–168, p. 145; Linda Pollock, *With Faith and Physic: The Life of a Tudor Gentlewoman, Lady Grace Mildmay 1552–1620* (London: Collins and Brown, 1993), pp. 132–3. When served with wine, Lady Mildmay notes, this tincture is "wonderfull good to stay all manner of bloody flux and subtle humours," and when "taken with conserve" it "conforteth much a weak stomach" (p. 133).

[59] For an account of this debate, see Lauren Kassell, "Of Cako, or the Medical Uses of Antimony," in Kassell, *Magic and Medicine in Elizabethan London: Simon Forman, Astrologer, Alchemist, and Physician* (Oxford: Oxford University Press, 2005), pp. 173–89.

years after its inception in 1616, and suggests a development in the interests of Wigges and/or the subsequent owner(s) of her book.[60]

The other extracts from this central portion of the book also date from the latter half of the seventeenth century. They are written in a different hand, a single cursive italic hand writing in pale brown ink. The hand is messy and hasty, and employs chymical symbols and abbreviations. The first of these extracts is entitled "A tretis of the most great … Philo[sopher] St. Dunstan Bishop of Canterbury of the [philoso]phors stone" (p. 449). It is an unacknowledged copy of the translation of the legendary "Book of St. Dunstan," first published in Lancelot Coelson's collection of chymical works, *Philosophia Maturata* (1668).[61] The extract opens with a brief account of St. Dunstan's life, and the treatise proper with a description of the ancient origins of chymistry.[62] In this treatise, chymistry is described as an effort to recreate and speed up the process by which precious metals are developed deep underground. The main principle behind these efforts is shown to be the extraction and unification of two principles within matter, variously called "Sol and Luna," red and white earth, and "their gold and silver" (p. 447).

Following this definition of chymistry is a translation from an unnamed source, dated 1627. This professes to be an eyewitness account of a number of operations on the Philosopher's Stone. The account, the author claims, is written in "plaine words" (p. 468), so that a "fool … may understand it" (p. 468) – it was, of course, a common complaint that chymical literature was (often by design) written in obscure, riddling language. Those authors who tried to target chymical literature at a female readership – the anonymous author of the first English translation of Flamel's *Exposition* (1624), for example – often criticized this obscurity,

60 There are recipes using antimony – including one for the 'blood of oil or antimony' – in Grace Mildmay's manuscript recipes: Linda Pollock, *With Faith and Physic*, p. 134. Dorothy Hudson collected notes on "The virtues of the Antimonial Cuppe" in her MS "Booke/ of resaytts ffor salfes/ and medessens Septemb[e]r the 23: 1629" (Oxford, Bodleian Library, MS Rawl.c.81, fols. 95^{v}–96).

61 *Philosophia maturata an exact piece of philosophy containing the practick and operative part thereof in gaining the philosophers stone: with the wayes how to make the mineral stone and the calcinations of mettals: whereunto is added a work compiled by St. Dunstan concerning the philosophers stone: and the experiments of Rumelius and preparations of Angelo Sala, all most famous chymists in their time* (London, 1668).

62 St. Dunstan (*d.* 988), Archbishop of Canterbury and former Abbot of Glastonbury, was reputed to have been in possession of the red and white powders of transmutation, and was attributed authorship of a book describing operations using these powders. The legend of Dunstan's book acquired renewed fame during the early modern period, particularly when Edward Kelley and John Dee claimed to have recovered the powders (Ashmole, *Theatrum Chemicum Britannicum*, sigs. A4v–B1r, p. 481; John Dee, *The Private Diary of Dr. John Dee, and the Catalogue of his Library of Manuscripts, from the original manuscripts in the Ashmolean Museum at Oxford and Trinity College Library, Cambridge* (London: Camden Society, 1842), p. 25).

favouring a "plain style" and the vernacular.[63] The recipe for multiplying the Stone is similarly practical, requiring the chymist to wear a curious set of protective "Armour" (p. 471) made of cotton wool and pigskin. This recipe, for the medicinal uses of the Stone, is straightforward, almost mundane in tone:

> Take the quantity of 4 graines and solve this in a pint of white wine, or renish wine but not in any hott wine, and put it into a great clear glass, and instantly it will colour the wine, almost a red as it selfe was, which is the brightest red in the world, let it stand … 4 days … then add to this a pint more of wine by degrees, till it be not so red, and stir it with a cleane stick, and so contineue poureing in the fresh wine untill it comes to the colour of Sol, which is a shining yellow … if it stand but 4 howers quiet, so soon as you see the white filme, let it run through a cleane lining cloath, or paper, and the white filme will stay be hind, and look like a pearle in the paper … of this golden water lett the party take for what desease soever a good spoonfull every morrow, and it will expel the desease by gentle sweat, for it neither purgeth nor vomits, but strengthen, and if the desease be of many years or a cronick, it will thenn be perhaps 12 dayes, otherwise but 24 hourse or 2 or 3 dayes: for all ulcers and out ward soares the place must be annoynted with the oyles of the stone it selfe. (pp. 469–70)

The latter procedure, we are informed, takes 9 days to accomplish; if a dose of the oil is taken first thing in the morning, "it will make ye feel as if one would fly" (p. 470).

The final excerpt from this central section is headed "A philosophicall worke" (pp. 478–84), and is again extracted from Coelson's *Philosophia Maturata* (1668). It details some of the key beliefs which underlie the chymical opus, and, in particular, the Paracelsian concept of the *tria prima* – the three principles present in all matter, namely Salt, Sulphur, and Mercury, or, as they are called in this work, "philosophical Niter," "subtile Salt," and "fixed Salt":

> The earth containes in it the seeds of all things and their operations. It is the center foundation and Mother of all things. Therein are great secrets; and the first begotten heavenly spirit of Nature is secretly shut up and hidden therein; Also in the center thereof lyes hidden a virgin Earth consisting in the 3 principles. If thou knowest how to separate them out of it and to joyne them againe philosophically thou shalt have the greatest treasure. (p. 478)

The excerpt moves on to instruct the reader in the best method to separate these principles from earth, the *prima materia*, or "first matter" from which the chymical opus proceeds. We are advised to take a portion of fresh earth, "which is sufficiently impregnated with the beams of the Sun and Moone and other stars" (p. 478), and to "divide it into eaquall parts measured" (p. 479). The three principles are then extracted by subjecting the *prima materia* to simple processes of "boyleing,

[63] *Nicholas Flammel, his exposition of the hieroglyphicall figures*, trans. Eirenaeus Orandus (London, 1624), sigs. A2v–A3r.

filtrating, evaporating, congealing" (p. 479), recipes for each of which are then given. The final outcome of this work is the Philosopher's Stone itself; this part of Coelson's book is missing from Wigges's manuscript.

Also belonging to this central portion of the book are a groups of accounts, made out in an italic hand. Employing an idiosyncratic system of abbreviations and symbols, the accounts detail ingredients and medicines supplied to neighbours, mostly women, but occasionally men. The cost of each item is noted and every receipt is dated; each account begins on a new page. These accounts are followed by another group of recipes for chymical compounds and medicines, most of which are in Latin. As with the accounts, the use of symbols and abbreviations and the hasty scrawl in which they are written would have made these entries all but illegible to anyone but the person responsible for writing them.

Towards the end of the volume, we return to general household receipts, and to the neat, secretary hand with which the book opened. These recipes begin with an introduction to the principles of sugar-craft: the first couple of recipes – for clarifying and refining sugar – are attributed to "Mo Wigges" and "Mrs Vernon." The remaining recipes are grouped in broad but overlapping sections: sweetmeats, lozenges, and comfits; preserves and conserves; sweet waters; powders; and perfumes. The final pages of Wigges's book feature a sequence of recipes for the manufacture of precious stones, including diamonds, sapphires, rubies, topaz, lapis lazuli, and emerald. These recipes are written upside-down, from the back of the book inwards. The hand is the same as that used for the chymical excerpts which fill the middle portion of the book – a hurried, yet confident italic, using a pale brown ink. These recipes require the use of minerals and mineral compounds; preparations that would have been purchased from visiting tradesmen, or perhaps imported from nearby towns and cities. They point to a technical sophistication beyond that required for simple distilled waters – although they could be tricky enough to prepare – and perhaps confirm the existence of a small-scale home industry. Again, it is quite possible that these recipes were collected by or for a woman: similar recipes for precious stones feature in women's printed receipt books, including, for example, Shirley's *The Accomplished Ladies Rich Closet of Rarities* (1694).[64] Sarah Wigges's book concludes with a neat table of contents, alphabetically arranged, written by the original amanuensis (pp. 609–18). Following the index, facing one last recipe for diamonds, the final binding leaf features an incomplete recipe for puff pastry, written upside-down. On the verso is a report, dated 1654, on efforts to find gold in Scotland.

Given the curious binding and arrangement of this book, it is impossible to determine how much of it was compiled under the guidance of Wigges herself. The latest hand in the book dates from the latter half of the seventeenth century, and

64 John Shirley, *The Accomplished Ladies Rich Closet of Rarities*, 4th edn (1694), pp. 171–92. See also Girolamo Ruscelli, *The secretes of the reuerend Maister Alexis of Piemont*, trans. William Warde (London, 1558), fols. 84v, 118–20, and *The seconde part of the Secretes of Master Alexis of Piemont*, trans. William Warde (London, 1560), fols. 16r, 30v.

the extract from the *Book of St Dunstan* presumably post-dates the publication of *Philosophia Maturata* (1668). It is tempting to assume that the chymical portions of the book, written in haste and with little concession to potential readers, are the work of someone else, possibly a son of the Wiggeses. But if 1616 is the date when Sarah Wigges began this book, then it is not inconceivable that the whole book was slowly compiled during her marriage to Richard Wigges, who may have taken an interest in his wife's studies, and that her chymical work was the basis of a home industry in which Sarah Wigges supplied medicines to friends and neighbours. The "conventional" recipes of housewifery in this book – puff pastry, rat poison, rose water, quince preserve, etc. – are arranged around the chymical material so that it is impossible to tell which came first. Furthermore, the entries from Basil Valentine are made in Wigges's own hand, and the medical recipes in this book include cabbalistic techniques and sympathetic magic as well as iatrochymistry. Did Sarah Wigges don an outfit of pigskin and cotton wool and stand beside a furnace 24 hours a day in imitation of some of the recipes contained in her manuscript? Probably not. But it is not inconceivable that she was interested in these topics because of her work as a housewife and healer, enthusiastic to learn more about the philosophical principles behind everyday processes like distillation, fermentation, and sublimation, and eager to know how else they might be applied. At the very least, I would suggest, the interests of Sarah Wigges informed the way in which any later owners used "hir Book" – there are no other marks of ownership – and that she encouraged a free, and, to her, probably quite natural, continuum between the philosophies of housewifery, medicine, and chymistry.

Conclusion

Writing in 1690, John Evelyn (1620–1706) recalls that the "Recreations" of women "were in the Distillatory, the knowledge of Plants and their Virtues, for the comfort of the poor Neighbours, and Use of the Family."[65] The stillroom (or "distillatorie") and the manuscript receipt book were two of the most important sites of female creativity in early modern England, and yet they have been largely forgotten to history. In part, this is because they are both ephemeral sites. Perhaps most importantly, they have been neglected because they were sites in which women "recreated" themselves and their worlds on a daily basis: recreating their homes, though the continuing cycle of feeding, preserving, healing, and washing; recreating their neighbours, through the distribution of foodstuffs and medicines,

---

[65] John Evelyn and Mary Evelyn, *Mundus muliebris: or, The ladies dressing-room unlock'd, and her toilette spread In burlesque. Together with the fop-dictionary, compiled for the use of the fair sex*, 2nd edn (London, 1690), sig. A4r. Some of the recipes of his wife, Mary Browne (c.1635–1709), are collected in London, British Library, Evelyn Papers MSS 51, 297, and 531. On Mary Evelyn, see Frances Harris, "Living in the Neighbourhood of Science: Mary Evelyn, Margaret Cavendish and the Greshamites," in *Women, Science and Medicine 1500–1700*, pp. 198–217.

and the circulation of receipts; and recreating themselves, as givers, receivers, and producers of knowledge.

Of course, much housework was sheer drudgery – it was hard, physically demanding, and repetitive work. No wonder Virginia Woolf, writing near the middle of the twentieth century, pointed to housewifery as a potential obstacle to the development of the woman writer, and to the "inner life" of early modern women.[66] But housewifery, as I have argued in this essay, also had the potential to be intellectually sophisticated, technically intricate and challenging, and imaginatively powerful. Housewifery could involve ideas that were interesting not simply in practical terms – as a means to an end – but for a certain aesthetic value, because at a theoretical level, they were beautiful and stimulating.

For a long time, it has been a largely unquestioned assumption that in early modern England, women existed at the margins of chymical and early scientific discourses and practices. But if we place women at the centre, rather than at the margins of the production and consumption of chymical knowledge, then the category of chymistry is reciprocally transformed. New themes assume greater prominence, and others fade into the background. Gold making – *chrysopoeia*, the transmutation of base metals into gold – becomes less important, and the status of precious stones as symbols of wealth and preservatives of health becomes more important. Instead of the search for a single Elixir of Life, there are many ongoing attempts for the achievable, tangible results that can be obtained from the quintessences of simples, balms, and compound medicines of manifold powers. Instead of multiplication or projection, distillation becomes the single most important stage in the chymical opus. Esoteric chymistry exists in a continuum with experimental chymistry, providing a framework through which practical tasks and daily acts of piety are understood and articulated. And the stillroom, a female preserve, stands alongside the laboratory as a centre of chymical practice and innovation.

[66] Woolf advanced this argument in the draft of her unfinished "Common History": see Juliet Dusinberre, *Virginia Woolf's Renaissance: Woman Reader or Common Reader?* (Basingstoke: Macmillan, 1997), pp. xxxi, xxxv.

Chapter 9
Cats on a Windowsill: An Alchemical Study of Marie de Gournay

Dorothea Heitsch

Qu'est ce qui mieulx ressemble chat en fenestres?
–C'est une chatte.[1]

Alchemy and Gender

Alchemy, an important part of the sciences in Europe until well into the seventeenth century, may be defined as the dream of the "homo faber," who by perfecting matter ultimately perfects himself.[2] In the course of this process, the alchemist assumes the place of time, and his oven becomes the earthly matter in which he brings about a return to primordial chaos and to cosmogony.[3] The occult art of the dissolution and transmutation of metals has several branches. The followers of practical alchemy search for the philosopher's stone. By liquefying the stone, they intend to obtain the panacea or quintessence, a universal remedy that restores strength and health to the human body. The stone also is said to convey marvelous powers, among them the gift of invisibility. The practitioners of mystical or philosophical alchemy endeavor to obtain spiritual gold with a view to purifying the soul in a transformation of the spirit. This ascetic quest from lead to gold theoretically leads to the discovery of spiritual treasures, intelligence, lightness, refinement, and illumination. As in practical alchemy, where the philosopher's

---

[1] Bruno Roy, ed., *Devinettes françaises du moyen âge* (Montréal: Bellarmin, Paris: Vrin, 1977), p. 90. "What resembles a male cat in a window best?–A female cat." (Translations are my own unless otherwise indicated.)

[2] According to some, the word "alchemy" may come from the Arabic 'el-kimya;' 'kimyâ' derives from 'khem,' "the black country," the name designating Egypt in Antiquity. Another etymology traces the word back to the Greek 'chyma,' "to fuse or cast metal." See Serge Hutin, *L'Alchimie* (Paris: Presses Universitaires de France, 2005 (1951)), p. 7 and Eric J. Holmyard, *Alchemy* (New York: Dover Publications, 1990 (1957)). For the role of alchemy in the Renaissance, see, for example, Jean-Marc Mandosio, "L'Alchimie dans les classifications des sciences et des arts à la Renaissance," in *Alchimie et philosophie à la Renaissance*, ed. Jean-Claude Margolin and Sylvain Matton (Paris: J. Vrin, 1993), pp. 11–41.

[3] Mircea Eliade, *Forgerons et alchimistes* (Paris: Flammarion, 1977), p. 145.

stone goes through a phase of black putrefaction, the individual here goes through a spiritual state of blackness, a negative state during which s/he measures his/her indignity, but which is necessary to his/her ultimate progression.[4] This so-called "ars magna" leads to recovering primordial dignity, the splendor and purity of prelapsarian life.[5]

It is the god Hermes or Mercury who is said to have revealed the art of alchemy. Consequently, alchemy often is symbolized by the figure of Hermes Trismegistus whose sexual dualism provides a useful means to describe an Aristotelian commonplace: all oppositions, sympathies, and antipathies found in the world result from the polarity of two complementary principles or universal forces, one active and masculine, the other passive and feminine. This is reflected in numerous tables of the elements, such as male–female, sperm–menstrual blood, active–passive, form–matter, soul–body, fire–water, warm/dry–cold/humid, sulphur–mercury, gold–silver, sun–moon, yeast dough–non risen dough.[6] According to many myths of creation, such opposites correspond to the principles into which an original hermaphroditic god divided; the coupling of the resulting two beings then produced the world. This union of the masculine generating and the feminine fertilized principle, of sun and moon, of man and woman thus becomes the ultimate explanation for everything. That is why, as has been stated, the rhetoric of alchemy is always gendered.[7]

The Paracelsian branch of alchemy spreads rapidly in sixteenth-century France.[8] In 1567, Jacques Gohory publishes the *Compendium de la philosophie et de la*

---

4 Hutin, *L'Alchimie*, p. 95.

5 Hutin, p. 99. There is also a religious aspect: "Les alchimistes ont abondamment commenté la parole évangélique: *si le grain ne meurt, il ne pourra porter de fruits*, qu'ils interprètent en disant que, de même que le froment doit se corrompre au sein de la terre, de même la matière de la Pierre doit passer par une phase de putréfaction. L'alchimie s'est ainsi annexé le domaine religieux" ("Alchemists have commented abundantly on the evangelical word: 'if the seed does not die, it cannot bear fruit,' which they interpret by saying that, just as the grain must decompose in the bosom/lap of the earth, in the same manner the material of the Stone must go through a phase of putrefaction. Thus, alchemy appropriated for itself the religious domain," p. 28).

6 Hutin, p. 32. The last binary refers to the alchemical theory that yeast acts as a ferment on dough as does the substance of the philosopher's stone that is added to baser metals so as to induce their transmutation into gold.

7 Kathleen Perry Long, "Salomon Trismosin and Clovis Hesteau de Nuysement: The Sexual Politics of Alchemy in Early Modern France," *L'Esprit créateur*, XXXV (2) (Summer 1995): 9–21 (9).

8 The presentations by Hugh Trevor-Roper, "The Court Physician and Paracelsianism," *Medicine at the Courts of Europe, 1500–1837*," ed. Vivian Nutton (New York, London: Routledge, 1990), pp. 79–94, and Allen Debus, *The French Paracelsians. The Chemical Challenge to Medical and Scientific Tradition in Early Modern France* (Cambridge: Cambridge University Press, 1991) have been elaborated by Didier Kahn who, following Lynn Thorndike's *History of Magic and Experimental Science* (New York: Columbia

médecine paracelsienne, accompanied by his commented edition of Paracelsus' *De vita longa*. Pierre Hassard d'Armentières translates *La grande, vraie et parfaite chirurgie* in 1568. At the same time, there is an increasing interest in alchemy as a spiritual or philosophical way to see the world as a series of conjunctions, a version which is often introduced and expounded upon by court physicians alongside their medical uses of this discipline. In the second half of the sixteenth century, this branch becomes an alternative to extremist Catholicism, particularly that of the League, and is favored by Protestants and moderate Catholics.[9] For all these reasons it is not surprising that Marie de Gournay (1565–1645), Montaigne's editor, would have had an interest in the art. As an early modern woman who desires to have a career as a writer, she can refer to female precursors in Europe as well as to contemporary colleagues like Anna Maria van Schurman. Yet her interest in domains that are considered masculine, that is, literary criticism, political treatises, pamphlets, and morality, does not allow her to easily find her personal style and professional role in the transition period between the sixteenth and seventeenth century, between Renaissance aesthetics and the constraints of Richelieu's language politics.[10]

These difficulties are reflected in the author's repeatedly tying writing to her corporality, most particularly in the image of androgyny.[11] On the one hand, she thus benefits from her friendship with Montaigne and her relationship with his work and the literary tradition. On the other hand, she may transfer accepted topoi and explore her own voice and position by dissolving traditional literary boundaries and by transmuting her literary persona. It is the connection to Montaigne that enables her to launch her career.[12] Consequently, in her novella *Proumenoir de Monsieur de Montaigne* (1594), the "Préface" to Montaigne's *Essais* of 1595, her manifestoes *Egalité des hommes et des femmes* (1622) and *Grief des dames* (1626), in her self-portraits *Apologie pour celle qui escrit* (1626), *Pincture de Moeurs* (1626), and *Vie de la Demoiselle de Gournay* (1641) as well as in several poems, Marie de Gournay construes her identity as a woman writer, by reiterating it as well as by

University Press, 1947–64), Vol. 5, p. 617, analyzes the "Paracelsian revival" in France in *Alchimie et Paracelsisme en France (1567–1625)* (Geneva: Droz, 2007), p. 137. For general studies on Paracelsus, see, for example, Walter Pagel, *Paracelsus* (Basel, New York: Karger, 1958) and the collection edited by Lucien Braun, *Paracelse* (Paris: A. Michel, 1980).

9 Kathleen Perry Long, "The Chemical Wedding in the Works of Clovis Hesteau de Nuysement," *Dalhousie French Studies*, 56 (2001): 27–35. See also Long's *Hermaphrodites in Renaissance Europe* (Aldershot, UK: Ashgate, 2006), pp. 110–11, p. 138.

10 For Marie de Gournay's publications on language, see Marie-Claire Thomine, "Les Traités linguistiques," in Marie de Gournay, *Oeuvres Complètes*, ed. Jean-Claude Arnould et al. (Paris: Champion, 2002), 2 vols., pp. 44–55.

11 I am using the term androgyny for my analysis, because it can encompass both the idea of the androgyne and the physical aspect of hermaphroditism. See Marian Rothstein, "Mutations of the Androgyne: Its Functions in Early Modern French Literature," *Sixteenth Century Journal* 34,2 (2003): 409–37 (410).

12 See, for example, Claude Blum, "L'Editrice des *Essais*," *Oeuvres Complètes*, 27–43.

trying out new mixed identities. How alchemical discourse assists her with this and then is transformed in the process will be presented in the following pages.[13]

Marie de Gournay and Alchemy

Marie de Gournay admits to having been interested in alchemy at the time of writing her *Pincture de Moeurs*:

> L'Alchimie est chez moy, mais non ses suittes folles;
> Tromper, dépenser gros, croire l'Art sans doubter,
> Attendre une Mer d'or, sans fin la trompeter:
> Aucun je n'ay trompé, j'ay faict peu de despense,
> J'attend peu, je dy moins, j'espere sans croyance.[14]
>
> (Alchemy is found at my home, but not its foolish consequences / Cheating, spending much, believing the Art without doubting, / Awaiting a Sea of gold, boasting of it endlessly: / I have deceived no one, I have spent little, / I expect little, I say less, I hope without believing.)

This interest is not astounding at a time when many intellectuals do more than dabble in the art. One of them is an acquaintance of the author. We know that after the publication of the *Proumenoir* and the 1595 edition of the *Essais*, Marie travels to the castle of Montaigne in the fall or winter of 1595. According to the *Pincture de Moeurs*, she goes with Jean d'Espagnet, the president of the Bordeaux parliament to whom she dedicates this poem, and his wife: "Nostre abord commença quand je fus à Montaigne: /Voir un mort au cercueil, sa fille et sa compagne, /Voyageant avec toy, qui menois de nouveau/Ta femme en leur Païs ton antique berceau" ("Our relationship began when I was at Montaigne/To see a dead man in his coffin, his daughter and his wife/Traveling with you who were once again/Taking your wife to their region, your venerable cradle").[15] Like his friend Michel de Montaigne earlier, Jean d'Espagnet will retire from public life in 1616 and then pursue natural philosophy and alchemy. Marie de Gournay will include a translation of this author's Latin verse in her work.[16]

Born in 1564, probably at Saint-Emilion, Jean d'Espagnet is sent by Henri IV to Labourd in the Basque country in 1609 in order to repress an epidemic of

[13] Some passages by François Secret should be mentioned here: "Mlle de Gournay, alchimiste," *BHR* XXXV (1973): 526–31. F. Secret's list of quotes from Marie de Gournay and some biographical information concerning Jean d'Espagnet provide a point of departure for my reading, because when I wrote this article, his short note was the most complete account available.

[14] *Oeuvres Complètes*, p. 1786. The fascination with alchemy will later be disavowed by the author (*Oeuvres Complètes*, p. 1786 n5).

[15] *Oeuvres Complètes*, p. 1783.

[16] "Traduction d'une inscription pour la statue du Pont-neuf. Du Latin de Monsieur le President d'Espagnet" (1626); the Latin original is added in 1634 (*Oeuvres Complètes*, p. 1830).

witchcraft that Pierre de Lancre describes in his book *Tableau de l'inconstance des mauvais anges* (1611). He directs the "Chambre de l'Edit" at Nérac, a tribunal composed of Catholics and Protestants that deals with problems between believers from both confessions.[17] His *Enchiridion Physicae restitutae* and *Arcanum Hermeticae Philosophiae Opus* are published anonymously in 1623 and translated into French by Jean Bachou in 1651. In the former, d'Espagnet explains that the world is like a hermaphroditic animal and of double nature, for it is of one and the other sex. Its superior and celestial part is active and masculine, whereas its inferior and elementary part is passive and feminine. The sphere of the earth is its womb where are received and nourished the fertile seeds of heaven: from the male comes life and vigor, and from the female corruption and death.[18] Jean d'Espagnet gives a definition of alchemy that is important in this context:

> 3. La science de faire la pierre philosophale, est une connoissance parfaite des operations de la nature, & de l'art touchant les metaux, dont la practique consiste à chercher les principes des metaux par resolution; et iceux principes estans rendus beaucoup plus parfaits qu'ils n'estoient pas auparavant les rallier derechef; afin qu'il en resulte une medecine universelle, tres-propre, & tres-efficace pour perfectionner les metaux imparfaits, & pour rendre la santé au corps indisposé de quelque sorte de maladie que ce soit.[19]
>
> (The science of making the philosopher's stone is a perfect knowledge of nature's operations, and of the art concerning metals, whose practice consists in looking for the principles of metals by resolution; these principles having been made much more perfect than they were before then are joined again; so that a universal medicine results from it, very proper and very efficient to perfect imperfect metals, and to give health to a body indisposed by any kind of illness.)

---

[17] For accounts of Jean d'Espagnet's life, see Didier Kahn, *Alchimie et paracelsisme en France (1567–1625)*, p. 529 and his article in Luc Foisneau, ed., *Dictionary of Seventeenth-Century French Philosophers* (London, New York: Thoemmes Continuum, 2008), pp. 438–41.

[18] Paragraph 227: "Le monde est comme un animal hermaphrodit, & de double nature; Car il est de l'un, & de l'autre sexe. La partie superieure; c'est à dire la celeste, est active, & masculine, & l'inferieure, & elementaire, passive, & feminine, le globe de la terre en est la matrice, où est receuë, & fomentée la semence feconde du Ciel; du costé du masle, procede la vie, & la vigueur, & du costé de la femme la corruption, & la mort." Jean d'Espagnet/Jean Bachou (trad.), *La Philosophie naturelle restablie en sa pureté, où l'on void à découvert toute l'oeconomie de la nature et où se manifestent quantité d'erreurs de la philosophie ancienne... avec le traicté de l'Ouvrage secret de la philosophie d'Hermez qui enseigne la matière et la façon de faire la pierre philosophale* (*Natural Philosophy Reestablished in its Pure Form, wherein One Sees Revealed the Entire Economy of Nature, and wherein are Made Manifest Many of the Errors of Ancient Philosophy...with the Treatise on the Secret Work of the Philosophy of Hermes who Taught about the Materials and Means of Creating the Philosopher's Stone*, Paris: E. Pépingué, 1651).

[19] *L'Ouvrage secret...*, cited in note 18, p. 258.

He proceeds to develop a recipe for the philosopher's stone, and insists that the apprentice alchemist, apart from a clear mind, solid judgment, and inclination for the study of natural philosophy, should have a pure heart, good manners, and fear of God, and should look for a companion with similar inclinations in order to then embark confidently on the task.[20] In her *Apologie pour celle qui escrit*, Marie de Gournay is far less optimistic in saying that no one knows the art and how to teach it, and that books describe it at the very most in allegorical terms.[21]

Of course, alchemy costs money, and detractors accuse Marie of having depleted her inheritance in order to spend it on expensive equipment. She explains: "A ce descry general des femmes studieuses, on adjouste en mon fait un poinct particulier, c'est de pratiquer l'Alchimie, qu'ils croyent en soy folie parfaicte" ("To that general condemnation of intellectual women, a particular point is added in my case–that is, my practice of alchemy, which they deem absolute folly in itself").[22] This is an accusation that she vehemently denies several times in the *Apologie*.[23] She even goes as far as to detail the cost and to indicate that she was given free access to the fire of a glass-maker close to her home.[24] Moreover, as she defends herself by alluding to Rudolph II of Habsburg, many modern emperors and kings have pursued alchemy as well as the most illustrious Frenchmen. In addition, she pursues, it is foolish to call foolish an art that is occult, whose secrets we do not know, and that cannot be taught.[25] She affirms that she is not even very

20 *L'Ouvrage secret*, pp. 261–2.

21 "…les sottes esperances de ces millions de millions, dequoy l'on attribue faussement la promesse aux Livres de cét Art, qui ne la proposent qu'allegoriquement en ceste mesure:…et s'abstienne outre plus, de l'estudier autre part que dans les Livres: puis qu'il est infaillible, que les hommes hors de là, n'offrent jamais de l'enseigner, que pour ce qu'ils ne la sçavent pas" (*Oeuvres complètes*, p. 1396). ("…those stupid hopes of the millions and millions that are falsely claimed to be promised in the books of that art, which present the promise only allegorically in these terms … and refrain, in addition, from studying anywhere else but in books. For it is infallible that people never offer to teach it outside of books, unless they do not know it." Richard Hillman and Colette Quesnel, *Apology for the Woman Writing* (Chicago and London: The University of Chicago Press, 2002), p. 127.

22 *Oeuvres Complètes*, p. 1395. Hillman and Quesnel, *Apology*, p. 127. See similarly "cet art-là, duquel on m'estime si coiffée…" ("that art, which they believe suits me so well") in "Bien-venue de Monseigneur le Duc d'Anjou," *Oeuvres Complètes*, p. 167.

23 For example: "Je diray donc, quittant cét intermede, pour renouer le fil de ma deffence, que ma mauvaise fortune ne vient pas de l'Alchimie, ny d'autre mien excès, et le puis prouver par plusieurs bouches et papiers notables: outre que je suis tres-religieuse à ne mentir point, et que je tiens les menteurs pour aussi mal sages qu'ils sont impurs" (*Oeuvres Complètes*, p. 1406). ("I will say, then, leaving this interlude to take up the thread of my defense again, that my ill fortune does not stem from alchemy or from any other excess of mine, and I can prove this by the authoritative testimony of many, oral and written, besides the fact that I am highly scrupulous about never lying and that I consider liars to be as poorly wise as they are impure" (Hillman and Quesnel, *Apology*, 135).

24 *Oeuvres Complètes*, p.1397. Hillman and Quesnel, *Apology*, pp. 128–9.

25 *Oeuvres Complètes*, p. 1396. Hillman and Quesnel, *Apology*, p. 127.

knowledgeable in alchemy, but ignorant of the most basic terms.[26] One reason for the disapproval that Marie de Gournay's interest incurred may be that at the time Paracelsian (alchemical) medicine competes with medicine in the Hippocratic-Galenic tradition, the rational medicine based on logic that is dominating most European universities. Paracelsianism, though in fashion, does have a reputation of charlatanism or witchcraft, and is even considered, in some cases, to be at least as revolutionary as Luther's doctrines.[27] In 1578, for example, Paracelsus' theses are condemned by the Sorbonne, 2 years before they are first put on an Index.[28] In 1624, 2 years before the publication of Marie's *Apologie pour celle qui escrit*, the Parlement of Paris condemns alchemy and in 1626, Heinrich Khunraths *Amphitheatrum Sapientiae Aeternae* is censored by the Sorbonne.[29]

If we believe Marie de Gournay, the pleasure of alchemy simply lies in observing the effects of fire on matter. To those who deride her efforts, she explains: "pour voir sous les degrez d'une tres-belle decoction, ce que deviendra la matiere que je tiens sur le feu: cette curiosité n'est-elle pas naturelle et saine?" ("[S]o that I may see, through the stages of a noble decoction, what the substance will become that I hold over the fire. Isn't that curiosity natural and healthy?").[30] Let us therefore emphasize the author's curiosity and define alchemy as the search for the missing component or half in an ideal fusion or relationship. Thus, she indulges in the myth of the "homo faber" who is perfecting matter while confirming personal perfection. The experience of totality attained in this way represents universal harmony, "coincidentia oppositorum." In such an organic world view, where everything is dissoluble and every metal is a compound, Marie assumes the place of time by changing nature. Accordingly, her alchemist's tools are the place of a return to primordial chaos, and she herself becomes similar to a divinity.

Alchemy and Writing

One of Marie de Gournay's matters of concern is the equality of men and women. This is an issue that she addresses in the context of her early novella or "histoire tragique" entitled *Proumenoir de Monsieur de Montaigne* in the form of a

26 "…je suis si vide de son intelligence, conduite et cabale vulgaire…" *Oeuvres Complètes*, p. 1396. ("…I am so devoid of the secret information, procedures, and mysteries regarding its vulgar form…" Hillman and Quesnel, *Apology*, p. 128).

27 H. Trevor-Roper, "The Court Physician and Paracelsianism," p. 79.

28 Didier Kahn, "Cinquante-neuf thèses de Paracelse censurées par la faculté de théologie de Paris, le 9 octobre 1578," *Documents oubliés sur l'alchimie, la kabbale et Guillaume Postel*, ed. Sylvain Matton (Geneva: Droz, 2001), pp. 161–78.

29 Allen Debus, *The French Paracelsians*, p. 71; Didier Kahn, *Alchimie et Paracelsisme en France (1567–1625)*, p. 30.

30 *Oeuvres Complètes*, p. 1398. (Hillman and Quesnel, *Apology*, p. 129). In 1641, she retracts her own statement by indicating that she has given up alchemy for some time (*Oeuvres Complètes*, p. 1398 nA).

digression. In subsequent years, she will remove the latter in order to develop it into an independent essay or manifesto *Egalité des hommes et des femmes*.[31] With this in mind, it is possible to maintain that some of her allusions to kinship with Michel de Montaigne, which are usually discussed under very different aspects, may have alchemical connotations and help her construe herself as a writer in her own right. In the "Préface" to the 1595 edition of the *Essais*, an account of her literary heritage and personal responsibility, she describes the closeness of her ties to the older writer by maintaining "for I am not myself except insofar as I am his daughter."[32] She reclaims the father-daughter relationship a number of times, stressing their similarity: "la nature m'ayant faict tant d'honneur, que sauf le plus et le moings, j'estois toute semblable à mon Pere: je ne puis faire un pas, soit escrivant ou parlant, que je ne me trouve sur ses traces" ("nature having done me so much honor that, except in the greatest and the least respects, I was wholly like my Father, I cannot take a step, whether in writing or speaking, without finding myself in his footsteps").[33] Not only here, but also in the "Epistre sur le Proumenoir de Monsieur de Montaigne," the author addresses Montaigne as "my father."[34] In the latter, she alludes to their conversation during a walk, she asks for suggestions concerning her writing, thinks about the nature of their relationship, and mentions "the power you have over me."[35] This text concerns the decision of a young woman to become a writer and to ask an older colleague and mentor for advice with regard to her choice of career.

Later in life, she recalls his offer of "affection et alliance," in the *Vie de la Demoiselle de Gournay*.[36] Indeed, the title that she already assumes in the 1594 edition of the *Proumenoir*, in both the long and short prefaces to the *Essais*, and that is on all the editions of the *Essais* that she oversees, is "fille d'alliance," a title

[31] See *Oeuvres Complètes*, pp. 1355–60.

[32] "[C]ar je ne suis moy-mesme, que par où je suis sa fille" (*Oeuvres Complètes*, p. 281). Richard Hillman and Colette Quesnel, *Preface to the Essays of Michel de Montaigne* (Tempe, AZ: Medieval & Renaissance Texts & Studies, The Renaissance Society of America, 1998), p. 29.

[33] *Oeuvres Complètes*, p. 327. (*Preface to the Essays of Michel de Montaigne*, p. 85).

[34] For passages in the long Preface, see, for example, *Oeuvres Complètes*, p. 281 ("leur Autheur mon Pere") and pp. 313, 314 ("mon Pere"); Hillman and Quesnel, *Preface to the Essays of Michel de Montaigne*, pp. 27, 75. For some passages in the Epistre, see *Oeuvres Complètes*, pp. 1282, 1283, 1287; Hillman and Quesnel, *Apology*, pp. 29, 32.

[35] "[L]'Empire que vous avez en moy" ("The power you have over me," *Oeuvres Complètes*, p. 1286); Hillman and Quesnel, *Apology*, p. 30. For an analysis of Montaigne's "empire," see Cathleen Bauschatz, "'Les Puissances de Vostre Empire:' Changing Power Relations in Marie de Gournay's *Le Proumenoir de Monsieur de Montaigne* from 1594 to 1626," *Renaissance Women Writers: French Texts/American Contexts*, ed. Anne R. Larsen and Colette Winn (Detroit, MI: Wayne State University Press, 1994), pp. 189–208.

[36] *Oeuvres Complètes*, p. 1863.

that is also given to her in Montaigne's *Essais*.[37] It has been translated as adoptive daughter, covenant daughter, or elective daughter and should certainly be seen in the context of the rhetoric of friendship and the rhetoric of reproduction, keeping in mind Montaigne's preference for spiritual over biological offspring.[38] In addition to mentioning that she has no other title to go by, Marie de Gournay speaks of "amitié élective," on which this alliance is built.[39] Etymologically, "alliance" can mean union by mutual agreement, a religious, political, or legal agreement, and a marriage link between two families. The *Dictionnaire de l'Académie* lists in addition the union of disparate, apparently incompatible elements, a rhetorical figure such as "se hâter lentement," an oxymoron. It is as "fille d'alliance" that Marie presents herself in her correspondence to Justus Lipsius.[40] The expression seems to be a way in literary circles to promote women writers, as does François Le Poulchre, seigneur de la Motte Messemé, for Marie Le Gendre.[41] In alchemical circles, according to Penny Bayer's essay in this collection, Jeanne du Port, Mme de la Martinville, and Quercitan's daughter all enter their profession in similar fashion, as does Elizabeth Jane Weston, whose alliance with Oswald Croll can also be read allegorically. Indeed, Lipsius will speak of Marie de Gournay as Montaigne's soul: "Quae ista est, vide & cognosce, filiam Michaelis Montani (ita se appellat) sed animo filiam, imo animam ejus ipsam" ("This is, see and understand, the daughter of Michel de Montaigne (that is how she calls herself),

---

37 *Le Proumenoir de Monsieur de Montaigne. Par sa fille d'alliance* from 1594–1607 (*Oeuvres Complètes*, p. 109). "Préface courte" (1611), "Préface longue" (1635), *Oeuvres complètes*, pp. 273, 275. "J'ay pris plaisir à publier en plusieurs lieux l'esperance que j'ay de Marie de Gournay le Jars, ma fille d'alliance..." Michel de Montaigne, *Oeuvres Complètes*, ed. Albert Thibaudet and Maurice Rat (Paris: Gallimard, 1962), II 17, p. 645 c; *The Essays of Michel de Montaigne*, trans. and ed. Michael A. Screech (London: Allen Lane, 1991), p. 751.

38 See Marc Schachter's chapter "Friendly Usurpations: Gournay and Montaigne" in *Voluntary Servitude and the Erotics of Friendship. From Classical Antiquity to Early Modern France* (Aldershot, UK: Ashgate, 2008), pp. 115–39 (p. 129).

39 "[J]e me pare du beau titre de ceste alliance, puisque je n'ay point d'autre ornement," (*Oeuvres complètes*, p. 281). For Marie's thoughts concerning elective affinities, see her "Epistre sur le proumenoir de Monsieur de Montaigne" (*Oeuvres complètes*, pp. 1284–5).

40 She mentions to Lipsius "un petit traité sur l'alliance de mon pere et de moy" (*Oeuvres complètes*, p. 1933).

41 Evelyne Berriot-Salvadore, "Marie Le Gendre et Marie de Gournay: A la manière de..." in *Le Lecteur, l'auteur et l'écrivain: Montaigne 1492, 1592, 1992, Actes du colloque international de Haïfa, Avril-Mai 1992* (Paris: Champion, 1993), pp. 237–51 (p. 237).

but daughter in spirit, or rather his soul itself").[42] In this way, Marie, Montaigne's daughter, becomes the philosopher's daughter, the alchemist.[43]

All the passages mentioned stress the thought-engendering power of a mentor, both in personal circumstances and on a literary level, in order to then affirm and legitimize the active role of Marie, the woman writer, in the transformation of inherited material. In the frame of the novella *Proumenoir*, the author mentions a free-flowing exchange with Montaigne concerning Plutarch's *Moralia*:[44] according to her, she told him the story before she wrote it down, thus alluding to the possibility of her mentor's having planned a possible companion piece. This is a strategy that Marie de Gournay frequently employs: we know that by mourning in public, a gesture that has solicited a variety of responses, she writes herself into the friendship of La Boétie and Montaigne.[45] She does this by presenting a – quite possibly fictionalized – act of gift giving, as has been explained by Jean-Claude Arnould. For had Marie really sent her novel to her mentor, she would not have mentioned this, not having received an answer from him; if the gift is fictitious, Montaigne's silence may be a simple gap in her strategy.[46] Accordingly, Marie de Gournay is conscious of being in a rather paradoxical situation: "having become daughter by social covenant and as the result of magical thinking, she owes more to the rhetorical construction of an artificially conceived nature [...] than she does to the workings of biological relations. She is a specially chosen friend in a world where female friendship with men appears to be something of a social anomaly."[47] The magical thinking alluded to by Kritzman is suggestive of the alchemical process, in which the state of mind can affect the state of matter.

How conscious Marie is of having to overcome the hurdle of being a woman is not only evident from the practical jokes that were played on her and that were retold with gusto, but on the textual level, for example in the later removed digression to the *Proumenoir*, where she says "Vous suffise donc, pauvres dames Romaines, que si Socrates eust esté femme on n'en eust pas bien parlé non plus

[42] Letter to Remalcus Robertus, 15 April 1597, cited by Günter Abel, "Juste Lipse et Marie de Gournay: autour de l'exemplaire d'Anvers des Essais de Montaigne," *BHR* XXXV (1973) : 117–29 (128).

[43] In addition, Marie uses the word "alliage," which is even closer to alchemical vocabulary, in order to describe relationships in her treatise "Que par necessité les grands esprits et les gens de bien cherchent leurs semblables" (That Great Minds and Good People necessarily look for their Equals") (*Oeuvres complètes*, p. 891, p. 898).

[44] "[T]ragiques accidens de l'Amour recitez par Plutarque" (*Oeuvres Complètes*, p. 1283); "the vicissitudes of love, in Plutarch" (Hillman and Quesnel, *Apology*, p. 29).

[45] Philippe Desan, "The Book, the Friend, the Woman: Montaigne's Circular Exchanges," in *Contending Kingdoms*, ed. Marie-Rose Logan and Peter Rudnytsky (Detroit, MI: Wayne State University Press, 1991), pp. 225–62.

[46] Marie de Gournay, *Le Proumenoir de Monsieur de Montaigne* (Paris: Champion, 1996), p. 6.

[47] Lawrence Kritzman, "Of Ashes Born: Montaigne's Surrogate Daughter," *The Journal of Medieval and Renaissance Studies* 1995 Fall (25:3): 425–6.

que de vous" ("May it suffice you, poor Roman ladies, that if Socrates had been a woman, he would not have been spoken well of any more than you").[48] Indeed, here as in the *Grief des dames*, she reiterates "C'est une femme qui parle" ("It's a woman speaking"), thus affirming her identity as a woman writer.[49] The latter text advocates the participation of women in conversation, that is, in social life and learning.[50] Adroitly, the author turns around and enriches with examples an antinomical statement by a male literary precursor, Charles Estienne. The latter claims in his *Paradoxes* (1553): "et s'il est vray ce que dict Aristote, que les personnes composées de chair plus noble et délicate sont de meilleur esprit que les autres, qui faict doute que la charnure de la femme ne soit plus tendre et mollette que celle de l'homme" ("and if what Aristotle says is true that people made of more noble and delicate flesh have a better mind than others, who can doubt that women's flesh is softer and more tender than men's?").[51] This is another instance of her strategically transforming male precursors' voices into arguments supporting her own cause. Moreover, Marie Meurdrac (end of the 16th century – before 1687), a fellow writer and initiate in alchemy, will in the 1666 preface to her *Chymie charitable & facile, en faveur des dames* not only allude to the difficulties that women face when they want to publish their thoughts and skills, but will also maintain "que les Esprits n'ont point de sexe; et que si ceux des femmes étaient cultivés comme ceux des hommes, et que l'on employât autant de temps et de dépenses à les instruire, ils pourraient les égaler" ("that minds are not gendered; and if those of women were cultivated like those of men, and if one used as much time and money to instruct them, they could equal them").[52]

In her *Egalité des hommes et des femmes*, Marie de Gournay criticizes the patchy education of women, seeing in it an exclusively sociological cause for the injustice between the sexes. Instead of defending women against male arrogance, she proposes to raise them to a level of equality with men. That her arguments are based on male authors should be interpreted in her favor, since they prove that women are capable of grasping these writings and of adapting them to their

---

48 *Oeuvres Complètes*, p. 1358. (Hillman and Quesnel, *Apology*, p. 57). For the practical jokes, I'll only mention the Racan episode and certain adventures surrounding the composition of *Vie de la Demoiselle de Gournay*. See, for example, Michèle Fogel, *Marie de Gournay. Itinéraires d'une femme savante* (Paris: Fayard, 2004), pp. 254–7 and pp. 16–8.

49 *Oeuvres Complètes*, pp. 283–4 and p. 1075. Hillman and Quesnel, *Preface to the Essays of Michel de Montaigne*, p. 35 and *Apology*, pp. 101–2.

50 I have discussed this elsewhere: "From Dialogue to Conversation: The Place of Marie de Gournay," in *Printed Voices: The Renaissance Culture of Dialogue*, ed. Dorothea Heitsch and Jean-François Vallée (Toronto: University of Toronto Press, 2004), pp. 113–33.

51 Charles Estienne, *Paradoxes*, ed. Trevor Peach (Geneva: Droz, 1998), p. 226 (("Pour les femmes." Declamation XXIV. "Que l'excellence de la femme est plus grande que celle de l'homme").

52 Marie Meurdrac, *La Chymie charitable et facile, en faveur des Dames* (1666), ed. Jean Jacques (Paris: CNRS Editions, 1999), p. 17.

own purposes, as in the case of Plutarch's *Mulierum Virtutes*.[53] Marie declares, like Plato and Agrippa before her, that sexual difference serves procreation only, because, after all, she explains, "there is nothing more like a cat on a windowsill than a female cat:"[54]

> Au surplus, l'Animal-humain n'est homme ny femme, à le bien prendre: les sexes estants faicts non simplement, ny pour constituer une differance d'especes, mais pour la seule propagation. L'unique forme et difference de cét Animal, ne consistent qu'en l'ame raisonnable: Et s'il est permis de rire en passant chemin, le quolibet ne sera pas hors de saison, lequel nous apprend; qu'il n'est rien plus semblable au chat sur une fenestre, que la chatte. L'homme et la femme sont tellement uns, que si l'homme est plus que la femme, la femme est plus que l'homme. L'homme fut creé masle et femesle, ce dit l'Escriture: ne comtant ces deux que pour un: et Jesus-Christ est appelé Fils de l'homme, bien qu'il ne le soit que de la femme: perfection entiere et consumée de la preuve de cette unité des deux sexes.[55]

> (Further, the human animal, taken rightly, is neither man nor woman, the sexes having been made double, not so as to constitute a difference in species, but for the sake of propagation alone. The unique form and distinction of that animal consists only in its rational soul. And if it is permitted to laugh in the course of our journey, the jest would not be out of season that teaches us that there is nothing more like a cat on a windowsill than a female cat. Man and woman are so thoroughly one that if man is more than woman, woman is more than man. Man was created man [male] and female – so says scripture, not reckoning the two except as one; and Jesus Christ is called Son of Man, although he is that only of woman – the whole and consummate perfection of the proof of this unity of the two sexes.)[56]

Marie refers to a quodlibet that did exist in her time and that is mentioned at the beginning of this essay. The quodlibet, a comic riddle, elicits a witty and unexpected repartee from the interlocutor, who cannot guess the correct answer unless he already has it.[57] In a rhetorical move, Marie disarms the ignorant reader, who supposedly would not agree with her stance, through the laughter of those who are in the know, at the same time conjuring up for her contemporaries a series of similar, often zesty riddles concerning cats. Apart from the fact that Marie owned a cat named Piaillon, to which Richelieu, according to Tallemant des

[53] See similarly Patricia F. Cholakian, "The Identity of the Reader in Marie de Gournay's 'Le Proumenoir de Monsieur de Montaigne' [1594]," in *Seeking the Woman in Late Medieval and Renaissance Writings*, ed. Sheila Fisher and Janet E. Halley (Knoxville: University of Tennessee Press, 1989), pp. 207–32.

[54] Plato, *Republic*, V.454 d–e. Heinrich Cornelius Agrippa, *De nobilitate et praecellentia foeminei sexus*, ed. R. Antonioli et al. (Geneva: Droz, 1990), pp. 49, 96.

[55] *Oeuvres Complètes*, pp. 978–9.

[56] Hillman and Quesnel, *Apology*, pp. 86–7.

[57] For a definition, see Bruno Roy, *Devinettes françaises du moyen âge*, p. 15.

Réaux, granted a pension,[58] the competent reader will remember two passages from Montaigne's *Essais*. In the first, the author describes his fascination with the cat's viewpoint during play, an observation that has stimulated a series of interpretative responses.[59] Montaigne also declares "…je dis que les mâles et femelles sont jettez en mesme moule; sauf l'institution et l'usage, la différence n'y est pas grande" ("I say that male and female are cast in the same mould: save for the education and custom the difference between them is not great").[60]

The treatise *Egalité des hommes et des femmes* begins with a critique of those people who cannot conceive that a great woman may name herself a great man by simply changing sex: "autant esloignez d'imaginer, qu'une grande femme se peust dire grand homme, le sexe simplement changé, que de consentir qu'un homme se peust eslever à l'estage d'un Dieu" ("They are as far from imagining that a great woman might style herself a great man, if her sex were simply changed, as from allowing that a man may raise himself to the level of a god").[61] The text ends with, among other things, Marie's affirming the impossibility of determining the gender of God.[62] Moreover, since God was conceived in woman, man cannot be

---

[58] Tallemant des Réaux refers to a dialogue between Richelieu and Boisrobert, during which Marie de Gournay was given a pension of 200 ecus, her servant was given 50 pounds, and her cat: "Il y a encore ma mie Piaillon," adjousta Boisrobert; "c'est sa chatte." – "Je lui donne vingt livres de pension," respondit l'Eminentissime, "à condition qu'elle auroit des trippes." – "Mais, Monseigneur, elle a chatonné," dit Boisrobert. "Le Cardinal adjousta encore une pistolle pour les chattons" ("'There is still my friend Piaillon,' Boisrobert added, 'That's her cat.' 'I will give her twenty pounds as a pension,' responded his Most Eminent, 'on the condition that she has tripe.' 'But, Monseigneur, she has given birth to kittens' said Boisrobert. The Cardinal added one pistole for the kittens," Tallemant des Réaux, *Historiettes* (Paris: Gallimard, 1960), Vol.1, p. 380.

[59] "Quand je me jouë à ma chatte, qui sçait si elle passe son temps de moy plus que je ne fay d'elle? Nous nous entretenons de singeries réciproques. Si j'ay mon heure de commencer ou de refuser, aussi a elle la sienne" (Michel de Montaigne, *Oeuvres Complètes*, II 12, p. 430 c); "When I play with my cat, how do I know that she is not passing time with me rather than I with her? We entertain ourselves with mutual monkey-tricks. If I have times when I want to begin or to say no, so does she" (*The Essays*, p. 505). For two examples of critical work on this topic, see Pierre Michel, "La chatte de Montaigne," *BSIAM*, no 29 (janv.-mars, 1964): 14–8; Jacques Derrida, *L'animal que donc je suis* (Paris: Galilée, 2006), pp. 18–8.

[60] Michel de Montaigne, *Oeuvres Complètes*, III.5, p. 875 b; (*The Essays*, p. 1016).

[61] *Oeuvres Complètes*, p. 966. (Hillman and Quesnel, *Apology*, p. 76).

[62] "Que si quelqu'un au reste est si fade, d'imaginer masculin ou feminin en Dieu, bien que son nom semble sonner le masculin, ny consequemment besoin du choix d'un sexe plustost que de l'autre pour honnorer ou relever l'Incarnation de son Fils: cestuy-cy montre à plein jour, qu'il est aussi mauvais Philosophe que Theologien" (*Oeuvres Complètes*, p. 986). "But further, if anyone is so dull as to imagine masculine or feminine in God–for although His name may seem to have a masculine sound to it, it does not follow that one sex needs to be chosen above the other to honor or exalt the incarnation of His Son–such a person shows in a plain light that he is just as bad a philosopher as he is a theologian" (Hillman and Quesnel, *Apology*, p. 94).

on a higher level than she is. This complicated equilibrium ultimately leads back to a composite image and to the original myth of a hermaphroditic human being. It has been noted that Marie de Gournay may present herself as an androgynous hero in the *Pincture des moeurs*, because the author's gender does not seem to be mentioned in this text.[63] Though it is certainly the case that she envisages an ideal of the whole human being, and even of the spiritual and intellectual androgyne, that is, to surpass gender-specific values and behavior patterns, these personae should also be read as referring to the alchemical tradition and ultimately to the Platonic one rather than as exclusive statements concerning the author's sexual preferences or her intending to actually be androgynous. The *Pincture de Moeurs* is the self-portrait of a 70-year-old lady who has made a virtue of necessity by not being avaricious, preferring instead the glory of a literary reputation, by being of a curious and open mind and interested in the natural sciences (alchemy), and by being a disinterested friend whose character flaws usually only harm herself. The *Apologie pour celle qui escrit* continues this turn of thought: not being able to keep up appearances, Marie de Gournay has lost her connections and now must defend herself against slander. Disinterested friendship – as well as disinterested writing – is thus no longer an option for her. The *Apologie* is a defense against such calumny and demonstrates a successful and necessary emancipation from conventions.

In the passages discussed above Marie de Gournay rejects the Aristotelian and Galenic notion of woman as passive and man as active. Her literary self-portrait is echoed in the *Essais*, where she is mentioned in a much disputed passage of "De la praesumption" ("On Presumption," II 17); it may also be she who is described in a short anecdote in "Que le goust des biens et des maux depend en bonne partie de l'opinion que nous en avons" ("That the Taste of Good and Evil Things depends in large part on the Opinion we have of them," I 14). The former passage presents Montaigne's hopes and love for her, the promise he sees in her, their friendship, and the young woman's good judgment.[64] The latter passage, according to some

---

63 Tilde Sankovitch, *French Women Writers and the Book. Myths of Access and Desire* (Syracuse, NY: Syracuse University Press, 1988), pp. 73–99: Gournay "makes her autoportrait into her myth and, conversely, fashions her myth through her autoportrait, effecting a complete coincidence between the two" (p. 73). She attempts a self-presentation "as a solid, clearly defined, fixed whole, that is, as a creature of myth much more than as a constantly evolving, changing, fundamentally ungraspable and fluid being" (p. 74). Yet at a closer look, gender is not only the basis of Gournay's *Apologie*, but is explicitly affirmed in the *Pincture*, as Sankovitch recognizes: "je suis bless*ée*," "sain*e*," "Je suis soigneu*se*, activ*e*, en mes desseins constant*e*, …, prévoyant*e*, nonchalant*e*, importun*e*" (p. 94).

64 "J'ay pris plaisir à publier en plusieurs lieux l'esperance que j'ay de Marie de Gournay le Jars, ma fille d'alliance, et certes aymée de moy beaucoup plus que paternellement, et enveloppée en ma retraitte et solitude, comme l'une des meilleures parties de mon propre estre. Je ne regarde plus qu'elle au monde. Si l'adolescence peut donner presage, cette ame sera quelque jour capable des plus belles choses, et entre autres de la perfection de cette trèssaincte amitié où nous lisons point que son sexe ait peu monter encores. La sincérité et la solidité de ses moeurs y sont desjà bastantes, son affection vers moy plus que sur-

readers, could be a reminiscence of Montaigne's visit at the castle of Gournay in Picardie in 1588 while he was attending the Estates General at Blois: "Quand je veins de ces fameux Estats de Blois, j'avois veu auparavant une fille en Picardie, pour tesmoigner l'ardeur de ses promesses et aussi sa constance, se donner du poinçon qu'elle portoit en son poil, quatre ou cinq coups dans le bras, qui luy faisoient craquetter la peau et la saignoient bien en bon escient" ("When I returned from those famous Estates of Blois, I had before seen a girl in Picardie who, to prove the ardor of her promises as well as her constancy, stabbed herself with her hairpin four or five times in her arm so as to break her skin and make herself bleed in good earnest").[65] If it is she who is being described, it is her unabated enthusiasm that is illustrated in this incident.

Readers have emphasized the eagerness with which she attaches herself to Montaigne, her sudden and impetuous affection that should surprise us because a temperate, moderate text like the *Essais* would have thus inflamed the imagination of a young girl who would have been unable to wholly appreciate it, since it is on older people usually that Montaigne exercises his full wisdom. Although he remarks the sharpness of her mind and the fire of her passion, Bonnefon maintains that her nature is sincere affection spoilt by false rhetoric, unflinching devotion unrecognizable behind exaggerated language.[66] Pierre Villey speaks of her poor fragile head suffering from the writing sickness and self-importance.[67] Anne

abondante, et telle en somme qu'il n'y a rien à souhaiter, sinon que l'apprehension qu'elle a de ma fin, par les cinquante et cinq ans ausquels elle m'a rencontré, la travaillast moins cruellement. Le jugement qu'elle fit des premiers *Essays*, et femme, et en ce siecle, et si jeune, et seule en son quartier, et la vehemence fameuse dont elle m'ayma et me desira long temps sur la seule estime qu'elle en print de moy, avant m'avoir veu, c'est un accident de très-digne consideration" (Michel de Montaigne, *Oeuvres Complètes*, II 17, p. 645 c). "I have been delighted to declare in several places the hopes I put in my adopted daughter Marie de Gournay who is loved by me with a more than fatherly love and included in my solitary retirement as one of the better parts of my being. She is the only person in the world I have regard for. If youth is any omen her soul will be capable of great things one day–among other things of that most perfect hallowed loving-friendship to which (so we read) her sex has yet been unable to aspire: the purity and solidity of her morals already suffice for this and her love for me is more than overflowing, such, in short, as to leave nothing to desire, if only the dread of my death (seeing that I was fifty-five when I first met her) were to torment her less cruelly. The judgement she made on my original *Essays*, she, a woman, in this century, so young, and the only one to do so in her part of the country as well as the known enthusiasm of her long love for me and her yearning to meet me simply on the strength of the esteem she had for me before she even knew me, are particulars worthy of special consideration" (*The Essays*, pp. 751–2).

65 Michel de Montaigne, *Oeuvres Complètes*, I 14, p. 60 c.

66 Paul Bonnefon, *Montaigne et ses amis*, Vol. II (Geneva: Slatkine Reprints, 1969 (1898)), pp. 333, 347, 359.

67 Pierre Villey, *Montaigne devant la postérité* (Paris: Boivin, 1935), p. 38: "Pauvre tête fragile, elle se grisa du rôle de fille désolée qui lui venait en partage" ("Poor fragile mind, she was drunk with the role of the disconsolate daughter which was her inheritance").

Uildriks underlines her impulsiveness and spontaneity as well as her rigidity and inability to consider her opponents' arguments.[68] Marie is a fighter who, according to Sainte-Beuve, being of too strong a personality and too sharp a character finally became a cantankerous and outmoded policeman of the old school.[69] According to Marie de Gournay's own words, the admiration she felt for the *Essais* and their author made her lose her head.[70] Above all, she mentions in her *Vie de la Demoiselle de Gournay* that she suffered from severe depression after she had mistakenly heard that Montaigne had died, thus depriving her of the possibility of his conversation and society.[71] Their meeting in Paris will be all that she ever dreamt of because, according to her, Montaigne offers her his friendship, which will become the point of departure for her career and for her increasingly independent life.[72]

Alchemical Images

In addition to what may be named Marie de Gournay's alchemical writing strategy, we find a number of images that could be described as specifically alchemical. In the case of the novella *Proumenoir de Monsieur de Montaigne*, in which she discusses arranged marriages, power relations, and the impossibility of a lasting union based

---

68 *Les Idées littéraires de Mlle de Gournay* (Groningen: Kleine, 1962), p. 21.

69 *Nouveaux Lundis* (Paris: C. Lévy, 1876), Vol. 9, pp. 393–4.

70 "L'admiration dont ils me transsirent" (*Oeuvres Complètes*, p. 280).

71 *Oeuvres Complètes*, p. 1863: "Tellement que sur la fin du terme de deux ou trois ans, qui se passa entre la première veue qu'elle eust du Livre et celle de l'Autheur, ayant receu comme elle luy vouloit écrire un faux advis qu'il estoit mort; elle en souffrit un déplaisir extreme: luy semblant que toute la gloire, la felicité et l'esperance d'enrichissement de son ame, estoient fauchez en herbe, par la perte de la conversation et de la societé qu'elle s'estoit promise d'un tel esprit" ("So much that at the end of two or three years that passed between the first glimpse she had of the Book and that of the Author, having received, when she wanted to write to him, a false note that he had died; she suffered from extreme sadness: it seemed to her that the glory, the felicity, and the hope for her soul's enrichment had been nipped in the bud by the loss of the conversation and society that she had promised herself from such a mind").

72 *Oeuvres Complètes*, p. 1863: "Il la vint voir et remercier dès le lendemain, luy presentant l'affection et l'alliance de pere à fille: ce qu'elle receut avec tant plus d'aplaudissement, de ce qu'elle admira la sympathie fatale du Genie de luy et d'elle: s'estant de sa part promis en son coeur une telle alliance de luy depuis la premiere inspection de son Livre: et cela sur la proportion de leurs aages, et l'intention de leurs ames et de leurs moeurs. Il sejourna huict ou neuf mois pardeçà continuant cette genereuse et philosophique amitié" ("He went to see her the next day, offering her the affection and kinship of father to daughter: which she received with even more approval as she marveled at the fateful sympathy of their two minds: having for her part promised herself in her heart such an alliance from him since her first reading his Book: and that despite their age difference and the intention of their souls and manners. He stayed nine or ten days there, continuing this generous and philosophical friendship").

on the passions, Marie goes so far as to perform an alchemical wedding between two corpses, their blood, or their liquids at the end of the plot: "Le corps tomba près de la Princesse, les playes joinctes, qui sembloient amoureusement s'entre-succer, et ce nouveau sang chaud et bouillant, vouloir r'animer l'autre par son infusion" ("The body fell at Alinda's side; the wounds, joining, seemed lovingly to welcome each other, and this new blood, hot and steaming, seemed to wish to reanimate the other by its infusion").[73] This memorable description of love beyond death with its final fusion of two blood-soaked corpses has been criticized for its bad taste, yet it is not only very much in tune with the images that one finds in the fashionable "histoires tragiques" of the time, but with it the author performs a transmutation of love into an operation reminiscent of the mixture of liquids in the melting pot. In addition, the text may allude to the end of essay "La Fortune se rencontre souvent au train de la raison" ("Fortune is often found in Reason's train"): "...que les bourreaux couperent ensemble leurs deux testes, laissant les corps tousjours pris en ce noble neud, et les playes jointes, humant amoureusement le sang et les restes de la vie l'une de l'autre" ("...that the executioners cut off both their heads at once, allowing their bodies to remain nobly entwined together, wound against wound, lovingly soaking up each other's life-blood").[74]

Marie de Gournay's work contains a few more alchemical images worth adding. In the *Bouquet de Pinde* we find among her poetry some Latin verses from 1626 on the hermaphrodite as well as their French translation:

Hermaphroditus
Cum mea me genitrix gravida gestaret in alvo,
Quid pareret fertur consuluisse Deos.
Est mas Phoebus ait, Mars foemina, Iunoque neutrum:
Cumque forem natus hermaphroditus eram.
Quaerenti lethum. Dicit Juno, occidet armis,
Mars cruce, Phoebus aquis: sors rata cuique fuit.
Arbor obumbrat aquas conscendo, decidit ensis
Quem tuleram, casu labor et ipse super,
Haesit pes ramis, caput incidit amne: tulique
Foemina, vir, neutrum, flumina, tela, crucem.

Hermaphrodite
Lors qu'en ses intestins la mere me porta,
Sur mon sexe incertain l'Oracle elle tenta.
Phoebus promit un fils pour heureuse nouvelle,
Mars predit que ce flanc couvait une femelle,
Junon, que cét enfant n'estoit fille ny fils,
Hermaphrodite aussi la lumiere je vis.

---

[73] In the versions after 1623, "infusion" is replaced by "meslange" ("mixture") (*Oeuvres Complètes*, p. 1375). (Hillman and Quesnel, *Apology*, p. 67).

[74] Michel de Montaigne, *Oeuvres complètes*, I.34, p. 220 b; *The Essays*, p. 250. See also Marie de Gournay, *Oeuvres complètes*, p. 1375nA.

Sur ma mort derechef l'Oracle elle reclame:
Junon dit que le glaive abregeroit ma trame,
Phoebus, que mon trespas aux ondes estoit deu,
L'advis de Mars porta que je serois pendu.
Le Ciel encore un coup accomplit leur presage.
Car montant sur un arbre au long d'un verd rivage,
Je glisse de mal-heur, mon chef trébuche en l'eau,
Mon pied reste surpris au fourchon d'un rameau,
Et ma dague en tombant de sa pointe me perce.
Quelle image de vie ou de fin plus diverse?
Masle, femelle, neutre, ayant roulé mes jours:
Dagué, pendu, noyé, ie terminay leur cours.[75]

(When my mother was carrying me in her womb,/Uncertain about my sex she consulted the Oracle./Phoebus promised a son for good news,/Mars predicted that her womb prepared a female,/Juno that this child was neither daughter nor son,/Thus I was born as Hermaphrodite./On my death afterwards she consulted the Oracle: /Juno said that the sword would shorten my life's thread,/Phoebus that my death would be due to the waves,/Mars opined that I would be hanged./ Heaven once more accomplished their prediction./For climbing a tree along a green river,/I unfortunately slip, I tumble into the water head first,/My foot rests trapped in the fork of a branch,/And my dagger, falling from its sheath, pierces me./What life or end would be more diverse?/Male, female, neuter, having lived my days: /Pierced, hanged, drowned I ended their course.)

This poem is interesting for a number of reasons. For one, the Latin text, whose source seems to be unclear, has recently been traced to Caspar Bauhin's *De hermaphroditorum monstrosorumque partuum natura*.[76] Bauhin (1560–1624) mocks a popular attribution to Antonio Panormitano and attributes it instead to Henrico Pulice Vincentino [Enrico Pulice] on the basis of his own source, Angelo Poliziano, who has a Greek version with his Latin translation that is cited by Bauhin.[77] The text is apparently translated by many humanists.[78] Second, the poem is interesting with regard to Marie's French rendering. The Latin text is composed in iambic hexameters of ten lines, the French translation is roughly twice as long with 18 lines in alexandrines, that is, heroic verse in pair rhyme with a regular change of masculine and feminine rhymes; this imitates the Latin scheme of having one accented syllable alternate with an unaccented one. Marie's French text follows the Latin original closely, the one problem being the rendering of "cruce"

[75] *Oeuvres Complètes*, p. 1814.

[76] *De hermaphroditorum monstrosorumque partuum natura. ex Theologorum, Jureconsultorumque, Medicorum, Philosophorum, et Rabbinorum sententia libri duo* (Oppenheim: Galleri, De Bry, 1614 (reprint of the 1600 Frankfurt edition)), B7v. (See Kathleen Long, *Hermaphrodites in Renaissance Europe*, p. 17.)

[77] B7v–B8 (Long, *Hermaphrodites*, 17–8).

[78] *Oeuvres Complètes*, p. 1814 nA.

as "pendu."[79] Third, the poem seems to be a well known piece. There is not only the Bauhin version, but Pierre Le Loyer (1550–1643) and Tristan L'Hermite (ca. 1600–1655) both write a sonnet based on the Latin text. Jean Loys (1553–1610) composes "L'Epitaphe d'un hermaphrodite prins du Latin" in 18 lines, like Marie de Gournay, but his version is less coherent, because he is less attentive to rhyme scheme, conjunctions, and general flow.[80]

Ovid's *Metamorphoses* IV, 285–388 tell us that Hermaphroditus was born male, but changed nature when entering the pool of the nymph Salmacis. Marie de Gournay, who may or may not have known any of the above cited French versions, chooses to translate the diverse origin and the manifold deaths of this androgynous being, all due to the will of three different gods. According to alchemical terminology, the hermaphrodite symbolizes a union of characters: the traits of the two sexes are joined in the same individual; male and female metals, the sulphurous and mercurial are married.[81] In this context, the hermaphroditic creature is the "rebis," the recreated thing or two-natured thing. The sex duality described in this being facilitates the experience of both male and female, presented as a complete experience of human existence. Whether Marie may above all apply this to the intellectual realm that has no limits, since the work of the mind can be done regardless of the sex of the worker, is an open question that already preoccupied her contemporaries.[82]

Another example of alchemical imagery found among Marie de Gournay's works is the witty poem "Sur quelque bain du Roy" ("On One of the King's Baths," 1626):

> L'Histoire dit qu'un grant Milord Anglois,
> Fut condamné par les severes loix:
> Parce qu'il fit une trame felonne,
> Contre son Roy pour ravir la Couronne.
> Le choix de mort ce bon Prince octroya,
> Dans le vin Grec le galand se noya.
> Que si jamais en la sotte entreprise,
> De cét Anglois je puis estre surprise,
> Si mon dessein sur le Throsne entreprend
> De Sainct Louys et de Charles le Grand;
> Je ne mourray comme ce lourd yvrongne,

---

79 Catharine Randall Coats proposes that "croix" and "gibet" are really synonyms in this context ("A Surplus of Significance: Hermaphrodites in Early Modern France," *French Forum* 19 (1994): 17–35 (p. 24)) and Kathleen Long proposes crucifixion or death at the cross (*Hermaphrodites*, p. 18).

80 All poems can be found in André Blanchard, *La poésie baroque et précieuse (1550–1650)* (Paris: Seghers, 1985), pp. 38, 52, 203. See also K. Long, *Hermaphrodites*, p. 181.

81 Jean-Pascal Percheron, *Le livre d'Or de l'alchimie* (Villeselve: Ramuel, 1998) and Lyndy Abraham, *A Dictionary of Alchemical Imagery* (Cambridge: Cambridge University Press, 1998).

82 See Michel Fogel, *Marie de Gournay*, pp. 200–202.

> Dans le vin Grec moins flambant que sa trongne:
> Mais si le chois du supplice est à moy,
> Je veux perir dans l'eau des bains du Roy.[83]

> (The story tells that a great English Lord/Was condemned by strict laws: /Because he wove a treacherous plot,/Against his King in order to ravish the Crown./The choice of death the good King imposed,/In Greek wine the scoundrel drowned./ If ever I am in such a stupid enterprise/Surprised as was this Englishman,/If my designs turn to the Throne/Of Saint Louis and Charles the Great; /I will not die like that clumsy drunkard,/In Greek wine less burning than his face: /But if I am to choose the punishment,/I want to perish in the waters of the King's bath.)

Marie may be retelling an anecdote found in Philippe de Commines' *Mémoires* I.7 and in François Rabelais' *Quart livre*, or she may simply endeavor to seek royal patronage.[84] The king's bath at the same time may refer to an alchemical operation to which philosophical mercury, sometimes called moon of the wise, is submitted when it assumes its final color in the course of its transmutation. Playing on the emotions involved in the relationship between poet and patron, Marie de Gournay here alchemically transforms the subservient gesture into a laugh. Her rebirth as phoenix, that is, court poet, is implied. In addition, Marie Meurdrac explains that among the three kinds of distillation the chymist can perform one is called distillation *per ascensum*: "[elle] se fait en plusieurs manières, selon la chose que l'on veut distiller. Si c'est Esprit de vin, elle doit se faire au Bain" ("it can be done in several ways, according to the thing which one wants to distill. If it is the Spirit of wine, it must be done in a bath").[85] With a view to this passage, we might imagine Marie de Gournay refined and distilled through the wine bath, unlike the scoundrel in the poem who simply sinks to the bottom of the cauldron.

To affirm Marie de Gournay's fascination with alchemy also leads to reinterpreting her reference to the cats on a windowsill. On the one hand, this image may refer to the complementary nature of the two sexes, an ideal that ultimately derives from the Platonic tradition. On the other hand, this union may touch on the chemical wedding, a mixture of materials in the melting pot rendered popular in the *Rosarium philosophorum* (1550).[86] Chemical nuptials are defined by the allegorical marriage of man and wife, king and queen, sulphur and mercury in the fire. The ultimate marriage is that of Adam and Eve: in hermetic symbolism they represent sulphur, salt, and philosophical mercury. Adam, in the beginning,

---

83 *Oeuvres Complètes*, p. 1828.

84 François Rabelais, *Quart livre*, ed. Mireille Huchon (Paris: Gallimard, 1998), p. 331: "…celluy milourt Anglois, auquel estant faict commendement pour les crimes des qulez estoit convaincu, de mourir à son arbitraige, esleut mourir nayé dedans un tonneau de Malvesie." ("…that English lord, to whom it was commanded that he should choose his manner of death for the crimes for which he was condemned, elected to die by drowning in a barrel of Malvasia" – Shakespeare fans might choose to translate this as "Malmsey" – See also *Oeuvres Complètes*, p. 1828nB.)

85 Marie Meurdrac, *La Chymie charitable*, p. 32.

86 Kathleen Long, *Hermaphrodites*, pp. 128–38.

is the only androgynous being that possesses male and female qualities. God then takes his feminine identity and separates sulphur from mercury. This androgyne consisting of Adam and Eve is represented in the alchemical symbol of the "rebis," which depicts harmony and perfection as it is achieved in the completed alchemical work and which echoes the originary hermaphroditic deity of hermetic lore. The androgynous "rebis" as well as androgynous Adam represent the stone – the ultimate goal of the alchemist.[87]

Such a chemical wedding is performed through the notion of "fille d'alliance," an alliance possibly sealed through a few drops of blood mentioned in Montaigne's essay I.14, and through the text of the *Essais* that Marie considers as touchstone for judging others[88] and that she describes as follows:

> Il se peut enfin nommer la quintessence de la vraye Philosophie, le thrône judicial de la raison: l'hellebore de la folie, le hors de page des esprits, et la resurrection de la verité morale et humaine; c'est à dire la plus utile et seule accessible: je laisse tousjours à part celle que Dieu nous communique par le don de l'Evangile, et de sa grace paternelle.[89]
>
> (It finally can be called the quintessence of true Philosophy, the judicial throne of reason: the hellebore of folly, the compensation of the intellect, the resurrection of moral and human truth; that is, the most useful and only accessible truth: always leaving aside the one that God gives us through the gift of gospel and by his paternal grace.)

Reading the *Essais* of Michel de Montaigne brings about rebirth or renewal on a higher level of existence in the competent reader, in precisely such a mind-changing experience as happened to Marie de Gournay.

Conclusion

Marie de Gournay is drawn to alchemy through her social connexions, through her curious mind, and through the opportunity it gives her to transmute Montaigne's persona and "magnum opus" for her own benefit. Her tireless efforts as an editor of Montaigne's *Essais* receive royal recognition in 1633 (and are crowned, so to speak, in the recent Pléiade edition).[90] Marie bursts onto the literary scene as the

[87] For a more precise analysis of the notion of 'rebis,' see Walter Pagel, "The Eightness of Adam and Related 'Gnostic' Ideas in the Paracelsian Corpus," *Religion and Neoplatonism in Renaissance Medicine* (London: Variorum Reprints, 1985), pp. 119–39 (p. 138).

[88] "Les Essais m'ont tousjours servy de touche, pour esprouver les esprits" (*Oeuvres complètes*, p. 281). Hillman and Quesnel, *Preface to the Essays of Michel de Montaigne*, p. 31.

[89] *Oeuvres complètes*, pp. 296–7.

[90] For the events surrounding the royal privilege granted in 1633, see Michèle Fogel, *Marie de Gournay*, pp. 276–9. For the choice of the 1595 edition overseen by Marie de Gournay rather than the Bordeaux copy as the text for the new Pléiade edition, see Michel de Montaigne, *Les Essais*, ed. Jean Balsamo, et. al. (Paris: Gallimard, 2007).

"fille d'alliance" who publishes a love story which, in its turn, will be alchemically transformed into discourses on equality, on the education of princes, and into poetry. Practical and, even more so, philosophical alchemy thus modify Marie's notion of the self. While much of alchemy echoes the Aristotelian and Galenic notions of man as active and woman as passive, other aspects of the art problematize this neat division. Marie de Gournay's use of alchemy is not merely an acceptance of gender roles in writing but a redefinition of those roles in much more complex and less distinct terms. As she sees, for example, teaching, friendship – and even social relations – as alchemical processes, alchemy helps her to form her literary style as well as her personality. In writing against the theories of radical imperfection that regard women as unfinished males, alchemical images and terms justify and legitimize her literary endeavor.

Chapter 10
Whither Childbearing: Gender, Status, and the Professionalization of Medicine in Early Modern France[1]

Bridgette Sheridan

Introduction

Before the seventeenth century, licensed midwives and surgeons in Paris traditionally learned their trade by working with an experienced practitioner—either through formal or informal apprenticeships. In this training, they focused primarily on practice—for example, delivering a child and treating external ailments of the body—rather than on medical theory. During the sixteenth and seventeenth centuries, aided by the growing publishing industry, some midwives and surgeons—especially those who served the royal court and the elite in Paris—were introduced to medical theory through books. By incorporating this theory into their practices and, in some cases, into their own medical writings, surgeons and midwives were able to challenge the notion that physicians were the only "learned practitioners." Physicians fought to maintain their status by differentiating their knowledge and practices from all other practitioners, including midwives and surgeons.[2] Physicians also played a role in surgeons' and midwives' certification,

---

[1] I presented an earlier version of this article at the Renaissance Society of America's Annual Conference in Cambridge, England (April 2005), where I received several comments and questions that helped me with revisions. I thank my fellow panelist, Elisabeth Wengler, for her careful reading and suggestions. Comments from our Chair, Elisa Rhodes, were also useful. In addition, I must thank Mara Amster, Christine Cooper, and Cynthia Klestinec, all of whom have given me extensive feedback. Stephanie O'Hara, translator extraordinaire, allowed me to cite her forthcoming translation of Bourgeois' manual. Her translations, as well as discussions with her about Bourgeois, have been invaluable. Jama Lazerow read a final draft of the article, and raised several helpful historical questions in addition to lending me his editorial eye. Finally, I am grateful, as always, to Margery Adams for her editorial assistance and her insights.

[2] In his discussion of the "medical marketplace," Roger French states, "The university doctors claimed that only their licence was complete, since it alone extended to the giving of internal medicines; and since they claimed that their own knowledge subsumed that of the various kinds of practice, they claimed control, too, over these other medical trades," Roger French, *Medicine Before Science: The Business of Medicine from the Middle Ages to the Enlightenment* (Cambridge: Cambridge University Press, 2003), p. 120. Physicians not only had to distinguish themselves from licensed practitioners, but they also had to

in part as a means to maintain their own status as the only "legitimate" practitioners of medicine. In the midst of competition for status in the medical community, care for women—especially during pregnancy and childbirth—became territory over which some midwives, surgeons, and physicians battled.

Scholars have written extensively on the dynamics of the relationship between physicians, surgeons, and midwives in early modern Europe.[3] In this essay, I focus

---

show the ways in which they were superior to popular unlicensed practitioners, such as monks, wise women, and herbalists. See: Susan Broomhall, *Women's Medical Work in Early Modern France* (Manchester: Manchester University Press, 2004), pp. 20–21; 45–51; Roger French, *Medicine Before Science,* pp. 118–26; Alison Klairmont Lingo, "Empirics and Charlatans in Early Modern France: The Genesis of the Classification of the 'Other' in Medical Practice." *Journal of Social History* 19/4 (1986): 583–603; Wendy Perkins, *Midwifery and Medicine in Early Modern France: Louise Bourgeois* (Exeter: University of Exeter Press, 1996), p. 2.

3 Historians Jacques Gélis and Mireille Laget dominate the literature written on the French case. See, for example: Jacques Gélis, Mireille Laget, and Marie-France Morel, *Entrer dans la vie* (Paris: Gallimard, 1978); Jacques Gélis, *L'arbre et le Fruit. La naissance dans l'occident moderne, XVIe—XIXe siècles* (Paris: Fayard, 1984). Trans. into English, *History of Childbirth: Fertility, Pregnancy, and Birth in Early Modern Europe,* trans. Rosemary Morris (Boston: Northeastern University Press, 1991); Jacques Gélis, *La sage-femme ou le médecin: Une nouvelle conception de la vie* (Paris: Fayard, 1988). Mireille Laget, "Childbirth in Seventeenth- and Eighteenth-Century France: Obstetrical Practice and Collective Attitudes," in *Medicine and Society in France: Selections from the Annales: E.S.C.*, 6, ed. R. Forster and O. Ranum (Baltimore: Johns Hopkins University Press, 1980), pp. 137–76; Mireille Laget, *Naissances: L'accouchement avant l'âge de la clinique* (Paris: Ed. du Seuil, 1982). Laget's work has clearly shaped the field as a relatively recent collection of essays by French scholars that was published in her memory indicates. See: *Naissance, enfance et éducation dans la France Méridionale du XVIe au XXe siècles: Hommage à Mireille Laget,* ed. Roland Andréani, Henri Michel and Elie Pélaquier (Montpellier: Université Paul-Valéry Montpellier III, 1999). For a more recent addition to the literature on France, see Lianne McTavish, *Childbirth and the Display of Authority in Early Modern France* (Aldershot, UK: Ashgate, 2005). For an early example of a general view on the subject, see Jean Donnison, *Midwives and Medical Men: A History of Inter-professional Rivalries and Women's Rights* (New York: Schocken Books, 1977). For work on early modern Germany, see: Lisa Forman Cody, "The Politics of Reproduction: From Midwives' Alternative Public Sphere to the Public Spectacle of Man Midwifery," *Eighteenth-Century Studies* 32/4 (1999): 477–795; Waltraud Pulz, "Aux origines de l'obstétrique moderne en Allemagne (XVIe–XVIIIe Siécle): Accoucheurs contre matrones?" *Revue d'histoire modern et contemporaine,* Mathilde LeMiére trans., Marie-France Morel, ed. 43/4 (1996): 593–617; Lynne Tatlock, "Speculum Feminarum: Gendered Perspectives on Obstetrics and Gynecology in Early Modern Germany," *Signs: Journal of Women in Culture and Society* 17/4 (1992): 760. Adrian Wilson has written extensively about the case in England. See, in particular, Adrian Wilson, *The Making of Man-midwifery: Childbirth in England, 1660–1770* (Cambridge, MA: Harvard University Press, 1995). Finally, for an excellent collection of scholarly essays that cover midwifery and professionalization in a variety of European countries, see: Hilary Marland, ed. *The Art of Midwifery: Early Modern Midwives in Europe* (London: Routledge, 1993).

on three seventeenth-century Parisian practitioners' lives and works in order to exemplify how this struggle played itself out in early modern Paris. The three practitioners, all of whom served the royal court, include the surgeon Jacques Guillemeau (1550–1613), the midwife Louise Bourgeois (1564–1636), and the surgeon and graduate physician Charles Guillemeau (1588–1656, Jacques Guillemeau's son). Both Louise Bourgeois and Jacques Guillemeau published birthing manuals in 1609 and were important contributors to a growing genre of published texts that focused on pregnancy and childbirth.[4] Jacques Guillemeau's son Charles published—along with surgical treatises—two polemical treatises that focused on the incompetence of midwives. One of these was aimed specifically at Louise Bourgeois. My analysis suggests that there was promise for these three practitioners to be accepted into—if not as colleagues, at least as junior members—the learned medical community, which consisted of university-trained physicians. All three were elite practitioners, serving the most exclusive population—the aristocracy and the haute bourgeoisie—in the realm, and thus had had greater access to learning and resources than the majority of midwives and surgeons in France at this time. And yet, while Jacques and, especially, Charles Guillemeau would gain entry into the realm of learned medicine, gendered dynamics played a pivotal role in ensuring that Louise Bourgeois would be marginalized in the medical community. Their story has broader implications for the history of the professionalization of surgery and midwifery in France. In foreshadowing the vicissitudes of the relationship among midwives, physicians, and surgeons, the case of Louise Bourgeois and the Guillemeaus offers a window onto the world of medical professionalization in seventeenth- and eighteenth-century Europe.[5]

---

[4] On the importance of the publication of vernacular texts on women to the changes in women's health care in sixteenth- and seventeenth-century France, see: Broomhall, pp. 127–55; Alison Klairmont Lingo, "Print's Role in the Politics of Women's Health Care in Early Modern France," in *Culture and Identity in Early Modern Europe (1500–1800): Essays in Honor of Natalie Zemon Davis*, ed. by Barbara Diefendorf and Carla Hesse (Ann Arbor: University of Michigan Press, 1993), pp. 203–21.

[5] Here, I am influenced by the notion of Edoardo Grendi's "exceptional normal" in history, when I argue that an examination of these exceptional practitioners' lives and works provides a broader understanding of the dynamics of professionalization in medicine in the early modern period. Paula Findlen describes it as follows: "The Italian social historian Edoardo Grendi famously described microhistory as the search for the "normal exception"—the kind of unique documentation that gives us a privileged viewpoint from which to examine aspects of society that are not, in fact, extraordinary but shed light on widespread social practices and cultural belief systems," Paula Findlen, "Two Cultures of Scholarship?" *Isis* 96 (2005): pp. 230–37, 233. I discovered this concept in Cathy McClive's work on early modern childbirth. McClive argues that, by examining an "exceptional" French legal case from 1666 concerning the difficulties in diagnosing whether a woman who was sentenced to be executed was pregnant, one can better understand the everyday anxieties and ambiguities that surrounded the process of childbirth in the early modern period. See Cathy McClive, "The Hidden Truths of the Belly: The Uncertainties of Pregnancy in Early Modern Europe," *The Society for the Social History of Medicine* 15/2

Further, it suggests the ways in which ideas about gender, or norms concerning masculinity and femininity, played a pivotal role in ensuring midwives' marginal status in medicine, and in defining who would have ultimate authority—midwives, surgeons, or physicians—over care for women.[6] I address these implications briefly in the conclusion. I begin by providing a brief background on the state of midwifery, surgery, and medicine in early modern France.

Professional Developments in Midwifery and Surgery in Paris

Before the seventeenth century, the rituals and events surrounding pregnancy and childbirth were a female domain. Men—even medical practitioners, priests, and husbands—rarely advised women on prenatal care and were only allowed into the birthing room under unusual circumstances. It was over the course of the sixteenth century that physicians and surgeons (both professions that were, with few exceptions, limited to men), influenced by scientific discoveries based on empirical evidence, began to challenge ancient medical theory through the "new

(2002): 209–27, esp. pp. 210–11. For more on Grendi's concept of "exceptional normal," see Carlo Ginzburg, "Micro-History: Two or Three Things that I know about it," *Critical Inquiry,* 20 (1993): 10–35, esp. p. 33.

[6] For a fuller discussion of the role of gender in the professionalization of medicine and surgery, see my forthcoming book, Bridgette Sheridan, *Gender and the Professionalization of Medicine: Midwives, Medical Men, and the* Querelle des Femmes *in Seventeenth-Century France.* In it, I investigate the role that conceptions of gender differences and the worth of women played in the professionalization of midwifery and surgery from the late sixteenth to the eighteenth century. I situate the changes within these trades in the context of the new value given to empiricism over ancient medical theory in the realm of medicine, and the philosophical debates concerning the moral and social worth of women known as the *querelle des femmes*. Over the course of the seventeenth century, gender difference—argued both by advocates for and against women—ultimately came to reinforce women's subordination. As science entered the birthing room, the ideal practitioner for women's health came to be defined as a knowledgeable medical practitioner. Midwives, because they were women, were eventually considered incapable of mastering the learning that becoming a medical practitioner required. My notion of gender is informed by Joan Scott's definition of gender and its usefulness as a category in studying the past. In her groundbreaking work, Scott analyzes and explores how gender is discursively constituted. As historian Kathleen Canning puts it, Scott understands gender to be "a system of meanings or symbolic order that signified relationships of power," Kathleen Canning, *Gender History in Practice: Historical Perspectives on Bodies, Class and Citizenship* (Ithaca: Cornell University Press, 2006), p. 9. See, also, Joan Scott, *Gender and the Politics of History* (New York: Columbia University Press, 1988), pp. 28–50. Gender, then, is not limited to understanding the dynamics between men and women (in this case surgeons/physicians and midwives), but is also an analytic category that can be used to understand the discursive realm of medicine and midwifery in early modern France.

science" of anatomy.[7] As medical men became increasingly interested in anatomy, women's bodies became subjects of scientific study. Legal authorities in France became more interested in childbirth and care for women in the sixteenth century. Because midwives provided care to the majority of women, they were often called to testify in cases concerning rape, illegitimate children, and illicit abortions. The legal authorities wanted to be certain that these midwives were reliable witnesses and that they would not collude with pregnant women who were seeking abortions. As a result, they began to require that midwives be licensed and regulated.[8] In Paris, the *Statuts et Reiglemens* that came into effect in 1560 provided a framework for the practice of midwifery. The document contained 25 clauses that detailed the necessary training and licensing procedures, along with a midwife's duties to her clients and to the state.[9] Physicians initially had little interest in midwifery since midwives' work did not appear to encroach upon their own. Surgeons, on the other hand, were attempting to elevate the status of their profession. Midwives were placed under surgeons' supervision, allowing surgeons to gain access to midwives' knowledge of birthing. In France, surgeons were the first in Europe to enter the birthing room and, while they did not take over the profession altogether—especially in rural areas—for a long time, they were quick to establish themselves as the preferred birthing attendants for women amongst the elite in Paris.[10]

Part of the reason for the erosion of the midwife's role in Paris was that women had fewer educational opportunities than men.[11] In 1630, one of the first schools

---

[7] Nancy Siraisi rightly points that physicians and surgeons continued to hold on to ancient medical ideas, even as they became more interested in human anatomy and participated more frequently in dissection (See Nancy G. Siraisi, *Medieval and Early Renaissance Medicine: An Introduction to Knowledge and Practice* (Chicago: The University of Chicago Press, 1990), p. 191. Nonetheless, as Mary Lindemann explains, ". . . with the rediscovery of Galen's texts on anatomy and the teaching of the Flemish physician Andreas Vesalius (1514–1564) at Padua in the 1520s, anatomy became increasingly central to medicine," Mary Lindemann, *Medicine and Society in Early Modern Europe* (Cambridge: Cambridge University Press, 1999), p. 71.

[8] Broomhall, p. 36.

[9] While the statutes were enforced rather spottily, this was not the case in Bourgeois' milieu, where midwives of her status certainly needed official training in order to be licensed and to practice. On the licensing of Parisian midwives, see Broomhall, 31–9. For more detail on the statutes of 1560, see: Richard Petrelli, "The Regulation of French Midwifery during the *Ancien Régime.*" *Journal of the History of Medicine and Allied Sciences* XXVI (1971): 276–92; Perkins, *Midwifery and Medicine,* pp. 3–5.

[10] Jean Donnison, pp. 10–11. Lianne McTavish argues that the displacement of midwives in France, indeed, began earlier than in other countries in Europe, though it was slow to catch on in rural and southern areas. See McTavish, p. 11.

[11] On the training and education of midwives in this period, see: Laurence Brockliss and Colin Jones, *The Medical World of Early Modern France* (Oxford: Clarendon Press, 1997), pp. 262–73; Donnison, pp. 1–20; Jacques Gélis, *La Sage-femme ou le Médecin*; Lindemann, pp. 116–19; Londa Schiebinger, *The Mind Has No Sex? Women in the Origins of Modern Science* (Cambridge, MA: Harvard University Press, 1989), pp. 102–12.

for midwives was established at the Hôtel-Dieu in Paris.[12] Even so, this school only allowed a small number of women to train in midwifery.[13] By 1638, the Hôtel-Dieu established that a surgeon had to be present at all deliveries. Most midwives, while criticized by medical men for their lack of expertise, were not taught new skills in birthing.[14] They were also not allowed to use new tools—such as forceps—that had come into use by surgeons. Not surprisingly, over the course of the seventeenth century, Parisian midwives began to experience difficulty keeping and increasing their clientele. Louis XIV encouraged the trend of hiring male birthing attendants when he appointed an *accoucheur*—a surgeon who specialized in childbirth—to deliver the children of his mistress in 1663 and of the queen in 1680. The trend became so powerful that, by the late seventeenth century in France, it seemed that even urban artisan women preferred an *accoucheur* to a midwife if they could afford to hire him.[15]

The struggle between surgeons and physicians for status in the medical hierarchy played an important role in men's entrance into the birthing room. Until the thirteenth century, barber-surgeons had been considered artisans rather than medical professionals, since they learned their skills through apprenticeship instead of by university education. In late thirteenth-century Paris, a number of surgeons abandoned barbery and apprenticed to practice surgery alone. They created a confraternity, the College of Saint-Côme, and insisted on wearing the same uniform as physicians. Still, they were largely excluded by physicians from the medical profession until the seventeenth century. By 1611, a group of surgeons had successfully organized a place of learning for surgeons on the margins of the faculty of medicine. Surgical training still focused on practice rather than

---

12 Jacques Gélis comments, "'Sortir de l'Hôtel Dieu' constitue une référence pour une sage-femme du XVIIe ou du XVIIIe siècle; 'la Maternité' est en effet pendant longtemps la seule veritable école d'obstétrique en Europe," in *La Sage-Femme ou le Médecin*, p. 56.

13 Perkins, p. 6.

14 In her examination of birthing manuals written by men in the early seventeenth century, Wendy Perkins writes, "It is striking that none of these books genuinely proposes improving education and training for prospective midwives." See Perkins, p. 102.

15 Indeed, as the practitioners that are discussed in this essay demonstrate, the issue of male versus female birthing attendants was actively debated among the elite. Louise Bourgeois comments on this extensively, especially the longer she is in practice. She says, for example, in a public letter that she wrote to her daughter who wanted to become a midwife, "Monsieur Honoré [an *accoucheur]* would know a lot about this. Countless coquettish women say that at births where the child presents well, they prefer for him to deliver them instead of a woman. This is the current trend," in Louise Bourgeois, *Various Observations Concerning Sterility, Miscarriages, Fertility, Birthing, and Diseases of Women and Newborn Children.* Trans. Stephanie O'Hara; ed. Alison Klairmont Lingo and Stephanie O'Hara. To be published by the Centre for Reformation and Renaissance Studies at the University of Toronto, in The Other Voice in Early Modern Europe: The Toronto Series. *Work in progress; do not cite without permission. Contact sohara@umassd.edu for further information.* See also, Brockliss and Jones, pp. 265–66.

theory, but it included demonstrations on cadavers, something new for surgeons. Surgeons began to challenge ancient medical theory using empirical evidence; this allowed them to claim in a more convincing manner that like physicians, they, too, were learned practitioners of medicine.[16] What followed was a long conflict over clients and expertise between surgeons and physicians, and between surgeons and barber-surgeons, which had as one of its consequences the diminishing of the role of midwives.

Physicians in this same period struggled to maintain their status as the most learned practitioners. Their knowledge of ancient medical theory meant that they were the only practitioners believed to understand the internal workings of the body. Ambitious French medical students would train in Paris or Montpellier in the early seventeenth century.[17] The education required was lengthy and rigorous; a physician-in-training theoretically had to spend 6 to 7 years at the faculty of medicine alone, undergoing several qualifying exams. In order to differentiate themselves from surgeons, physicians emphasized that their art involved an understanding of medical literature and did not include any manual care of the patient, including bloodletting and operations. For manual care, physicians relied on licensed practitioners—such as midwives, barbers, surgeons, and apothecaries—who were deemed as below physicians in the medical hierarchy. And yet, the designed educational program for physicians was not always followed, and exceptions were often made to the length of time a candidate was required to study at university.[18] This likely contributed to surgeons' belief that they could gain the respectability and status of physicians, despite surgeons' less rigorous schooling.[19] But surgeons also needed a larger clientele in order to compete with physicians. In part, they turned to midwifery to increase the scope of their practice and their clientele.

The struggle for supremacy in the medical hierarchy intensified over the course of the seventeenth and eighteenth centuries as physicians began to be squeezed by surgeons.[20] As their reputation for expertise in birthing grew, surgeons began to have their own female clientele for both illnesses and birthing.[21] The fact that surgeons began to care for women throughout their pregnancy, including delivery,

---

16 On training and education of surgeons in this period, see: François Lebrun, *Se soigner autrefois: Médecins, saints et sorciers aux XVIIe et XVIIIe siècles* (Paris: Éditions du Seuil, 1995), pp. 37–46; Lindemann, pp. 109–16; Siraisi, pp. 153–93.

17 Françoise Lehoux, *Le Cadre de vie des médecins Parisiens aux XVIe et XVIIe Siècles* (Paris: Éditions A. & J. Picard, 1976), pp. 11–2.

18 Brockliss and Jones, pp. 175–6; Lehoux, pp. 12–3.

19 In addition, Mary Lindemann explains that there was great diversity in the training that surgeons received in this period. Some studied medical theory extensively and, as she says: "Certainly, in many places, the time spent becoming a surgeon exceeded that for a physician," Lindemann, p. 112.

20 For an analysis of medical corporatism from the sixteenth to the end of the eighteenth century, see Brockliss and Jones, pp. 170–229; pp. 480–552.

21 On the rise of the *accoucheur*, see Brockliss and Jones, pp. 610–17; Gélis, pp. 291–327.

meant that they threatened midwives' practices. Yet the concern for physicians was that surgeons began to treat women's illnesses, thus encroaching on physicians' territory. By the eighteenth century, midwives became a pawn for both physicians and surgeons in this struggle.[22] Rather than viewing midwifery as a branch of the medical community, physicians and surgeons considered midwives to be a group of manual practitioners who needed to be regulated and controlled. Thus, the question of who would control midwives and the industry of women's health care was bound up in the battle for supremacy in the medical hierarchy.[23] It was in the context of the early struggle for control over care for women, particularly among the elite, that the Guillemeaus and Louise Bourgeois practiced.

Pathways to Medicine in Early Modern Paris

Jacques Guillemeau (1550–1613)

The son of a royal surgeon, Jacques Guillemeau was born in Orléans in 1550.[24] Not only was Guillemeau's father a surgeon, but so was his uncle. While little is known about his early childhood, it is clear that his father had determined early in his life that Jacques would follow in his footsteps by becoming a surgeon. Guillemeau began his apprenticeship as an adolescent in Orléans. In 1571, at the age of 21, Guillemeau moved to Montpellier—a city renowned for the study of medicine—to continue his training.[25] In all likelihood aided by his father and his uncle, Jacques Guillemeau was successful in making important and powerful contacts in the French medical community very early in his career. For example, in Montpellier, he studied with Laurent Joubert, physician to the king and author of several medical treatises, including one on care for women. He also befriended

---

22 Though this struggle began in the seventeenth century, it was at full tilt by the eighteenth century. For an excellent analysis of the way in which midwives became the pawn of both physicians and surgeons in the eighteenth century, see Nina Ratttner Gelbart, *The King's Midwife: A History and Mystery of Madame du Coudray* (Berkeley: University of California Press, 1998), esp. pp. 36–44.

23 Bridgette Sheridan, "Childbirth, Midwifery, And Science: The Life and Work of the French Royal Midwife Louise Bourgeois" (PhD dissertation, Boston College, 2002), pp. 153–98.

24 For a detailed account of both Jacques and Charles Guillemeau's careers, see: François Poulain, "La Vie et L'Oeuvre de Deux Chirurgiens: Jacques Guillemeau (1550–1613) et Charles Guillemeau (1588–1656)" Thesis, Université de Montpellier, 1993.

25 Males typically began their apprenticeships with a master-surgeon as young adolescents, working for a number of years before they were considered journeymen. They were then to travel to other places in order to gain more experience working with new masters. See Lindemann, p. 111.

the young doctor-in-training Jean Héroard, who was later to become Louis XIII's personal physician.[26]

Guillemeau moved to Paris in 1573, which marked the beginning of a long and important relationship between Guillemeau and his new master Ambroise Paré (1510–1590). Paré was renowned for his innovations in surgery as well as for his work in obstetrics.[27] He served under four French kings: Henri II, François II, Charles IX, and Henri III. An army surgeon in the midst of the wars of religion, Paré gained a wealth of experience patching up soldiers on the battlefield. Trained as a barber surgeon, he did not know Latin. In 1554, Paré became a member of the College of Saint-Côme and thus became a master surgeon. While he published a small treatise on obstetrics in 1549, it was not until 1573, when he published a more extensive treatise on the subject, that he became a recognized authority on childbirth.[28] As Paré's favorite student, Guillemeau was able to assist at the autopsy of King Charles IX at the young age of 24, launching him into an elite club of the great surgeons and anatomists of his time.[29] While he traveled as part of the king's army during the French Wars of Religion, Guillemeau eventually settled in Paris and remained one of Paré's closest colleagues and friends.[30]

Guillemeau's connection to Paré, as well a host of other physicians and surgeons, led to his promotion to the grade of ordinary surgeon to King Henri III. Like Paré, Guillemeau was a member of the corporation of surgeons of Saint-Côme and he was invested in elevating the status of surgeons by publishing medical treatises on surgery, anatomy, and birthing.[31] Guillemeau's first foray into print was when he translated Paré's works from French into the learned language of Latin, so that they would be considered worthy of study not only by fellow surgeons, but also by physicians. In 1581, prior to publication, the medical faculty of Paris called into question whether Guillemeau could have been capable of translating the text, because he was only a surgeon.[32] In the end, even though the medical faculty maintained that Guillemeau was not the translator, editions were

---

[26] Poulain, pp. 26–8.

[27] On the life of Paré, see: Francis R. Packard, *Life and Times of Ambroise Paré [1510–1590]: With a New Translation of his Apology and an Account of his Journeys in Divers Places* (New York: Benjamin Blom, Inc., 1971).

[28] Ambroise Paré, *Deux Livres De Chirurgie: I. De la generation de l'homme, et maniere d'extraire les enfants hors du ventre de la mère, ensemble ce qu'il faut faire pour la faire mieux et plustost accoucher, avec le cure de plusiers maladies qui lui peuvent survenir* (Paris, André Wechel, 1573).

[29] Poulain, pp. 32–5.

[30] Paule DuMaître refers to Paré as Guillemeau's "spiritual father" in "Autour d'Ambroise Paré: Ses Élèves, Ses Amis," *Histoire des Sciences* Médicales XXX/3 (1996): 354.

[31] Brockliss and Jones, pp. 104–5.

[32] Françoise Lehoux credits the translation to Guillemeau's friend, the physician Jean Hautin (Lehoux, p. 452). François Poulain believes that while Guillemeau was likely assisted by Hautin, he probably played some role in translating the text. See Poulain, pp. 57–60.

published that attributed the translation to Guillemeau. This attribution not only benefited Guillemeau, but also elevated the status of all surgeons.

Guillemeau went on to publish his own works, including a treatise on diseases of the eye, an anatomical table, and a treatise on surgery that depicted all of the latest surgical methods and instruments. By the time that he published his manual on birthing in 1609,[33] Guillemeau had successfully established himself in both the medical and publishing world. Guillemeau's manual was, in part, informed by his years of experience assisting at deliveries at the Hôtel-Dieu in Paris. In the preface, Guillemeau explained that he had gathered together both what he had observed in 40 years of practice along with the fruits of ancient and contemporary medical theory. Thought to be the most innovative of all of his works, with this manual Guillemeau successfully broke into the world of medicine. That is, the manual helped to solidify his reputation as a learned, rather than simply a skilled surgeon. The publication of a newly revised collection of his works in 1612[34] assured his standing as a significant contributor to the production of medical knowledge in the sixteenth and seventeenth centuries.

Guillemeau played an integral role in advancing surgeons' status in the medical community of early modern France. The protégé of the most innovative surgeon of the time, Ambroise Paré, Jacques Guillemeau advanced the cause for surgeons as learned practitioners by publishing books on anatomy and childbirth, two areas of medicine where surgeons could successfully compete with physicians. Further, Guillemeau's knowledge of Latin meant that he was able to read medical texts that many surgeons could not, thus granting him the respect of many physicians and surgeons. Though he died in 1613, before many surgeons had taken up delivering women in childbirth, the publication and success of his birthing manual were indicative of the growing trend toward surgeons rather than midwives as birthing attendants.

Louise Bourgeois (1563–1636)

Just as Jacques Guillemeau hoped to elevate the status of surgeons, Louise Bourgeois hoped to elevate the status of midwives. And yet, Bourgeois's career path shows that midwives would have an even more difficult time gaining entry into the realm of learned medicine than would surgeons. Louise Bourgeois was born in 1563, about the time that Jacques Guillemeau was beginning his apprenticeship in

[33] Jacques Guillemeau, *De l'heureux accouchement des femmes, où il est traicté du gouvernement de leur grossesse, de leur travail naturel et contre nature; du traictement es tant accouchées et de leurs maladies* (Paris, N. Buon, 1609).

[34] Jacques Guillemeau, *Oeuvres de chirurgie de Jacques Guillemeau, chirurgien ordinaire du roy et juré à Paris, avec les pourtraicts de toutes les parties du corps humain et des instruments necessaries au chirurgien, augementée et mises en un et enrichies de plusieurs traictez, pris des leçons de Mr. Germain Courtin, Docteur en medicine* (Paris: Nicolas Buon, 1612).

Orléans. Like Guillemeau, little is known about her childhood, except that she grew up in the Paris suburb of Saint-Germain. Judging by her father's property holdings, her family was fairly well off and would have been considered part of the growing bourgeois class.[35] She probably received the basic education—reading, writing, and needlework—for young women of her time whose families could afford it. At the age of 21, in 1584, Bourgeois married Martin Boursier, a barber-surgeon for the king's army. Her husband was already well established in his profession by the time Bourgeois married him. While not a famous surgeon in his own right, Martin Boursier spent 20 years training with Paré. Jacques Guillemeau and Bourgeois's husband would certainly have known one another, since they trained with Paré at the same time. By 1589, she and her husband had three children and were living a comfortable life in Saint-Germain. Had Paris and its environs continued to be a stable and peaceful place to live, it is likely that Bourgeois would have raised her children and perhaps assisted her husband with his practice. But this was not to be. In her writings, Bourgeois explained that she took up midwifery out of necessity when her family fortune was lost during the siege of Paris by Henri IV's armies in 1589.[36]

Bourgeois published an account of how and why she became a midwife, which provides a unique glimpse into a midwife's career in this period. Her entry into the occupation of midwifery differed significantly from Guillemeau's entry into surgery. Unlike Guillemeau, Bourgeois did not take up her profession because it ran in the family. Guillemeau began his apprenticeship in surgery as an adolescent; Bourgeois was 31 years old when she began her training in midwifery. Further, whereas Guillemeau considered Paré his mentor and advisor, Bourgeois claimed no mentors, nor did she reference any past midwives as models for her own career. Bourgeois must have trained with another midwife, but she never mentioned her. While there was no formal schooling in midwifery available, Bourgeois was unusual in that she was able to study Paré's work on childbirth. She explained that her husband, a surgeon who had trained with Paré, could also help her learn the necessary skills of midwifery.[37] Bourgeois understood the kind of midwifery where practice was complemented by medical theory, as different—namely, better—than the traditional practice of midwifery. It was Bourgeois's connection to the medical world—through books and through her husband—that made her unique, and incidentally, threatening to other midwives. After studying and

[35] Achille Chéreau, *Esquisse historique sur Louise Bourgeois Dite Boursier, sage-femme de la Reine Marie de Médicis* (Paris: L'Union Médicale, 1852), p. 8.

[36] In her description of how she became a midwife, Bourgeois explained that after her family had lost everything, it was ultimately the fear of seeing her children in need that convinced her to take up midwifery. See Louise (Boursier) Bourgeois, "Comment j'ay apprins l'art de sage-femme." In: *Observations diverses sur la sterilité, perte de fruict, foecondité, accouchements et maladies des femmes, & enfants nouveaux naix, amplement traitées, et heureusement praticquées par L. Bourgeois dite Boursier* (Paris: H. Ruffin, 1652), II, p. 88.

[37] Bourgeois, *Observations diverses,* II, p. 88.

practicing midwifery for nearly 5 years, Bourgeois became a certified midwife in 1598. At this time, the licensing board for midwives consisted of one physician, two surgeons, and two midwives. Bourgeois writes:

> Thus I was sent to see two midwives, Mesdames Dupuis and Peronne. They fixed a day when I could meet both of them. They asked me what my husband's profession was, and when I told them, they did not want to receive me as a midwife. Or at least Madame Dupuis did not, for she said to the other woman, "Good God, my friend, my heart tells me this won't do us any good, since she's a surgeon's wife. She'll get along with the physicians like purse-cutters at a fair. We must accept only artisans' wives, who don't understand anything about our affairs."[38]

Madame Dupuis clearly felt that Bourgeois was an ally of physicians and surgeons, and therefore a threat to midwives. Despite Madame Dupuis's views, Bourgeois passed her examination on November 12th 1598 and was granted a license to practice.[39]

Just 3 years after she was certified, Bourgeois attained the status of Royal Midwife for Queen Marie de Médicis in 1601. Bourgeois's explanation of how she was appointed to the position of royal midwife shows the ways in which medical, social, and political connections were all vital to the making of this midwife's career.[40] Similar to Guillemeau, Bourgeois's familial connections to the elite were important in establishing her career. Guillemeau's close relationship with Paré was assuredly the key factor in Guillemeau's later successes. Bourgeois, on the other hand, had to rely on her own connections to aristocratic women, in addition to husband's and her own connections to medical men. Indeed, in order to obtain her position, Bourgeois had to be officially approved by several royal physicians and 12 aristocratic women.[41] Bourgeois went on to serve Marie de Médicis at the births of all of the royal children and at the same time was able to establish a successful and thriving midwifery practice.

In the early 1600s, the occupation of midwifery was exceptional in that women were accorded some measure of expertise and authority. But Louise Bourgeois was not a typical seventeenth-century midwife. A midwife at first out of necessity, Bourgeois was able to turn her circumstances into an opportunity to raise the status of her profession. Her position as royal midwife not only considerably raised her own and ultimately her family's status, but she gained access to public life through the publication of her experiences at court and her midwives' manual. She was the author of several published works, including a three-volume manual on midwifery that includes her advice and remedies for illnesses and problems associated with

---

[38] Bourgeois, *Various Observations,* II.

[39] Perkins, p. 17.

[40] For an analysis of Bourgeois's appointment process, see Sheridan, "Childbirth, Midwifery, and Science," pp. 35–47.

[41] Louise (Boursier) Bourgeois, *Observations diverses,* p. 131.

pregnancy.[42] The only manual of its era written by a woman, Bourgeois's book provides a unique view into the practice of midwifery in the seventeenth century. Bourgeois was unusual because of her knowledge of medical theory and because she was a published expert on the subject of birthing.

The Birthing Manuals

It was a particular historical moment—when science and men began to enter the birthing room—that allowed for Bourgeois and Guillemeau to rise to the position of published authors who were renowned for their knowledge and expertise in care for women. Jacques Guillemeau and Louise Bourgeois were indebted to many of the same medical men, were both present at the birth of Louis XIII, and were practitioners to the elite in Paris and its suburbs; they crossed paths on a regular basis. While they did not acknowledge one another in their writings, there is no evidence that indicates anything different than an amicable, if distant, professional relationship with one another. While their birthing manuals were published at nearly the same time, influenced by the same expert on childbirth—Ambroise Paré—and written in the same city, they were addressed to different audiences and were aimed at fulfilling different purposes.

Jacques Guillemeau had included some of his advice on childbirth in his surgical treatises, but he believed that the complexity of birthing warranted its own treatise.[43] While his manual included advice for midwives, he emphasized in his preface that he wrote the manual for young surgeons-in-training who planned to specialize in childbirth. Acknowledging that not all surgeons would know Latin or Greek, he wrote his manual in French so that it would be widely accessible.[44] In his manual, Guillemeau made the case that surgeons were uniquely trained to help women during pregnancy and delivery, particularly those involving complications. At this time, surgeons, unlike midwives, were not general practitioners in caring for women during their pregnancies. The primary role for a surgeon in childbirth was to intervene when deliveries went awry. And yet, Guillemeau argued that even when a child was born without intervention by either a surgeon or a midwife, the mother and child would need assistance upon the child's arrival that only a surgeon was qualified to provide. For example, the child could be extraordinarily weak or its head could be misshapen, or the woman's womb could be malformed. However,

---

42 Louise (Boursier) Bourgeois, *Observations diverses sur la sterilité, perte de fruict, foecondité, accouchements et maladies des femmes, & enfants nouveaux naix, amplement traitées, et heureusement praticquées par L. Bourgeois dite Boursier* (Paris: H. Ruffin, 1652). This edition contains all three volumes of her manual. The first volume was published in 1609, the second in 1626, and the third in 1626.

43 James (sic.) Guillemeau, *Child-birth or, The Happy Deliverie of Women. Wherein is set down the Government of Women* (Amsterdam: Theatrvm Orbis Terrarvm Ltd., 1972), fol. ¶ 3v.

44 James (sic.) Guillemeau, *Child-birth or, The Happy Deliverie of Women,* fol. ¶¶ v.

he wrote, many midwives and family members, because of their willfulness, failed to call upon a surgeon in these situations, to the peril of the laboring woman and the child.[45] He believed that all surgeons should learn medical theory, and that it was in the realm of childbirth above all where surgeons could be seen as medical experts. Nonetheless, Guillemeau stressed the importance of surgeons' empirical training over theoretical knowledge in the realm of birthing, suggesting the superiority of surgeons over physicians when it came to childbirth.

Bourgeois's manual was the first manual written by a midwife for midwives. The midwife, unlike the surgeon, provided care to the parturient woman throughout her entire pregnancy, delivery, and post-delivery period. Midwives' primary charge was to provide comfort to women giving birth and to ensure safe deliveries of their children. In order to do this, midwives had to mediate many different relationships: between woman and husband, woman and birthing attendants, woman and surgeon, husband and surgeon, and birthing attendants and surgeon. Bourgeois understood the role of the midwife as fluid: a midwife would provide care as well as medical recipes, and if need be, she would also use techniques in order to save the life of the mother and child. On the other hand, Bourgeois was not afraid to recommend other practitioners—physicians and/or surgeons—if they could provide the best care.

In her manual, Bourgeois focused on what to do for pregnant and laboring women in the case of an emergency. Yet, in her preface, she emphasized the importance of making the basic skills of midwifery accessible to all practitioners and parturient women. In Guillemeau's manual, he described the course of a normal pregnancy, but in his preface focused on how a surgeon's intervention could save women's lives. The differences in the prefaces can be explained by the writers' sense of who they believed to be the most important caretakers for women. Guillemeau, invested in the notion of surgeons as the most senior caretakers for women, spent as much time on normal as abnormal deliveries, since most young surgeons would be unfamiliar with what a normal delivery entailed. Bourgeois, writing for literate midwives, focused on particularly difficult problems for women throughout her manual, as these were the situations midwives may not normally have learned how to manage, given their limited access to both anatomy and medical theory. Yet she also emphasized the importance of patience and nonintervention—the time-honored traditions in midwifery.

Both Guillemeau and Bourgeois devoted a portion of their work to the duties and responsibilities of the midwife. In his second volume, Guillemeau explained midwives' traditional role throughout history, their role in preparing a woman for delivery, and their responsibilities during a normal delivery. Guillemeau therefore acknowledged midwives' place in the birthing room, but he defined clear boundaries between midwives' roles and the role of medical men in childbirth. Guillemeau began his brief history of midwifery by stating that most women delivered

[45] James (sic.) Guillemeau, *Child-birth or, The Happy Deliverie of Women*, fol. ¶ 2v.

without the need for any intervention whatsoever.[46] Thus, according to him, the midwife's primary role in childbirth required very little skill. Her most important responsibilities were to keep the laboring woman calm and to be patient so as to let nature do its work. While he acknowledged that childbirth was often painful, he stressed that women should try to remain calm and patient throughout labor. Guillemeau concluded with the assurance that the pain most women experienced in childbirth, while unpleasant, was ordained by God because of women's original sin.[47] Claiming that it was unusual to find a midwife who would be skilled enough to handle complications during delivery, Guillemeau strongly recommended that the midwife call in a surgeon or a physician at the first sign of trouble.[48]

Bourgeois also addressed midwives' roles and responsibilities, discussing at length what a midwife must do for a woman in a normal delivery. Similar to Guillemeau, Bourgeois indicated that during normal deliveries midwives must be patient and let nature take its course. Yet her compassion for the pain that women experienced was evident throughout her description of a midwife's responsibilities. She emphasized the tremendous amount of work involved in birthing a child, and therefore encouraged midwives to be gentle and kind to the laboring woman. Midwives were to walk the fine line between assuaging the anxiety and pain of a laboring woman and remaining in control of the birthing process.[49]

In addition, Bourgeois addressed a midwife's responsibility when she was called to deliver a woman before term or when the woman was at term with a difficult labor.[50] She included several observations based on her own experience, and suggested remedies and techniques that a midwife could employ in order to ensure a safe delivery. Unlike Guillemeau, Bourgeois assumed that midwives could handle difficult situations as long as they had experience. Still, she encouraged midwives to defer to physicians and surgeons if necessary for the good of the patient. For example, in one of her observations Bourgeois explained that a woman who was about 7 months pregnant bled whenever she experienced any emotion. When she was put to bed the bleeding would stop, but once she stood up, the blood flowed profusely. Bourgeois explained that unless a midwife had experience in delivering a woman with this problem, as Bourgeois did, she should defer to a surgeon or a physician.[51] Bourgeois was adamant that the lives of the mother and child were the priority in a delivery.

As the publication of both Bourgeois's and Guillemeau's manuals shows, the beginning of the seventeenth century was a time when the subject of birthing

---

46 Jacques Guillemeau, *De la grossesse et accouchement des femmes: du governement dicelles et moyen de survenir aux accidents qui leur arrivent, Ensemble de la nourriture des enfans* (Paris: Abraham Pacard, 1620), II, p. 153.

47 See Guillemeau, *De la grossesse*, II, pp. 168–9.

48 Guillemeau, *De la grossesse,* II, p. 188.

49 Bourgeois, *Observations diverses,* II, pp. 150–84.

50 Bourgeois, *Observations diverses,* I, pp. 48–61.

51 Bourgeois, *Observations diverses*, I, pp. 31–3.

belonged to both surgeons and midwives. Guillemeau believed that midwives could manage deliveries, as long as there were no complications. In difficult deliveries, midwives were obligated to call in and defer to a surgeon, according to Guillemeau. Bourgeois believed that midwives could manage both uncomplicated and complicated deliveries, as long as they were willing to consult with physicians and surgeons in situations that were beyond their skills. Guillemeau died shortly after he published his work on childbirth, just as Bourgeois entered the public domain as a published author and a famous midwife; she was at the height of her career. Guillemeau likely seemed unthreatening to Bourgeois since it was clear that the work he published on childbirth would be his last. In addition, Paré had long since passed away. With these two famous birthing experts gone, Bourgeois seemed the likely successor to be the foremost birthing practitioner in Paris (even if, or as she hoped, *because* she was a woman). Learned in medical knowledge and practiced in her art, Bourgeois exemplified a new kind of midwife; one she hoped would become part of the expanding medical community. While Bourgeois was certainly successful for many years following the publication of her manual, the tension over who would have authority in the birthing room was growing. A brief look at Jacques's son Charles Guillemeau's career helps to illustrate the way this tension among practitioners manifested itself in early modern Parisian society.

Charles Guillemeau (1588–1656)

Just as Jacques Guillemeau was destined to follow in his father's footsteps, so also was Charles Guillemeau destined to become a surgeon like his father. Indeed, Jacques Guillemeau had promised Henri IV that he would pass on his skills to his eldest son who would also serve the king.[52] By 1612, at the age of 24, Charles Guillemeau had already achieved the rank of royal surgeon. While he was not quite as prolific as his father, Charles published several surgical treatises. He also augmented his father's manual on childbirth, most notably by adding to it a polemic against midwives.[53] Like his father, Charles was interested in elevating surgeons' status in the medical hierarchy. For example, in 1614, he was one of several surgeons of Saint-Côme who lectured on anatomy to fellow surgeons, much to the dismay of medical faculty in Paris.[54] Yet Charles was in some ways more ambitious than his father; he wanted to be more than just a royal surgeon. By 1618, he had managed to obtain the post of provost of the College of surgeons in Paris. At this time, surgeons—especially those in powerful positions like Charles—supervised the certification of midwives and exercised a great deal of control. For example, in 1618, Charles forbade one physician to proceed with the admission of a midwifery

52 Guillemeau, "Au Roi," in *Les Oeuvres de Chirurgie* (Paris: N. Buon, 1612).

53 Charles Guillemeau, "Traicté des Abus qui se Commettent sur les Procedures de l'Impuissance des Hommes & des Femmes," in: Jacques Guillemeau, *De la grossesse et accouchement des femmes: du governement dicelles et moyen de survenir aux accidents qui leur arrivent, Ensemble de la nourriture des enfans* (Paris: Abraham Pacard, 1620).

54 Brockliss and Jones, p. 222.

candidate because there was no priest or senior midwife present. The disgruntled physician complained that this was unwarranted, especially since two surgeons and two midwives were present.[55] Here Charles asserted surgeons' control over midwives at the same time as he demanded respect for surgeons from physicians. By 1625, Charles Guillemeau had surpassed his father in rank by attaining the position of premier surgeon to the king.

Despite the progress that surgeons had made in gaining legitimacy as learned practitioners, in 1609 the Parlement of Paris found in favor of physicians when they prevented surgeons from establishing themselves as official faculty of medicine.[56] This ruling may have convinced Charles Guillemeau that obtaining a medical degree would help his career. While the surgeons of Saint-Côme did establish their own place of learning, they were not officially part of the faculty of medicine. By 1626, Charles had successfully passed his exams and obtained all of the privileges of a graduate physician.[57] In order to obtain a medical license, Charles had to swear that he would no longer consort with surgeons.[58] Nonetheless, even after he obtained these privileges, he retained his position as premier surgeon to the king. His credentials as both premier royal surgeon and graduate physician meant that he was in an ideal position to claim expertise in all medical matters, be they concerned with medical theory or with practice. Perhaps this was why Charles Guillemeau was the one to write the remonstrance that ultimately ended Louise Bourgeois's career.

On June 5th 1627, the Princess Marie de Bourbon-Montpensier—Gaston d'Orléans's wife and Louis XIII's sister-in-law—died a week after giving birth to a girl. As was customary, Marie de Médicis ordered that an autopsy be performed by five physicians and five surgeons. The short report—less than a page long—implied that the cause of death was a piece of placenta attached to the womb that had become gangrenous. Removal of the placenta would have been the midwife's job. Bourgeois took this to be a direct implication of blame and immediately wrote back a public response to these physicians and surgeons.[59] Shortly thereafter, a defense

---

55 Lehoux, p. 448.

56 Brockliss and Jones, p. 222.

57 Poulain, pp. 182–3.

58 Practicing both physic and surgery was generally not allowed at this time. Brockliss and Jones gave the example of Jacques D'Amboise, who had become a member of the corporation of Saint-Côme while he was a bachelor of medicine. When the Paris Faculty learned of this, they made him swear to not practice surgery or belong to the company of Surgeons of Saint-Côme under the penalty of expulsion (Brockliss and Jones, p. 214). At least one medical student was unhappy about Guillemeau's admission into the realm of physic. François Lehoux cites a journal entry from a medical student, who upon hearing of Guillemeau's licensing, wrote that he was horrified that physicians would be thrown in with illiterate men, like surgeons, who do not even know Latin. See Lehoux, p. 2.

59 Louise Bourgeois, *Apologie de Louise Bourgeois Dite Bourcier sage femme de la Royne Mere du Roy, & de feu Madame. Contre le Rapport des Medecins* (Paris: Chez Melchior Mondiere, 1627).

of the surgeons and physicians who performed the autopsy was written by an anonymous author, now assumed to be Charles Guillemeau.[60]

In Bourgeois's response to the autopsy report, she wanted to do more than deny responsibility for the princess' death; she wanted to show that she was skilled and learned enough in the matter of birthing to be able to prove her innocence. In doing so, Bourgeois used both her skills based on experience and her knowledge of medical theory. Bourgeois showed that, like the physicians and surgeons who wrote the autopsy report, she understood anatomy, physiology, humoral theory, and the possible causes and effects of gangrene. It is striking how Bourgeois used physicians' and surgeons' own knowledge, language, and position of authority against them. Citing medical knowledge that had traditionally belonged to physicians and increasingly belonged also to surgeons, she claimed to prove that the death of the princess was the fault of the princess' physicians.[61] It was, by her charge, the princess' physicians who should have attended to her illness before she even went into labor. Bourgeois also cited the ways in which her skills in midwifery and knowledge of women's health were a resource to both midwives and medical men. She affirmed her midwifery skills by citing her record of 34 years of experience in Paris. Further, she claimed expertise in medicine by declaring that her writings had been published and translated into several languages for which she received thanks from "the greatest Physicians in Europe, who profited from reading my books."[62]

Charles Guillemeau's response to Bourgeois is an indication of the increasing ease with which surgeons and physicians were able to challenge the age-old notion that the birthing room was the midwife's domain. Guillemeau attacked Bourgeois's expertise in an area that midwives were traditionally presumed to be superior to medical men: the care of the female patient and the practical skills involved in the successful delivery of a woman. Though he mocked Bourgeois's attempts to cite ancient authorities against the physicians and surgeons, he did allow for the possibility that Bourgeois may have been correct in her explanations of medical problems, such as whether or not a retained placenta alone could cause

[60] *Remonstrance à Madame Bourcier touchant son Apologie contre le Rapport que les medecins ont faict de ce qui a causé la mort deplorable de Madame* (Paris: J. Jacquin, 1627). Though the author of this *Remonstrance* is not included in the text, the copy that I looked at from the Bibliothèque Nationale includes Charles Guillemeau's name handwritten on the document. See also Poulain, pp. 183–5; François Rouget and Colette H. Winn, "Introduction," to *Récit Véritable de la Naissance de Messeigneurs et Dames Les Enfans de France, Instruction a ma Fille, et Autres Textes* (par Louise Boursier), Genève: Droz, 2000, p. 21.

[61] Bourgeois cited both ancient and contemporary surgeons and physicians—including Galen and Hippocrates—to support her claims and to prove midwives' superior knowledge in the realm of birthing. For a fuller analysis of the princess' death and these texts, see Sheridan, "Childbirth, Midwifery, and Science," pp. 130–50.

[62] Bourgeois, *Apologie,* p. 15. Translation is my own.

gangrene.[63] Instead, Guillemeau claimed that it was Bourgeois's incompetence in providing basic care to the princess during labor that caused the princess' death. For example, Guillemeau noted that the cause of the gangrene could be something other than a retained piece of the placenta. He suggested that it could also be any one of the following: too much pressure on the uterus to extract the placenta, rough treatment throughout the delivery, or binding the abdomen too tightly after the birth.[64] Guillemeau thus implied that, whatever the cause of the gangrene, it was clearly the midwife's fault, as she would have been responsible for any of these procedures. Accusing her of ineptness in basic care was an effective strategy; there could have been no greater blow to Bourgeois's authority and reputation. Bourgeois's precarious position at court—much more true by 1627 than it had been in 1609, given her connection to the increasingly unpopular Marie de Médicis—combined with increasing arguments in favor of men's role in birthing and women's health, meant that Bourgeois was unable to maintain her role as an authority on childbirth and midwifery at the royal court. We have almost no information about Bourgeois's life from this point until her death in 1636.[65]

As this story demonstrates, as early as 1627, birthing for the elites in France was no longer an all-female affair. True, physicians and surgeons had made their way into the birthing room as trusted birthing attendants only among the aristocracy and the upper bourgeoisie. Still, even if most women were still attended by midwives, physicians and surgeons were increasingly understood to be the experts on women's health. This was a result of, in particular, the improved education and training of physicians and especially surgeons. Coupled with an increase in physicians' and surgeons' published treatises on women's health, midwives gradually began to lose their position as the authorities in the birthing room.

Conclusion

The early seventeenth century in Paris was a moment of opportunity for surgeons (male) and midwives (female) to forge their way into the burgeoning medical community. Both occupations had always emphasized the importance of experience and observation in treating their clientele. At a time when medical men were beginning to question ancient medical theory, it seemed possible that midwives and surgeons might find a place for themselves in the medical hierarchy. Because

[63] Charles Guillemeau, *Remonstrance,* pp. 4–6.

[64] Charles Guillemeau, *Remonstrance,* p. 11.

[65] The general consensus of several historians who have written about Bourgeois is that she retreated from the court at the time of the princess's death. See, for example: Chéreau, p. 28; Rouget and Winn, p. 21. Wendy Perkins goes so far as to say, "What is beyond doubt is that Bourgeois's career, amongst the aristocracy at any rate, ended here [with the princess's death]." Perkins, p. 25. Though Bourgeois's records of her clientele have not been found in order to prove this, there is also no indication that she attended more births at court.

midwives had always provided care for women, Louise Bourgeois imagined that this would continue to be true. Bourgeois practiced midwifery when there was a window of opportunity for some women to acquire the skills and knowledge of a learned medical practitioner. Bourgeois felt that by learning the tools of medicine, she could become the model for a new kind of midwifery: a profession that valued (male) medical science but also maintained the traditional (female) features of midwifery such as patience, caring, and empathy. Furthermore, and importantly, Bourgeois emphasized that women should care for other women because it was improper for men to view women's bodies. The taboo against men seeing women's bodies was an oft-cited reason for keeping men out of the birthing room.[66]

And yet, as the story of Bourgeois's dismissal from the royal court indicates, her vision of a "new kind of midwife" was one that did not come to fruition. While women were allowed to participate in the production of medical knowledge for some time, the gendered nature of medical professionalization meant that their participation in medicine was curtailed. Once men gained the experience that women had in caring for women, they were able to challenge arguments such as those that focused on the immorality of men viewing women's bodies. Thus, while men gained the experience that traditionally only women possessed, women did not in turn come to be regarded as scientific practitioners. Further, male surgeons and physicians were able to claim that new skills in birthing, believed to ensure safe delivery of mother and child, belonged exclusively to medical men. Just as Ambroise Paré, Jacques Guillemeau, and Charles Guillemeau had hoped, surgeons were able to successfully raise their status in the medical profession by reorganizing their guild, revamping their educational program, and claiming expertise in the realm of birthing. Midwives, on the other hand, were forced into licensing and regulation by both legal authorities and medical men as a means of controlling their actions rather than improving their education. Their limited educational program did not elevate the profession of midwifery. While the struggle for supremacy between surgeons and physicians continued, midwives were eventually contained outside of the medical hierarchy.

[66] For more on the trope of modesty in defending female practitioners, see Sheridan, "Childbirth, Midwifery, and Science," pp. 153–98.

Chapter 11
Touching and Telling: Gendered Variations on a Gynecological Theme

Kirk D. Read

Childbirth for women at the turn of the sixteenth century was at once life-giving and life-threatening; to bring children into the world was to put oneself in danger. Birthing children of the mind through writing and publishing was an equally perilous enterprise for women in a society that marked all of their reproductive capacities, both biological and intellectual, with shame and suspicion. An investigation of the writings of both men and women surrounding childbirth can prove fruitful regarding the limits and possibilities of women's expression, both of the body and the spirit.

The perception of childbirth as a dangerous event in the life of early modern women is the subject of no little debate, and the language and arguments used for framing the polemic are instructive in and of themselves. Lianne McTavish is wont to question overly dire statistics. She sees the exaggeration of reports on maternal mortality as participating in a transhistorical misogynistic tradition of condemning midwives' incompetency. She says of recent historians of medicine, "By undertaking careful archival research, they have undermined longstanding assumptions about early modern childbirth. It is no longer possible to presume that female midwives were incompetent, women had no control over conception, and birth itself was extremely dangerous."[1] McTavish responds to the conventional and repeated wisdom of scholars such as Lawrence Stone who generalize broadly from what seems like much of the cautionary, hyperbolic literature from the early modern period. "For women, childbirth was a very dangerous experience, for midwives were ignorant and ill trained, and often horribly botched the job, while the lack of hygienic precautions meant that puerperal fever was a frequent sequel."[2] Commensurate with such predictions is the speculation of B.M. Willmott

---

[1] Lianne McTavish, *Childbirth and the Display of Authority in Early Modern France* (Aldershot, UK: Ashgate, 2005), p. 8.

[2] Lawrence Stone, *The Family, Sex, and Marriage in England 1500–1800* (New York: Harper & Row, 1977), p. 79. For countervailing argument and evidence in a variety of European examples, see Roger Schofield's "Did the Mothers Really Die? Three Centuries of Maternal Mortality in 'The World We Have Lost,'" in *The World We Have Gained: Histories of Population and Social Structure* (New York: Blackwell, 1986).

Dobbie, whose prose betrays not only the general mystery of the birthing process in the early modern era, but our knowledge of its history from that time to the present:

> An enquiry into family structure in previous centuries reveals evidence of the high price in women's lives of replenishment of the population. It could not be otherwise, for when Nature failed in her task, or was thwarted by such adversities as pelvic deformity or malpresentation, attempts to help were mostly fumbling in the dark, literally and metaphorically, and well-meant interference was almost certain to introduce infection, so often fatal.[3]

Dobbie's characterization of Mother Nature "failing in her task" in the context of bumbling early modern midwives is, in itself, fodder for a rich discussion of gender and contemporary gynecological rhetoric about the past. While that metacritical study is not the focus here, it does serve to contextualize the work of McTavish and others who seek to put into question the assumptions that such characterizations validate. To be sure, however, Dobbie's suppositions participate fully in the highly gendered discourse of this era that François Rouget and Colette Winn describe as clearly polemic:

> C'est dans le dernier tiers du XVIe siècle que s'amorce le fameux conflit entre les practiciennes et les 'hommes d'art' opposant les femmes, fortes de leur expérience mais ignorantes des principes élémentaires de l'anatomie et de l'hygiène, qui refusaient de céder le monopole dont elles avaient joui jusque-là dans le domaine obstétrical, aux hommes, qui souvent n'avaient qu'une connaissance théorique des mécanismes de la parturition.[4]
>
> (It is in the final third part of the sixteenth century that begins the famous conflict between female practitioners and the 'men of science' opposing these women who were fortified by their experience but ignorant of basic principles of anatomy and hygiene and refused to give up the monopoly they had theretofore enjoyed in the realm of obstetrics over men who often had only theoretical knowledge of the mechanics of birthing.)

Of concern to me here are the ways in which anxiety over the woman's body in birth inflects this polarized debate. Rouget and Winn continue: "Le respect des traditions mais aussi les préjugés et les tabous, notamment la pudeur et la peur qu'avaient les femmes d'être souillée, ne cessaient d'alimenter le fameux débat sur 'l'indécence aux hommes d'accoucher les femmes'" ("Respect for tradition but also

---

[3] B.M. Willmott Dobbie, "An Attempt to Estimate the True Rate of Maternal Mortality, Sixteenth to Eighteenth Centuries," Medical History, 26 (1982): 79.

[4] François Rouget and Colette Winn, "Introduction" to Louise Boursier, *Récit veritable de la naissance de messeigneurs et dames les enfans de France; Instruction à ma fille et autres textes* (Geneva: Droz, 2000), p. 16. All translations are my own unless otherwise noted.

prejudices and taboos, notably modesty and women's fear of being sullied, did not cease from fueling the famous debate on the 'indecency of men assisting women in childbirth,'" 17). If Dobbie raises the specter of well-intentioned birth attendants "fumbling in the dark," so do I here take up the veiled and anxious discourse around who is privileged to fumble about; how early modern birth attendants approached their mission; and how their writing defended their decisions and livelihood.

Not surprisingly, Louise Boursier, whom Wendy Perkins hails as "the foremost female health worker in France," plays a crucial role here.[5] Midwife to the Parisian elite of her day, including, on six occasions, Marie de Médicis, Boursier sets the scene in her *Observations diverses* of 1609:

> … je me trouvais un jour à l'accouchement d'une honnête demoiselle de mes bonnes amies, de laquelle le mari était absent; elle était assistée de trois ou quatre de ses amies, lesquelles me demandèrent l'état de son accouchement, je leur dis que l'enfant venait mal, mais que je l'aurais, aidant Dieu, sans danger de la mère ni de l'enfant; elles me prièrent d'avoir agréable de la faire voir au chirurgien; pour leur décharge, je leur accordai, pourvu qu'elle ne le vît point, d'autant que je savais que cela était capable de la faire mourir d'appréhension, et de honte. Je la persuadai de se glisser aux pieds de son lit. Je mis le chevet au milieu du lit et abattis le tour du lit du côté qu'il devait passer, et aux pieds: il la toucha comme je parlais, elle ne le vit point, et accoucha sans artifice ni aide, que de Dieu et de la nature.[6]
>
> (… I found myself one day at the birthing of a proper lady known to my good friends whose husband was absent; she was attended to by three or four of her friends who asked me about the progress of the birth. I told them that the child was coming with difficulty but that I would receive it, God willing, without danger to the mother nor to the child; they asked me kindly if I would consent to having her seen by a physician; to assuage their fears, I consented, provided that she not be allowed to see him, for I knew that this could cause her to die of apprehension or shame. I persuaded her to slide to the foot of the bed. I put the pillow in the middle and built up the bed on the side where he would approach, as well as down by her feet. He touched her while I spoke, she never laid eyes on him and gave birth without any special intervention or help, either from God or nature.)

Such anecdotes are one of the most compelling features of the midwife's or physician's manual. Nestled in among Petrarchan sonnetry in the dedications,

---

5 "Between 1601 and 1609 she was midwife to Marie de Médicis, queen of France, delivering all six of her children. Her rise to prominence was in fact meteoric: having passed the official examination only in 1598, she had by 1601 delivered the future Louis XIII and was assured of a successful, influential career." Wendy Perkins, *Midwifery and Medicine in Early Modern France: Louise Bourgeois* (Exeter: University of Exeter Press, 1996), p. 1.

6 Louise Boursier, *Observations diverses sur la stérilité* … ed. Françoise Olive (Paris: Côté femme, 1992), p. 187.

classical and folkloric allusions, herbal remedies and tips on everything from dry skin and vomiting to paternity and multiple births, the eyewitness account is what turns the pages. *I saw, I attended, I saved.* These are the terms that lend respect and veracity. Boursier's story here is a particularly poignant one for what it says about the state of the increasingly medicalized view of childbirth. It betrays the moment where attending to women's reproduction and birthing was literally slipping from the midwife's hands.[7]

Boursier's narrative is couched clearly in an atmosphere of mistrust regarding women's capacities to oversee births, particularly in the case of difficult ones. In consenting to her client's wishes to have a doctor present, she must stage an elaborate deception so that the birthing woman hears her, but is touched by the man behind the screen: "il la toucha comme je parlais, elle ne le vit point, et accoucha sans artifice ni aide, que de Dieu et de la nature" ("He touched her while I spoke; she never laid eyes on him and gave birth without any special intervention or help, either from God or nature"). She talks reassuringly and he touches. Boursier, related as she was through marriage to some of the most renowned surgeons of her day, is not overly begrudging; but we do sense in the "sans artifice ni aide"—meaning that no extraordinary measures were needed that would have required a doctor—that this was something that could have been handled (pun intended) between women. Louise Boursier reminds her daughter and the reader in her *Instruction à ma fille*:

> Advisez ma fille, ce que vous pouvez estre plus que moy: estant petite fille de Phanerote, disciple de Lucine, maistresse de Mercure, à cause que Lucine l'a assujetty à vostre mere. Vous estes née dans l'exercice que ceste sage m'a monstré … Vous n'en manquerez nullement, d'autant que vous estes enfant de famille, un Docteur en medecine est mary de vostre soeur, vostre mary fait son cours pour l'estre, l'un de vos freres est Pharmacien, vostre pere est Chirurgien, et moy sage-femme; le corps de la medecine est entier dans nostre maison.[8]
>
> (Consider, my daughter, that you can become even greater than I: being granddaughter of Phanerote, disciple of Lucina, mistress of Mercury because Lucina put her in your mother's service. You are born into the work that this wise woman showed me … You can't hardly fail, being a child in such a family, your sister's husband is a doctor of medicine, your own husband is studying to be one, one of your brothers is a pharmacist, your father is a surgeon, and I, a midwife; the entire medical establishment is represented in our household.)

---

[7] Of insight in this realm of investigation, particularly with regard to the example of Louise Boursier is Wendy Perkins' study, *Midwifery and Medicine in Early Modern France*; Rouget and Winn's edition of Boursier's *Récit véritable* is highly useful with regard to primary work by Boursier and biography. Of interest as well is the more universal study of women and medicine by Evelyne Berriot-Salvadore, *Un Corps, un Destin: La femme dans la médecine de la Renaissance* (Paris: Champion, 1993).

[8] Rouget and Winn, 124.

Louise Boursier's husband, Martin Boursier, studied under Ambroise Paré and became one of the king's surgeons. Boursier indulges both her actual lineage so redolent of medical acumen, and, more importantly, her female mythological forebears whom she uses to establish her credibility as a midwife. And for good reason, it would appear.

Professional medical men were increasingly implicating themselves into the process of childbirth; the written record of their advice regarding their profession reflects not only the fact of their involvement, but a certain anxiety regarding the tensions between men and women, surgeons and midwives, that clearly marked this period of transition.[9] One can explore more closely this phenomenon through a shared narrative, a story taken up by the surgeon Jacques Guillemeau in his *De l'heureux accouchement des femmes* of 1609 and interpreted differently by another writer with more literary pretentions, Catherine des Roches, in her first published works, *Les Oeuvres*, of 1578. The story that both retell is that of Agnodice, the mythic first woman physician who attended to the women of Athens, fearful for their reputations lest they be seen and touched by men. The story came to both authors through Hyginus, a second-century Latinist as published in his *Fabulae*. Their respective approaches to this tale are the stuff of gendered authorship: What do they include? Why? Who constitutes their putative readership? What's at stake?

Hyginus and (Women's) Hygiene

Hyginus embeds his story in a chapter entitled "Inventors and their Inventions" wherein a variety of discoveries and inventions are discussed: wine, pruning, the needle, bronze, lead, arms, and then somewhat incongruously, herbs, which lead to a reference to Chiron, son of Saturn (first to use herbs in the medical art of surgery), Apollo (first to practice in the art of treating eyes) and Asclepius, his son, who purportedly began the art of clinical medicine. The story of Agnodice follows.

[9] Of primary importance to this discussion—and of some help in my conception of a title for this essay—is the work of Caroline Bicks on Shakespearean midwives: "What distinguishes the early modern midwife from the other women of the birthroom, however, is the fact that she was recognized as a sanctioned shaper of men's, women's, and children's bodies. Although any birth attendant was theoretically privy to a new mother's secrets, the midwife had an acknowledged duty to handle bodies and interpret their secrets. Given that European men had participated in making the midwife an integral part of their countries' institutional structures and less tangible cultural operations, her tales and touch posed a particular challenge to male claims about women's bodies and children's origins—and to the masculine identities that those claims helped underwrite." Caroline Bicks, *Midwiving Subjects in Shakespeare's England* (Aldershot, UK: Ashgate, 2003), p. 12. See also Lianne McTavish's cautionary interpretation of this issue as discussed in my introduction, where she warns against an overly polemicized debate according to gender.

> The ancients didn't have obstetricians, and as a result, women because of modesty perished. For the Athenians forbade slaves and women to learn the art of medicine. A certain girl, Hagnodice, virgin, desired to learn medicine, and since she desired it, she cut her hair, and in male attire came to a certain Herophilus for training. When she had learned the art, and had heard that a woman was in labor, she came to her. And when the woman refused to trust herself to her, thinking that she was a man, she removed her garment to show that she was a woman, and in this way she treated women. When the doctors saw that they were not admitted to women, they began to accuse Hagnodice, saying that 'he' was a seducer and corruptor of women, and that the women were pretending to be ill. The Areopagites, in session, started to condemn Hagnodice, but Hagnodice removed her garment for them and showed that she was a woman. Then the doctors began to accuse her more vigorously, and as a result the leading women came to the Court and said: 'You are not husbands, but enemies, because you condemn her who discovered safety for us.' Then the Athenians amended the law, so that free-born women could learn the art of medicine.[10]

Hyginus then quite characteristically shifts gears and plunges straight away into a list of other inventions: compasses, statuary, astrology, dye, musical pipes, and so forth. This "invention," as it were, is far more elaborated than any other items in Hyginus's chapter; it seems to carry a lot more weight. His attention betrays a conscious and concerted attention to the issue of women's health and the anxieties attached to it. Hyginus introduces this "invention" or origin story as being about female obstetricians. Yet it is curious to note how he has the Athenian women characterize it within his narrative: "'You are not husbands, but enemies, because you condemn her who discovered safety for us'" ("Vos coniuges non estis sed hostes, quia quae *salutem* nobis inuenit eam damnatis").[11] In a gesture reminiscent of Aristophanes's *Lysistrata*, where sex is withheld for peace, the Greek women rise up and command the patriarchy into submission; the drama of their proclamation mirrors the drama of the central acts of disrobing and discovery. It is not hard to see the connections to the anxieties of covering, uncovering ("illa

[10] Hyginus, *The Myths of Hyginus*, ed. and trans. Mary Grant (Lawrence: University of Kansas Publications, 1960). The identity of the author Hyginus remains subject to ardent debate. Mary Grant seems clear that he was not the commonly accepted C. Julius Hyginus, freedman of Augustus and librarian of the Palatine Library, but paints an ample portrait of the author, based upon evidence from the text itself and contemporary sources. The recent French edition, edited by Jean-Yves Boriaud (Paris: Les Belles Lettres, 2003), still accepts this attribution of Hyginus as a learned freedman, friend of Ovid, erudite and close to the seats of power in contrast to Grant (relying heavily on H.J. Rose's critical edition) who sees evidence in this early work of little more than "a mere schoolboy, and not a very alert one at that" (Grant, p. 3). In any case, it appears clear that the text of the *Fabulae* (known in the original, presumably, as *Genealogiae*) was a type of reference for writers wishing to utilize Greek and Roman myths in some way (Grant, p. 4).

[11] English translation, Grant, p.176; Latin original, Hyginus, *Fabulae*, ed. Peter K. Marshall (Munich: K.G. Saur, 2002), pp. 196–7.

tunica sublata ostendebat se feminam esse" and "tunicam alleuauit et se ostendit feminam esse"), hiding and revealing, suffering and healing so crucial to the story I began with by Louise Boursier.

Of particular relevance to this investigation is the thoroughgoing work of Helen King, whose study of the historical Agnodice (Agnodike to this Hellenist) focuses heavily on the act of "anasyrmos," the gesture of lifting of the garments to reveal the lower part of the body.[12] King shows this gesture to be highly charged and enumerates its many meanings, whether to drive away evil forces, to invite fertility, to provoke laughter, to make oneself sexually available, to shame men in retreat in battle, to prove one's sexual identity or, as in the case among women, to show solidarity. For the purposes of this study, it is these latter two impulses that take precedence, though the wartime scenario—literally, "Is this where you cowards are running back to, back to your mother's womb?"—has some poignancy if we remind ourselves again of Aristophanes's *Lysistrata*, in which women's sexual power is wielded with remarkable, transformative effect, though presumably to opposite ends. King aptly remarks the context in which the story of Agnodice is told: Hyginus's "quis quid inuenerit"—more literally, who discovered what—with an emphasis on *covering* and *un-covering*. To find out how this was played out in the early modern France, we turn first to physician Jacques Guillemeau.

A Surgeon's Handling of Hyginus

Guillemeau's retelling of Hyginus is included at the beginning of Book II of his medical treatise wherein he devotes 13 pages to the duties of midwives (the entire book is 200 pages long). If the percentage of time spent on women's role as practitioners at childbirth is relatively small, it might be explained in the rhetoric of danger and precariousness with which he approaches his subject:

> Or comme ainsi soit que la plus grande maladie que les femmes puissent avoir, est celle des neuf mois, dont la crise & guarison se faict par leur accouchement: Il ne faut point douter que telles femmes ne se soient addonnees & exercees aux accouchemens des femmes, & qu'il y en a eu de tout temps.[13]
>
> (Now since the greatest disease that women can have is that of the nine Moneths, the Crisis and cure whereof consists in their safe deliverie: we must not doubt, but that there have been some women addicted thereto, and practized therein, in all ages…)[14]

[12] Helen King, "Agnodike and the Profession of Medicine," Proceedings of the Cambridge Philological Society, 32 (1986): 53–77.

[13] Jacques Guillemeau, *De l'heureux accouchement des femmes, où il est traicté du gouvernement de leur grossesse, de leur travail naturel et contre nature; du traictement es tant accouchées et de leurs maladies* (Paris, 1609), p. 146.

[14] Jacques Guillemeau, *Child-birth or, The Happy Deliverie of Women*, anonymous translation (London, 1612), p. 81.

The audience is clearly marked as the fraternity of surgeons who must come to terms with the sorority of midwives, as it were, "addonnee & exercees" to the work that men were gradually taking over.

Guillemeau retells the story with clear emphasis on the crisis in women's health:

> …la necessité, maistresse des arts, a contrainct les femmes, les unes avec les autres d'apprendre & practiquer la Medecine: car se trouvans affligees & atteintes de plusieurs maladies en leurs parties honteuses, estans destituees de tous remedes: à faute de quoy plusieurs languissoient, & mouroient miserablement, n'ont osé se descouvrir, & deceler leur mal, qu'à elles-mesmes estimans cela deshonneste.[15]

> (necessitie, (the mistresse of Arts) hath constrained women, to learne and practise Physicke, one with an other. For finding themselves afflicted, and troubled with divers diseases in their naturall parts, and being destitute of all remedies, (for want whereof many perished, and died miserably) they durst not discover, and lay open their infirmities, to any but themselves, accounting it to be dishonest.[16]

It is not surprising that Hyginus's characterization of women "perishing for modesty" came to mind. The "discovering" and "laying open" here of infirmities is clearly related to women's genitalia, the site of childbirth, to be sure, but also of intercourse, desire, shame, pollution, and the ever-threatening licentiousness of women's exposed bodies—the "parties honteuses"—to which we will shall return. Guillemeau's version sticks closely to the myth as told by Hyginus; his is a fairly faithful rendering of the tightly constructed drama of Agnodice's desire for learning: the physical transformation of her hair and clothes; her uncovering of herself to the doubting Athenian women; her subsequent development of an enthusiastic following; the Athenian men's accusation of transvestism and debauchery—ironically that she might be a man posing as a woman; the second "discovery" as her raised tunic proves them wrong; the charge of greater concern, that of studying and practicing as a woman; the Athenian women's uprising and condemnation of the men's objections; and finally, the revising of Athenian law to allow women to study medicine.

Two discrepancies are noticeable and significant. First, it is telling that in Guillemeau's version, Agnodice is said to return from medical school (as it were) to practice first upon a woman characterized as "afflicted in her shameful parts": "ayant esté advertie qu'il y avoit quelque femme *malade en ses parties honteuses*, alla vers elle, pour luy offrir son service: Ce que la malade recusa (sic), estimant que ce fust un homme" (Guillemeau, 144, my emphasis; "having notice of a certaine woman that *was troubled in her naturall parts*; she went unto her, and made proffer of her service; which the sicke party refused, thinking she had been a man," *Child-*

15 Guillemeau, *De l'heureux accouchement*, 143–4.

16 *Child-birth*, 80.

birth, 80) This is indeed how he introduced the idea of midwifery: a profession borne out of women's shame. Hyginus's description of Agnodice's first client was, we may remember, unattached to shame ("et feminam *laborantem audisset ab inferiore parte*"); the "laborantem" does not necessarily suggest the labor of childbirth, as would "parturire." Yet it is somewhat ironic that it would suggest, indeed, "suffering under bodily affliction," but also "a state of being troubled or anxious;" in this case, Guillemeau is seen layering the narrative with the specter of shame and embarrassment more with respect to *himself* than to the woman. Guillemeau appears too troubled or anxious to call it like it is—this "inferiore parte"—without invoking the shamefulness of the woman's vagina and uterus.

Interesting as well is the way in which the two authors describe the climax of the story wherein the Athenian women speak out against the unreasonable injunctions against women's participation in medicine. From Hyginus, who gives them direct speech: "'You are not husbands, but enemies, because you condemn her who discovered safety for us'" (Grant, 176; "Vos coniuges non estis sed hostes, quia quae salutem nobis inuenit eam damnatis," Marshall, 197); and from Guillemeau: "qu'elles ne les tenoient aucunement pour leurs maris & amis, mais pour ennemis, de vouloir condamner celle qui leur donnoit la santé" (Guillemeau, 145; "that they did not account them, for their husbands, and friends, but for enemies; that they would condemne her, which restor'd them to their health," *Child-birth*, 80). Hyginus tells his story in the context of inventors and inventions, people who discover. Agnodice is therefore the actor, the discoverer, the first woman gynecologist, who invents women's safety. Hyginus's women's speech is direct; Guillemeau's is reported. Guillemeau's text remains one about healing and restoring health, a medical view of everything pertaining to women's well-being; the intensity of the Athenian women's dramatic declaration is diminished by the indirect discourse, their voices silenced. Agnodice remains in some ways transvested for Guillemeau. He makes no plea for changes in the laws of early modern France to allow women to practice medicine; for all of the drama that the transvesting narrative affords, Guillemeau's tale is not meant to empower women to become doctors, but to remind men, the "we" in his text (the ubiquitous and unquestionably masculine "on"), that women may well continue to lay claim to this burgeoning profession.[17]

All the better, the reader might well surmise, from the description of bedside fumbling about in the dark that he describes in his "Au Lecteur":

[17] For a contemporaneous example of the battle of the sexes and professions that was played out in print, one need only consult the reports of surgeons regarding the death of Marie de Bourbon Montpensier, 5 days after giving birth while attended by Louise Boursier. The report implicates Louise Boursier as negligent, a charge to which she replies in her *Fidelle relation de l'accouchement, maladie et ouverture du corps de feu MADAME*. For both see Rouget and Winn's modern edition of Boursier's *Récit Véritable*, Appendices I & II, pp. 97–120.

> Or pour la dexterité, il n'y a rien de comparaison avec les autres o(pe)rations: car il ne se faict aucunes oeuvres en Chirurgie, où il ne soit necessaire de voir clair, soit par la lumiere, qui nous est donnee du jour, ou de la chandelle, & que la partie que l'on traicte & manie, ne soit apparente & manifeste à l'oeil. Au contraire, en ceste operation, tant pour la presence de ceux qui assistent, que pour la crainte que pourroit avoir la femme, l'on est contrainct de cacher seulement l'entrée par laquelle il faut mettre la main, puis icelle y estant mise, il faut chercher l'enfant en quelque situation qu'il soit, sans le pouvoir voir…[18]
>
> (Now for the dexteritie: there is no comparision betweene this and other practises; for there be no workes to be done in Chirurgery; where it is not necessary, to have the benefit either of daylight or candle light, and the part which is to be handled, and dressed must be apparent and laid open to the eye. Whereas contrariwise in this worke as well by reason of the company present, as also, least the woman should be afraid, the very entrance, whereby hee should put in his hand, they are constrained to hide: and then his hand being there, he must search for the child (howsoever it be placed) not being able to see it.)[19]

Guillemeau's text suggests the challenge of men practicing upon women in a society fearful of women's exposure or discovery in public: here we have the physician's version of what it was like to attend to a birth such as the one described by Louise Boursier from the beginning of this essay; Guillemeau betrays the compromised nature of this fumbling delivery himself. There is nowhere to look without fear or shame, and yet Guillemeau bravely flaunts the social proscriptions, reaches in and touches, delivers. Tellingly, while Guillemeau is often suspicious of midwives' competency in their vocation because of their gender, he does bring them on the scene in his manual when it comes to the "internal exam" to verify pregnancy:

> … un signe aussi bien certain est recogneu par la Sage-femme, en mettant son doigt dedans le col de la matrice, duquel elle touchera le col interieur d'icelle: si la femme est grosse, elle la trouvera si exactement fermee, que la pointe d'une esguille n'y pourroit pas entrer, il sera mollet neantmoins, & sans estre accompagné d'aucune dureté, lequel pareillement sera retiré en haut, s'estant raccourcy retroussé à raison du corps de la matrice qui s'est resserree en soy, pour embrasser la semence, ce qui est cause que ladite Sage-femme n'y peut toucher que difficilement.[20]
>
> (…another certaine signe may be perceived by the Midwife, who putting up her finger into the wombe to touch the inner orifice thereof, if the woman be with child she shall finde it so close shut, that the point of a needle will scarse enter therein, yet soft, and without any hardnesse, which also will bee drawn upward being shrunke and as it were trussed up, because the body of the Matrice doth gather it selfe together to embrace the seed, which is the reason that the Midwife can very hardly come to reach it with her finger.)[21]

---

18 Guillemeau, e i.

19 *Child-birth*, 7b.

20 Guillemeau, 10.

21 *Child-birth*, 7.

Such intimate knowledge of the woman's cervix is best recounted, it would appear, with a woman's probing finger in mind. What Guillemeau mitigates for, ever so circuitously here, is safer delivery. His rhetoric of "shameful parts," however, suggests that while the birth of the child may be inevitable, the birth of truly enlightened knowledge and safety regarding women's reproduction may be a ways off.

Agnodice as Medical and Literary Gyn-Ecologist

Turning to Catherine des Roches's retelling of the myth of Agnodice, one finds illuminating counterpoint. Inserted in a poetic collection whose themes betray an enthusiastic appraisal of women's community and their literary and domestic lives, this Agnodice becomes a touchstone for women's health and knowability in a way far beyond the scope of Guillemeau.

Catherine des Roches is no physician; she is, however, in the more generous and radical sense of the term, an avid gyn-ecologist (with thanks to Mary Daly).[22] Her version of the Agnodice myth appears in the context of a woman writer coming to terms with bodies of writing, writing bodies, and all of the rich attendant allusions to safety, patriarchal control, and sisterhood that we have observed so far in Louise Boursier and Jacques Guillemeau. Her Agnodice is told by an author who has eschewed births of living children in favor of children of the spirit. As she says to her mother in the preface to the volume that includes the Agnodice:

> J'ay seulement pensé de vous monstrer comme j'employe le temps de ma plus grande oisiveté, et vous supplie humblement (ma mere) de recevoir ces petits escrits qui vous en rendront tesmoignage; si vous en trouvez quelques-uns qui soient assez bien nez, avoüez-les s'il vous plaist pour voz nepveux, et ceux qui ne vous seront agreables, punissez-les à l'exemple de Jacob qui condemna la famille d'Isachar pour obeir à ses autres enfans.
>
> (I have only thought of showing you how I employ my idle time, and humbly beseech you (my Mother) to receive this little collection of writing that bears witness to you; if you find some of them well enough conceived, please acknowledge them as your very own progeny, and those that you do not find

22 The radical connection that Mary Daly makes in her groundbreaking work between women's physical and intellectual and spiritual health is most pertinent to this discussion, though perhaps worthy of elaboration elsewhere: "This book is primarily concerned with the mind/spirit/body pollution inflicted through patriarchal myth and language on all levels … Phallic myth and language generate, legitimate, and mask the material pollution that threatens to terminate all sentient life on this planet. The title *Gyn/Ecology* is a way of wrenching back some wordpower. The fact that most gynecologists are males is in itself a colossal comment on "our" society. It is a symptom and example of male control over women and over language, and a clue to the extent of this control." Mary Daly, *Gyn/Ecology* (Boston: Beacon Press, 1978), p. 9.

> agreeable, punish them in the same way Jacob condemned the family of Issachar to serve his other children.)[23]

Catherine des Roches presents her writings to her own mother as the fruits of her scholarly labor. The "nepveux" of whom she speaks is a play on her mother's birth name, Neveu, felicitously combined with the latinate *neveux* (from *nepotes*) or descendants.[24] What Catherine des Roches gives birth to is a broad-ranging collection of dialogues, sonnets, occasional poems, dedications, epitaphs, a theatrical piece, and the retelling of several biblical and mythological tales. It is a large family she has spawned. The favorite daughter, for my purposes here, is her 177-line verse rendition of the tale of Agnodice.

Her mother Madeleine des Roches has previously shown herself predisposed to literary rather than flesh-and-blood grandchildren; indeed her Ode 1, included in this joint publication, presents one of the most unglamorous and cranky diatribes against wedlock and motherhood one could imagine:

> Noz parens ont de loüables coustumes,
> Pour nous tollir l'usage de raison,
> De nous tenir closes dans la maison
> Et nous donner le fuzeau pour la plume.
>
> Trassant noz pas selon la destinée,
> On nous promet liberté et plaisir:
> Et nous payons l'obstiné desplaisir,
> Portant le dot sous les loix d'Hymenée.
>
> Bientost apres survient une misere
> Qui naist en nous d'un desir mutuel,
> Accompagné d'un soing continuel,
> Qui suit tousjours l'entraille de la mere.[25]
>
> (Our parents have laudable customs
> To deprive us of the use of our reason:
> They lock us up at home
> And hand us the spindle instead of the pen
>
> Conforming our steps to our (female) destiny,
> They promise us liberty and pleasure:
> But we reap continuous displeasure,
> When we lose our dowry to the laws of Marriage.

---

23 Catherine des Roches, *Les Oeuvres* (1578), ed. Anne R. Larsen (Geneva: Droz, 1993), p. 185. Translation, Anne R. Larsen, *Madeleine and Catherine des Roches: From Mother and Daughter* (Chicago: University of Chicago Press, 2006), p. 87.

24 See Larsen's edition of *Les Oeuvres*, p. 185, n. 11.

25 *Oeuvres*, 86–7.

Then soon after comes a new misery,
Born within us of mutual desire,
Accompanied by those continuous cares
That always burden the mother's womb.)[26]

Real progeny seem like the end of a raw deal, wherein bright women are robbed of their study time (giving up the pen for the distaff, an image that her daughter will take up directly in her poem "A ma quenoille") and burdened with the inequitable rules and duties of marriage. One might imagine a far warmer depiction of the arrival of a child than her "misere/qui naist en nous d'un desir mutuel" followed by constant worry by a mother reduced to a burdened gut. One might also imagine a more tempered depiction, given the embeddedness of her poem within the works of her very own, cherished daughter; history suggests however, that Catherine was fully aware of the hardships of the married, childbearing life, a path she chose to avoid to the bafflement and consternation of a multitude of suitors, but not, presumably, of her mother.[27]

Who then, does Agnodice become for Catherine des Roches? Agnodice arrives as a stranger to rescue the Athenian women who are condemned to a life robbed of learning as a consequence of the death of Phocion and the anger of Envy. Envy induces all husbands to become tyrants, forbidding their wives to read books thereby sapping them of the desire or force of will to live. To one such victim she growls:

Car en despit de toy j'animeray les ames 61
Des maris, qui seront les tyrans de leurs femmes,
Et qui leur deffendant le livre et le sçavoir,
Leur osteront aussi de vivre le pouvoir.[28]

(For to spite you, I'll incite
Husbands to become the tyrants of their wives;
By keeping learning and books from them,
They'll take away their very desire to live.')[29]

---

[26] Larsen, *From Mother and Daughter*, 53.

[27] See the judgments of the family friend Estienne Pasquier as he ruminates over Catherine des Roches's reticence in matters of marriage: "Il n'y a qu'une chose qui me déplaise en ceste maison, qu'estant la fille belle en perfection tant de corps que d'esprit, riche de biens, comme celle qui doit estre l'unique heritiere de sa mere, requise en mariage par une infinité de personnages d'honneur, toutes-fois elle met toutes ces requestes sous pied; resolue de vivre & mourir avec sa mère" ("There is but one thing that displeases me in this household, that the daughter, possessed of a perfect beauty of both body and soul, wealthy (as she is her mother's sole inheritor), all the same, she refuses all suitors, resolved to live and die with her mother"). Estienne Pasquier, Letter to Monsieur Pithou, Seigneur de Savoye (Book VI, Letter 11 of his *Lettres familières*) in Anne R. Larsen's edition of Madeleine and Catherine des Roches, *Les Missives* (1586) (Geneva: Droz, 1999), pp. 348–9.

[28] *Oeuvres* 1578, 335–440.

[29] Larsen, *From Mother and Daughter*, 124–5.

Des Roches thus embellishes the Hyginus tale at the onset by positing the source of women's torment, not as the pangs of labor, nor the onset of some gynecological disorder, but as a physical reaction to the privation of their vocational, or better, literary aspirations. The decree causes a physical malaise that soon afflicts the spiritually bereft women:

> Les dames aussitost se trouverent suivies 73
> De fiebvres, de langueurs, et d'autres maladies;
> Leur faisoit supporter incroyables tourmens.
> Aymant trop mieux mourir que d'estre peu honteuses 76
> Contant aux Medecins leurs peines langoureuses,
> Les femmes (o pitié!) n'osoient plus se mesler
> De s'aider l'une l'autre; on les faisoit filler.[30]
>
> (The women soon found themselves beset
> By fevers, faintness, and other illnesses,
> Envy forced them to bear incredible torments.
> They preferred death to the shame of
> Telling the (male) Doctors about their debilitating troubles.
> The women (what a pity!) did not dare
> To help one another, they were made to spin.)[31]

The "tourmens" and "peines langoureuses" are quite clearly references to the women-and-knowledge boilerplate text from Genesis, that the torments of labor are a reminder of woman's original sin, the sin of desire for knowledge whose consequences are likewise linked to her reproductive capacities.

> Enter Agnodice.
> Ceste Dame, cachant l'or de sa blonde tresse, 92
> Aprist la medecine, et s'en feit grand maistresse.
> Puis se resouvenant de son affection,
> Voulut effectuer sa bonne intention, 95
> Et guerir les douleurs de ses pauvres voisines[32]
>
> (This young woman, hiding the gold of her blond locks,
> Learned medicine, and became quite expert at it.
> Then, remembering her original intent,
> She wanted to carry out her plan
> To heal the sufferings of her poor sisters)[33]

Agnodice returns and the crucial scene "self-disclosure" or "self-discovery" is enacted:

---

30 *Oeuvres*, 336.

31 Larsen, *From Mother and Daughter*, 126–7.

32 *Oeuvres*, 336.

33 Larsen, *From Mother and Daughter*, 126–7.

Agnodice, voyant leur grande chasteté,
Les estima beaucoup pour ceste honnesteté;
Lors descouvrant du sein les blanches pommes rondes,
Et de son chef doré les belles tresses blondes,
Monstre qu'elle estoit fille, et que son gentil cueur
Les vouloit delivrer de leur triste langueur.
Les Dames admirant ceste honte naïsve,
Et de son teint douillet la blanche couleur vive,
Et de son sein poupin le petit mont jumeau,
Et de son chef sacré l'or crepelu tant beau,
Et de ses yeux divins les flammes ravissantes,
Et de ses doux propos les graces attirantes,
Baiserent mille fois et sa bouche et son sein,
Recevant le secours de son heureuse main.[34]

(Agnodice, seeing their great chastity,
Esteemed them all the more for their virtue,
And uncovering then the white round apples (of her bosom),
And the beautiful blond tresses of her golden head,
Showed that she was a maiden, and that her kind heart
Wished to deliver them from their sad predicament.
The Ladies admiring her innocent modesty,
And the lively whiteness of her soft complexion,
And the little twin mounts of her adorable breasts,
And the beautiful golden shine of her blessed head,
And the ravishing flames of her divine eyes,
And the engaging gracefulness of her sweet words,
Kissed a thousand times both her mouth and her breast,
As they received help from her blessed hands.)[35]

The story here becomes ever more lyrical, ecstatic, and erotic; the women of Athens are delivered from their "langueur"—the illness induced by the privation of learning—into a state of delirious contentment. In contrast to Hyginus and Guillemeau (and most poignantly, perhaps, to Boursier), the woman's body is touchable, and knowable in a way that flies in the face of accusations of licentiousness: des Roches participates fully in the rhetoric of love poetry, and of the blazon in particular as she delineates the woman's body in all its glorious detail. She lingers specifically on the breast, "les blanches pommes rondes" (the white round apples) reiterated in "son sein poupin le petit mont jumeau" (the little twin mounts of her adorable breasts) illuminated by the "flammes ravissantes" (ravishing flames) of her heavenly countenance. The scene culminates in rapture as the Athenian women kiss her mouth and breast while receiving the help of her blessed hand.

Other possible allusions from the ancient world attest ever more suggestively to a view to women's empowerment and community. In Greek myth, Baubo, in an

[34] *Oeuvres*, 337.

[35] Larsen, *From Mother and Daughter*, 127, 129.

attempt to relieve the torment of grief, was said to have joked with the bereaved goddess Demeter by painting a face on her stomach and then pulling her dress over her head and dancing. The anger and anguish that the Athenian women express is clearly fueled by grief over their neglected sisters. The sisterhood of the goddess Diana surrounded by her nymphs is clearly another reference, especially given the physical descriptions: Diana is the chaste female figure *par excellence* whose very existence relied on the exclusion of men for her survival (and when you got too close, you got eaten by your own dogs…). Helen King remarks this possible allusion to the original Agnodice, placing it squarely in the context of Hyginus's work. In Fabula 189, he retells the story of Procris, a woman, who cuts her hair and dons a tunic and challenges and beats her husband in a hunt. He asks for the javelin and the dog that Diana had given her in exchange for money; she asks instead for sex and reveals herself posthaste as a woman: "tunicam leuauit et ostendit se feminam esse et coniugem eius" (King, 61). The utopian gynaceum that des Roches depicts is rich with the erotic potential of her ancient predecessors, here to the exclusion of men.

Such a contrast we have here to the plight of Guillemeau whose *unhappy* hand gropes about blindly in the dark, ashamed both for himself and for his patient. Des Roches's women, on the other hand, have found not only health and safety, but a renaissance in letters rendered through this particular climactic moment, an act that would be impossible, inappropriate, indeed unspeakable, by Agnodice's male counterpart. Agnodice arrives and is given this excited welcome by women thanks to the fact that they have at last a healer who, with no sense of impropriety or shame, can touch them. When word gets around that Agnodice is attending to these women to their obvious well-being and delight, the same scene of revelation is enacted for the male authorities who, in a fantasy of stunning conversion, stand in mute, awed acceptance:

Depuis qu'elle eut parlé, oncq une seulle voix
Ne s'esleva contre elle; ains toute l'assistance
Monstroit d'esmerveiller ceste rare excellence;
Ils estoient tous ravis, sans parler ny mouvoir,
Ententifs seulement à l'ouyr et la voir.
Comme l'on voit parfois apres un long orage,
R'asserener les vents, et calmer le rivage.[36]

(After she had spoken, not a single voice
Was raised against her; on the contrary, the entire audience
Marveled at her rare excellence;
Everyone was filled with wonder, and no one moved or made a sound,
Attentive only to hearing and seeing her.
In like manner one sometimes sees, after a long storm,
The winds die down, and the waves become calm.)[37]

[36] *Oeuvres*, 339.

[37] Larsen, *From Mother and Daughter*, 131

And so Catherine des Roches dispenses with the scene wherein Agnodice is condemned and then subsequently defended by her Athenian sisters; in her version, Agnodice's compelling oratory on her own behalf stuns the men into submission. The storm of controversy surrounding women attending to women is calmed entirely by one learned and persuasive woman. Agnodice singlehandedly transforms the Envy-tainted society that has banished women from books and learning and begins the work of repairing wounded minds and bodies. Agnodice is the midwife of children of both the body and the spirit. The labor is difficult and noble and cherished for women in a society suspicious and highly proscriptive, a society that links women's unworthiness constantly to the messiness, the shame, and the mutable nature of their bodies. And so Agnodice arrives to dispel such mythologizing and indeed to turn such opinion on its head: perhaps women are worthy and capable *because* of this ability to reproduce.

Facing the Blank Page and Women's Reproductivity

I hope to have demonstrated that the retelling of the myth of Agnodice by a physician, Jacques Guillemeau, and an early modern female poet, Catherine des Roches, means different things for the authors and constituencies concerned. Guillemeau's version is retold in the context of a sincere coming-to-terms with the anxieties and exigencies surrounding women's health at the time; he is not immune to the illogical, silly, and ultimately dangerous proscriptions against men's "illumination" with regard to women's health—he does not use the tale of Agnodice, however, to propose education for women that would allow them to take over his role. He is interested in producing responsible midwives who know when to call the doctor. Catherine des Roches, on the other hand, extols the glories of women as at once (re)producers, midwives, and physicians as a metaphor for protecting women's livelihood in the realm of letters. Their ecstatic enthusiasm comes in equal measure to the immense oppression we saw quite clearly and sadly drawn in her mother's first ode.

To conclude, I would direct us to a document of keen interest to this discussion from a contemporaneous translation of Guillemeau's text. It is the anonymous translator's epistle wherein he feels compelled to defend himself for having brought such delicate material to light. It is he who makes the most eloquent bridge between literary and anatomical production one could imagine. His anxiety is everywhere apparent:

> Thus far hath the Authour pleaded for him selfe, whom while I Translate, least the fault be translated upon me, I will speake somewhat for my selfe, before I be accused, there be no bodie to speake for me: If therefore it be thought prejudiciall, either to the literarie common-wealth of Physicke, that I have exported and made common a commoditie, which the learned would have had private to themselves: or if I have been offensive to Women, in prostituting and divulging that, which they would not have come to open light, and which beside cannot be exprest in such modest terms, as are fit for the virginitie of pen and

> paper, and the white sheetes of their Child-bed. I must (as well as I can) defend my selfe from these imputations, and shew my care to keep both learning and modestie illibate, and inviolable … As for women (whom I am most afraid to offend) they must be content to have their infirmities detected, if they will have helpe for them, which I wish might not come to any eare or eye, but to those which they themselves would have acquainted therewith, and as well for their sakes, as mine owne satisfaction: I have endevoured to be as private and retired, in expressing al the passages in this kind as possibly I could.[38]

The translator thus declares himself appropriately concerned with bringing "to open light" the woman's body with all of the attendant discourse of shame and licentiousness: prostitution, divulging, violation. He is in concert with Guillemeau in this way, and he appears not to shy from promoting a sort of public-health message of his own that encourages women to benefit from this wisdom and swallow the inevitable shame: his prose is potentially life-saving. It is the arresting image of the virgin pen and the white sheets of childbed that remain with us, however. The productive pen must spill ink to express itself; no childbed sheets remain white for very long.

It is a document created for feminist critic Susan Gubar's discovery and delectation. Her groundbreaking work on women's creativity in nineteenth- and twentieth-century literature, most notably "'The Blank Page' and the Issues of Female Creativity," airs women's dirty laundry, as it were, and sees in both the stained sheets of the virgin's wedding bed and those that emerge shockingly pristine in the case of her lapsed sisters, a history of women—their bodies, their beds, and their books—as perpetually interwoven.

> Because of the forms of self-expression available to women, artistic creation often feels like a violation, a belated reaction to male penetration rather than a possessing and controlling. Not an ejaculation of pleasure but a reaction to rending, the blood on the royal marriage sheets seems to imply that women's paint and ink are produced through a painful wounding, a literal influence of male authority. If artistic creativity is likened to biological creativity, the terror of inspiration for women is experienced quite literally as the terror of being entered, deflowered, possessed, taken, had, broken, ravished—all words which illustrate the pain of the passive self whose boundaries are being violated.[39]

Guillemeau and his translator are clearly dealing with the post-virginal woman's body, yet the ravishing of which Gubar writes is entirely consonant with the extreme trepidation with which male physicians approached the woman's body during birth. As for the translator's virgin pen—well, never has a case of phallic anxiety been more clearly construed. He as well fears the wrath of accusations

---

38 "Translator's Preface," in Guillemeau, *Child-birth*, p. 2.

39 Susan Gubar, "'The Blank Page' and the Issues of Female Creativity" in Elizabeth Abel (ed.), *Writing and Sexual Difference* (Chicago: University of Chicago Press, 1982), p. 80.

for the improper use of his instrument. Alas, ink must be spilled in order to save women's lives, says he. Again, from Gubar:

> This model of the pen–penis writing on the virgin page participates in a long tradition identifying the author as a male who is primary and the female as his passive creation—a secondary object lacking autonomy, endowed with often contradictory meaning but denied intentionality. Clearly this tradition excludes woman from the creation of culture, even as it reifies her as an artifact within culture. It is therefore particularly problematic for those women who want to appropriate the pen by becoming writers.[40]

Des Roches's experience is radically transformative of this notion of creativity as issuing from wounding or phallic penetration. The Athenian women greet Agnodice—the discoverer of their safety, the guardian of their health—with deep sensual, if not sexual, pleasure at the rediscovery of their learned selves, not far removed from the ejaculation of pleasure of which Gubar writes, yet utterly feminized: Catherine has, in effect, called upon Agnodice to lead her mother out of the misery of marriage and childbirth and shown light on a powerful, supportive, grateful, ecstatic community of women, free at last to touch and to tell.

---

40 Gubar, 70.

Bibliography

Primary Sources

Agrippa, Heinrich Cornelius. *De nobilitate et praecellentia foeminei sexus*. R. Antonioli et al., eds. Geneva: Droz, 1990.

———. *De Occulta Philosophia*. Cologne, 1533.

———. *Of vanitie and uncertaintie of Arts and Sciences*. Trans. James Sanford. London: John Daye, 1589.

———. *Three Books of Occult Philosophy*. Trans. J[ames] F[rench]. London, 1651.

Alberti, Leon Battista. *The Family in Renaissance Florence*. Bk. III. Renée Neu Watkins, ed. and trans. Illinois: Waveland Press, 1994.

Allestree, Richard. *The Ladies Calling*. London, 1673.

Ariosto, Ludovico. *Satire e rime, nuovamente ordinate e corredate di note con in fine: L'erbolario, Le lettere, Le poesie attribuite all'autore e I carmi latini*. Trieste: Sez. letterario-artistica del Lloyd austriaco, 1858.

Aristotle. *Generation of Animals*. In *The Complete Works of Aristotle*. Ed. Jonathan Barnes. Princeton, NJ: Princeton University Press, 1984.

Artis Auriferae. Basel, 1572.

Ashmole, Elias. *Theatrum Chemicum Britannicum*. London, 1652.

d'Aubigné, Théodore Agrippa. *Les Tragiques*. *Oeuvres*. H. Weber, ed. Paris: Gallimard, 1969.

Bacon, Francis. *The Advancement of Learning*. Ed. G.W. Kitchin. London: J.M. Dent & Sons Ltd., 1973; Totowa, NJ: Rowman and Littlefield, 1974.

———. *Selected Writings of Francis Bacon*. Introduction by Hugh G. Dick. New York: Modern Library, 1955.

Bacon, Roger. *The Mirror of Alchimy*. London, 1599.

Bauhin, Caspar. *De corporis humani fabrica* ... Basel: Sebastianum Henricpetri, 1590.

Bourgeois, Louise (Boursier). *Apologie de Louise Bourgeois Dite Bourcier sage femme de la Royne Mere du Roy, & de feu Madame. Contre le Rapport des Medecins*. Paris: Chez Melchior Mondiere, 1627.

———. *Observations diverses sur la stérilité, perte de fruict, foecondité, accouchements et maladies des femmes, & enfants nouveaux naix, amplement traitées, et heureusement praticquées par L. Bourgeois dite Boursier*. Paris: H. Ruffin, 1652.

———. *Observations diverses sur la stérilité, perte de fruits, fécondité, accouchements et maladies des femmes et enfants nouveau-nés suivi de Instructions à ma fille*. Françoise Olive, ed. Paris: côté-femmes, 1992.

———. *Récit véritable de la naissance de messeigneurs et dames les enfans de France* [Instruction à ma fille, et autres textes]. F. Rouget and C. Winn, ed. Geneva: Droz, 2000.

Bruno, Giordano. *Le Cena De Le Ceneri* [*The Ash Wednesday Supper*, 1584]. Ed. and trans. Edward A. Gosselin and Lawrence S. Lerner. Toronto, Buffalo, and London: University of Toronto Press, Renaissance Society of America Reprint Texts 4, 1977, reprint 1995.

Bry, Theodor de, *America tertia pars memorabilem provinciae Brasiliae historiam continens…* Frankfurt: M. Becker, 1605.

Campanella, Tommaso. *Astrologicorum Libri VI. In quibus Astrologia, omni superstitione Arabum & Iudæorum eliminata, physiologicè tratatur, secundùm S. Scripturas, & doctrinam S. Thomæ, & Alberti, & summorum Theologorum; Ita ut absque suspicione mala in Ecclesia Dei multa cum utilitate legi possint.* Lugduni, 1629.

———. *The City of the Sun.* In *Ideal Commonwealths*. Henry Morley, ed. New York: Colonial Press, 1901.

Carpi, Jacopo Berengario da. *Isagogae breves, perlucidae ac uberrimae in anatomiam humani corporis*. Bologna: Benedictus Hector, 1523.

Cavendish, Margaret. *Philosophical and Physical Opinions* (London, 1663). "To his Excellencie the Lord Marquis of Newcastle."

———. *Observations upon Experimental Philosophy*. London, 1666.

Cervantes, Miguel de. *Don Quijote de la Mancha*. Ed. Francisco Rico. Madrid: Crítica, 1998. Vol. 1.

Clifford, Anne. *Lives of Lady Anne Clifford Countess of Dorset, Pembroke, and Montgomery (1590–1676) and of her parents summarized by herself.* J.P. Gilson, ed. London: Roxburghe Club, 1916.

———. *The Diary of Anne Clifford, 1616–1619: A Critical Edition*. Katherine O. Acheson, ed. London: Garland, 1995.

A Closet for Ladies and Gentlewomen. London, 1608.

Coelson, Lancelot. *Philosophia maturata an exact piece of philosophy containing the practick and operative part thereof in gaining the philosophers stone: with the wayes how to make the mineral stone and the calcinations of mettals: whereunto is added a work compiled by St. Dunstan concerning the philosophers stone: and the experiments of Rumelius and preparations of Angelo Sala, all most famous chymists in their time*. London, 1668.

Copie d'une letter escripte a Monsieur du Chesne d'une Docte demoiselle de france. Denmark: Copenhagen, Royal Library MS. 1792.

Cortese, Isabella. *I Secreti de la Signora Isabella Cortese: Ne'quali si contengo cose minerali, medicinali, artificiose, e Alchimique, & molte de l'arte profumatoria, appartenenti e ogni gran Signora*. Venice: Giovanni Bariletto, 1574.

———. *I secreti della Signora Isabella Cortese*. Chicca Gagliardo, ed. Milan: La Vita Felice, 1995.

Coste, Hilarion de. *Les Eloges et vies des reynes, des princesses, et des dames illustres en piété, en courage & en doctrine, qui ont fleury de nostre temps, & du temps de nos Peres*. Paris: Cramoisy, 1647.

De Alchimia opuscula complura veterum philosophorum [...] *Rosarium Philosophorum Secunda Pars*. Frankfurt: Cyriac Jacob, 1550.

De arte cabalistica [On the Art of the Kabbalah]. Hague, 1517.

de Leon, Moses. *The Zohar*. Pritzker Edition. Daniel C. Matt, trans Stanford: Stanford University Press, 2004.

Dee, John. *Elements of Geometrie of the most auncient Philosopher Euclide of Megara*. Trans. Sir Henry Billingsley. London, 1570.

———. *John Dee on Astronomy: Propaedeumata Aphoristica (1558–1568) Latin and English*. Ed. and tr. Wayne Shumaker. Berkeley: University of California Press, 1978.

———. *Monas Hieroglyphia*. Trans. C.H. Josten. Journal of the Society for the Study of Alchemy and Early Chemistry (1964): 199–200.

———. *The Private Diary of Dr. John Dee, and the Catalogue of his Library of Manuscripts*. From the original manuscripts in the Ashmolean Museum at Oxford and Trinity College Library, Cambridge. London: Camden Society, 1842.

Descartes, René. *Discourse: On the Method of Rightly Conducting Reason and Seeking Truth in the Sciences*, [*Discours de la Méthode pour bien conduire le raison et chercher la Verité dans les sciences*], 1637. Trans. John Veitch. In *The Method, Meditations, and Philosophy of Descartes*. New York: Tudor Publishing Co., 1901.

Digby, Kenelm. *Choice and Experimented Receipts in Physick and Chirurgery*. London, 1668.

Discours philosophical. Paris: Bibliothèque Mazarine MS 3681 (2679), no 22.

Dodoens, Rembert. *A Niewe Herball: Or, Historie of Plantes*. Trans. Henry Lyte, 4 edns, 1578–1619.

Epistola Nobilissime Matrone de Martinvilla ad Dom Quercitanum + 1609. Copenhagen: The Royal Library, MS 1776.

Espagnet, Jean d'. *L'Oeuvre secret de la Philosophie d'Hermès, précédé de la Philosophie naturelle restituée*. Paris: Denoel, 1972.

———. *La Philosophie naturelle restablie en sa pureté, où l'on void à découvert toute l'oeconomie de la nature et où se manifestent quantité d'erreurs de la philosophie ancienne... avec le traicté de l'Ouvrage secret de la philosophie d'Hermez qui enseigne la matière et la façon de faire la pierre philosophale*. Jean Bachou, trans. Paris: E. Pépingué, 1651.

———. *Miroir des Alchimistes*. Sl, 1609.

Estienne, Charles. *De dissection partium corporis humani libri tres*. Paris: Simon Colinaeus, 1545.

———. *Maison Rustique*. Richard Surflet, trans. London, 1600.

———. *Paradoxes*. Trevor Peach, ed. Geneva: Droz, 1998.

Fanshawe, Ann, and Anne Halkett. *The Memoirs of Anne, Lady Halkett and Ann, Lady Fanshawe*. John Loftis, ed. Oxford: Clarendon Press, 1979.

Ficino, Marsilio. *De vita coelitùs comparanda*. In *Three Books on Life*. Carol V. Kaske and John R. Clark, ed. and trans. Tempe, AZ: Medieval and Renaissance Texts and Studies, The Renaissance Society of America, 1998.

Fitzherbert, John. *Fitzharberts Booke of Husbandrie*. London, 1598.

Flamel, Nicholas. *Nicholas Flammel, his exposition of the hieroglyphicall figures*. Eirenaeus Orandus, trans. London, 1624.

French, John. *The Art of Distillation*. London, 1651.

Gerard, John. *The Herball or Generall Historie of Plantes*. London, 1597; revised edition, Thomas Johnson in 1633

Gesner, Conrad. *The Treasure of Euonymus*. London, 1559.

Gournay, Marie de. *Apology for the Woman Writing*. Richard Hillman and Colette Quesnel, tr. Chicago and London: The University of Chicago Press, 2002.

———. *Bouquet de Pinde*. M. Bertelà, ed. Ravenna: Longo, 1995.

———. *Fragments d'un discours féminin*, E. Dezon-Jones, ed. Paris: Corti, 1988.

———. *Oeuvres Complètes*. Jean-Claude Arnould et al., eds. Paris: Champion, 2002, 2 vols.

———. *Preface to the Essays of Michel de Montaigne*. Richard Hillman and Colette Quesnel, trans. and ed. Tempe, AZ: Medieval and Renaissance Texts and Studies, The Renaissance Society of America, 1998.

———. *Le Proumenoir de Monsieur de Montaigne*. Paris: Champion, 1996.

———. *Textes relatifs à la calomnie*. C. Venesoen, ed. Tübingen: Narr, 1998.

Guillemeau, Jacques. *Child-birth or, The Happy Deliverie of Women*. Anonymous translation. London: A. Hatfield, 1612.

———. *De la grossesse et accouchement des femmes: du governement dicelles et moyen de survenir aux accidents qui leur arrivent, Ensemble de la nourriture des enfans*. Paris: Abraham Pacard, 1620.

———. *De l'heureux accouchement des femmes, où il est traicté du gouvernement de leur grossesse, de leur travail naturel et contre nature; du traictement es tant accouchées et de leurs maladies*. Paris: Buon, 1609.

———. *Oeuvres de chirurgie de Jacques Guillemeau, chirurgien ordinaire du roy et juré à Paris, avec les pourtraicts de toutes les parties du corps humain et des instruments necessaries au chirurgien, augementée et mises en un et enrichies de plusieurs traictez, pris des leçons de Mr. Germain Courtin, Docteur en medicine*. Paris: Nicolas Buon, 1612.

———. *Child-birth or, The Happy Deliverie of Women. Wherein is set down the Government of Women*. Amsterdam: Theatrvm Orbis Terrarvm Ltd., 1972.

Hariot, Thomas. *Admiranda narratio, fida tamen, de commodis et incolarum ritibus Virginiae ... Anglico scripta sermone à Thomas Hariot*. Ed. and illus. by Theodor and Johann Theodor de Bry. Frankfurt: de Bry, 1590.

Hartman, George. *The True Preserver and Restorer of Health*. London, 1682.

Hermetica. Trans. and ed. Brian P. Copenhaver. Cambridge: Cambridge University Press, 1992.

Hoby, Margaret. *Diary of Lady Margaret Hoby, 1599–1605*. Dorothy M. Meads, ed. London: George Routledge & Sons, 1930.

———. *The Private Life of an Elizabethan Lady: The Diary of Lady Margaret Hoby, 1599–1605*. Joanna Moody, ed. Stroud: Sutton, 1998.

Howard, Alathea. *Natura exenterata: or Nature unbowelled by the most exquisite anatomizers of her*. London, 1655.

Huarte de San Juan, Juan. *Examen des esprits pour les sciences*. Biarritz: Atlantica, 2000.

Hyginus. *Fabulae*. Peter K. Marshall, ed. Munich: K.G. Saur, 2002.

———. *The Myths of Hyginus*. Mary Grant, trans. and ed. Lawrence: University of Kansas Publications, 1960.

Johnson, Thomas. *The Herball or Generall Historie of Plantes*. London, revised edition, 1633.

Jonson, Ben. *The Alchemist*. Elizabeth Cook, ed, 2nd edn. London: A & C Black, 1995.

Jonstonus, Joannes. *An History of the Wonderful Things of Nature*. London, 1657.

Kent, Elizabeth. *A choice manuall, or rare and select secrets in physick and chyrurgery collected, and practised by the Right Honourable, the Countesse of Kent, late deceased*. London, 1653.

La Toyson d'Or. Oxford: Bodleian Library, Ashmole MS 1395.

The Ladies Cabinet Opened. London, 1639.

The Ladies Cabinet Enlarged and Opened. London, 1654

Lambsprinck. *De Lapide Philosophico Libellis*. Frankfurt: Luca Jennis, 1625.

Le Moyne de Morgues, Jacques. *America, Brevis narratio eorum quae in Florida Americae provincial Gallis acciderunt…* Ed. and illus. by Theodor and Theodor Johann de Bry. Frankfurt: de Bry, 1591.

Léry, Jean de. *History of a Voyage to the Land of Brazil*. Ed. Janet Whatley. Berkeley: University of California Press, 1990.

Les Amadis en France au XVIe siècle. Paris: Editions Rue d'Ulm/Presses de l'Ecole Normale Supérieure, 2000.

Lodge, Thomas. *The Complete Works of Thomas Lodge*. Edmund Gosse, ed. Glasgow: Hunterian Club, 1883.

Machiavelli, Niccolò. *Il principe*. Ed. Luigi Firpo. Turin: Einaudi, 1984.

Magnus, Albertus. *De Spiritu & Respiratione*. *Opera Omnia*, XI, ed. Borgnet. Paris: Louis Vivès, 1890.

Maier, Michael. *Atalanta fugiens*. Kassel: Bärenreiter-Verlag, 1964.

———. *Atalanta fugiens*. Trans. and ed. Joscelyn Godwin. Grand Rapids: Phanes, 1989.

———. *Symbola Aureae Mensae Duodecim Nationum*. Frankfurt: Luca Jennis, 1617.

Markham, Gervase. *The English Huswife*. London, 1615.

Meurdrac, Marie. *La Chymie charitable et facile, en faveur des Dames* (1666). Jean Jacques, ed. Paris: CNRS Editions, 1999.

Mikrokosmographia: a description of the body of man: together with the controversies and figures thereto belonging / collected and translated out of all the best authors of anatomy, especially out of Gaspar Bauhinus and Andréas Laurentius. Helkiah Crooke, ed. London: printed by R.C. and are to be sold by Iohn Clarke, 1651.

Montaigne, Michel de. *Oeuvres Complètes*. Albert Thibaudet and Maurice Rat, eds. Paris: Gallimard, 1962.

———. *Essais*. Pierre Villey, ed. Paris: Presses Universitaires de France, 1978.

———. *The Essays of Michel de Montaigne*. Michael A. Screech, trans. and ed. London: Allen Lane, 1991.

———. *Les Essais*. Jean Balsamo, et. al ed. Paris: Gallimard, 2007.

Nicholas of Cusa. *Opera*. Paris, 1514; rpt. Frankfurt: Minerva, 1962.

Orlebar, Diana Astry. "Diana Astry's Recipe Book." Bette Stitt, ed. *The Publications of the Bedfordshire Historical Record Society* 37 (1957): 83–168.

Ovid (Publius Ovidius Naso). *Metamorphoses*. Rolfe Humphries, trans. Bloomington: Indiana University Press, 1963.

———. *Metamorphoses*. William S. Anderson, ed. Leipzig: Teubner, 1985.

Paracelsus (Theophrastus Bombast von Hohenheim). *Archidoxa*. Kracow: 1569.

———. *Archidoxa. De tinctura physicorum; de occulta philosophi*. Strasburg: 1570.

———. *The Hermetic and Alchemical Writings*. A.E. Waite, ed. and trans. London: J. Elliott, 1894.

———. *Selected Writings*. Ed. Jolande Jacobi. Bollingen Series XXII. Princeton: Princeton University Press, 1951/1979.

Paré, Ambroise. *Deux Livres De Chirurgie: I. De la generation de l'homme, et maniere d'extraire les enfants hors du ventre de la mère, ensemble ce qu'il faut faire pour la faire mieux et plustost accoucher, avec le cure de plusiers maladies qui lui peuvent survenir*. Paris, André Wechel, 1573.

———. *Des Monstres et prodiges*. Jean Céard, ed. Geneva: Droz, 1971

Partlicius, Simeon. *A new method of physick: or, A short view of Paracelsus and Galen's practice*. London, 1654.

Partridge, John. *The Treasurie of Hidden Secrets*. London, 1633.

Pasquier, Estienne. *Lettres familières* [1586]. D. Thickett, ed. Geneva: Droz, 1974.

Pico della Mirandola, Giovanni. *Commentary on a Poem of Platonic Love*. Trans. Douglas Carmichael. New York and London: University Press of America, 1986.

———. *Disputationes Adversus Astrologiam Divinatricem*. (1493–94, first edition 1496) Ed. Eugene Garin. Florence: Vallechi, 1952.

———. *Opera Omnia*. Basel, 1572.

———. *Oration: On the Dignity of Man*. Trans. Elizabeth L. Forbes. *The Renaissance Philosophy of Man*. Ed. Ernst Cassirer, Paul O. Kristeller, and John H. Randall, Jr. Chicago: The University of Chicago Press, Phoenix Books, 1948.

Petrarch, Francesco. *De ignorantia* [*On his own ignorance and that of many others*]. Hans Nachod, trans. *The Renaissance Philosophy of Man*. Ed. Ernst Cassirer, Paul O. Kristeller, and John H. Randall, Jr. Chicago: The University of Chicago Press, Phoenix Books, 1948.

———. *Secretum*. Trans. Davy Carozza and H. James Shey. New York: Peter Lang, 1989.

Plato. *Republic*. Robin Waterfield, trans. Oxford: Oxford University Press, 2008.

———. *Republic*. In *The Collected Dialogues of Plato*. Edith Hamilton and Huntington Cairns, ed. New York: Bollingen Foundation, 1961.

Platt, Hugh. *Jewell House of Art and Nature*. London, 1594.

La poésie baroque et précieuse (1550–1650). André Blanchard, ed. Paris: Seghers, 1985.

Pomponazzi, Pietro. *De immortalitate animae*. Trans. William H. Hay II, rev. John H. Randall, Jr. *The Renaissance Philosophy of Man*. Ed. Ernst Cassirer, Paul O. Kristeller, and John H. Randall, Jr. Chicago: The University of Chicago Press, Phoenix Books, 1948.

Postel, Guillaume. *De Orbis terrae Concordia: libri quatuor...* Basel: Oporinus, 1544.

———. *De la Republique des Turcs, et là ou l'occasion s'offrira, des meurs et loy de tous Muhamedistes...Histoire et considération de l'origine, loy et coustume des Tartares, Persiens, Arabes, Turcs...* Poitiers: Chez E. de Marnef, 1560.

———. *Les très merveilleuses victoires des femmes du nouveau monde*. Geneva: Slatkine Reprints, 1970.

Primaleón. Marín Pina, María Carmen, ed. Alcalá: Centro de Estudios Cervantinos, 2001.

Quercitan's Daughter's Letters. London: British Library, Sloane MS 693.

Rabelais, François. *Quart livre*. Mireille Huchon, ed. Paris: Gallimard, 1998.

Remonstrance à Madame Bourcier touchant son Apologie contre le Rapport que les medecins ont faict de ce qui a causé la mort deplorable de Madame. Paris: J. Jacquin, 1627.

Ricettario galante. Del principio del secolo XVI. Olindo Guerrini, ed. Bologna: Gaetano Romagnoli, 1883.

Roches, Catherine des. *Les Œuvres* [1578]. Anne R. Larsen, ed. Geneva: Droz, 1993.

Rodríguez de Montalvo, Garci. *Amadís de Gaula*. Ed. Juan Manuel Cacho Blecua. Madrid: Cátedra, 1987–1988.

Rosarium philosophorum. Oxford: Bodleian Library, Ashmole MS 1459.

Rosarium Philosophorum: Ein Alchemisches Florilegium des Spätmittelaltes, Faksimile des illustrierten Estausgabe Frankfurt 1550. Joachim Telle, ed. Weinheim: VCH Verlagsgesellschaft, 1992.

The Rosary of the Philosophers. Adam McLean, ed. Edinburgh: Magnum Opus Sourceworks, 1980.

Ruscelli, Girolamo. *The seconde part of the Secretes of Master Alexis of Piemont*. William Warde, trans. London, 1560.

———. *The secretes of the reuerend Maister Alexis of Piemont*. William Warde, trans. London, 1558.

Salutati, Coluccio. *De laboribus Herculis*. Ed. Berthold L. Ullman. Zürich: Artemis Verlag, 1951.

Secreti diversi e miracolosi. Raccolti dal Falloppio... Venice, Zaltieri, 1588.

Sefer Yetzirah: The Book of Creation in Theory and Practice. Revised edition, ed. Aryeh Kaplan. San Francisco: Weiser Books, 1997.

Shelley, Mary. *Frankenstein*. New York: W.W. Norton, 1995.

Shirley, John. *The Accomplished Ladies Rich Closet of Rarities*. 4th edn, 1694.

Speght, Rachel. *The Polemics and Poems of Rachel Speght*. Barbara Kiefer Lewalski, ed. Oxford, Oxford University Press, 1996.

Staden, Hans. *Americae tertia pars memorabilem provinciae Brasiliae historiam continens, Germanico primum sermone scriptam à Ioanne Stadio…*Theodor and Johann Theodor de Bry, ed. and illus. Frankfurt: Matthias Becker, 1592, then 1605.

Stuart, Arbella. *The Letters of Arbella Stuart*. Sara Jayne Steen, ed. Oxford: Oxford University Press, 1995.

Tallemant Des Réaux, Gédéon. *Historiettes*. Antoine Adam, ed. Paris: Gallimard, 1960, Vol.1.

Thevet, André. *André Thevet's North America*. Roger Schlesinger and Arthur P. Stabler, ed. Montreal: McGill-Queen's University Press, 1986.

Thornborough, John. "A Letter of Chemistry." London, British Library, Sloane MS 814.

———. "A Letter of Chemistry." London, British Library, Sloane MS 1799.

Trismegistus, Hermes. *The Theological and Philosophical Works of Hermes Trismegistus, Christian Neoplatonist.* John David Chambers, trans. Edinburgh: T. & T. Clark, 1882.

———. *Hermetica*. Trans. Brian P. Copenhaver. Cambridge: Cambridge University Press, 1992.

Trismosin, Solomon (pseudo.). *Splendor Solis*. London: K. Paul, Trench, Trubner and Co., 1921.

The Turba Philosophorum or Assembly of the sage. A.E. Waite, ed. and trans. London: George Redway, 1896.

Valla, Lorenzo. *Dialogue on Free Will*. Charles E. Trinkaus, Jr., trans. *The Renaissance Philosophy of Man.* Ed. Ernst Cassirer, Paul O. Kristeller, and John H. Randall, Jr. Chicago: The University of Chicago Press, Phoenix Books, 1948.

Valverde de Amusco, Juan. *Historia de la composicion del cuerpo humano…* Rome: Salamanca and Lafrery, 1556. Republished as *Anatomia del corpo humano*. Rome: Salamanca and Lafrery, 1560.

Vaughan, Thomas. *Aqua Vitæ: Non Vitis*. London, British Library, Sloane MS 1741.

Vaughan, Thomas. *Aqua Vitæ: Non Vitis: Or, The radical Humiditie of Nature: Mechanically, and Magically dissected By the Conduct of Fire, and Fermen*t. Donald R. Dickson, translator. Tempe, AZ: Arizona Center for Medieval and Renaissance Studies, 2001.

———. *Magia adamica or the antiquitie of magic*. London, 1650.

Vesalius, Andreas. *De Humani Corporis Fabrica*. Basel: I. Oporini, 1543.

Villanova, Arnald de. *Opus Aureum*. Frankfurt, 1604.

Walker, Anthony. *The Holy Life of Mrs Elizabeth Walker*. London, 1690.

———. *The Vertuous Wife: or, the Holy Life of Mrs Elizabeth Walker*. London, 1694.

Wigges, Sarah. *Her Book*. London, Royal College of Physicians, MS 654.

The worke of Neptis communicated to Quercitanus. Scotland: University of Glasgow, Ferguson MS 163.

Zohar. Kabbalah Centre International. http://www.kabbalah.com/k/index.php/p=zohar.

Secondary Sources

Abel, Günter. "Juste Lipse et Marie de Gournay: autour de l'exemplaire d'Anvers des Essais de Montaigne," *BHR* XXXV (1973): 117–29.

Abraham, Lyndy. *A Dictionary of Alchemical Imagery*. Cambridge: Cambridge University Press, 1998.

Allen, Sally G. and Joanna Hubbs. "Outrunning Atalanta: Feminine Destiny in Alchemical Transmutation," *Signs*, 6, 2 (1980): 210–29.

Angenot, M. *Les Champions des Femmes*. Montréal: Les Presses de l'Université du Québec, 1977.

Archer, Jayne. "Women and Alchemy in Early Modern England," unpublished PhD dissertation. University of Cambridge, 2000.

———. "The Queens' Arcanum: Authority and Authorship in *The Queens Closet Opened* (1655)." *Renaissance Journal* 1.6 (June 2002).

———."'Rudenesse it Selfe She Doth Refine': Queen Elizabeth I as Lady Alchymia." *Goddesses and Queens: The Iconography of Elizabeth I*. Ed. Annaliese Connolly and Lisa Hopkins. Manchester: Manchester University Press, 2007. pp. 45–66

Arnold, A. James, ed. *Monsters, Tricksters, and Sacred Cows: Animal Tales and American Identities*. Charlottesville: University of Virginia Press, 1996.

Arnould, J.-C. *Marie de Gournay et l'Edition de 1595 des Essais de Montaigne*. Paris: Champion, 1996.

The Art of Midwifery: Early Modern Midwives in Europe. Hilary Marland, ed. London: Routledge, 1993.

Ashe, Geoffrey. *Mythology of the British Isles*. London: Methuen, 1990.

Avalle-Arce, Juan Manuel. *Amadís de Gaula: El primitivo y el de Montalvo*. México: Fondo de Cultura Económica, 1990.

Barthes, Roland. *Le Degré zero de l'écriture*. Paris: Seuil, 1953.

Bauschatz, Cathleen. "'Les Puissances de Vostre Empire:' Changing Power Relations in Marie de Gournay's *Le Proumenoir de Monsieur de Montaigne* from 1594 to 1626." *Renaissance Women Writers: French Texts/American Contexts*. Anne R. Larsen and Colette Winn, ed. Detroit, MI: Wayne State University Press, 1994. pp. 189–208.

Bausi, Francesco. "Machiavelli and Caterina Sforza." *Archivio storico italiano* (1991) disp. IV: 887–92.

Bausum, Henry S. "Edenic Images of the Western World: A Reappraisal." *South Atlantic Quarterly* (Autumn 1968): 672–87.

Bayer, Penny. "From Kitchen Hearth to Learned Paracelsianism: Women and Alchemy in the Renaissance." In *"Mystical Metal of Gold": Essays on Alchemy and Renaissance Culture*. Stanton J. Linden, ed. Brooklyn, NY: AMS Press, 2007.

———. "Jeanne du Port, Alchemist Daughter of Joseph du Chesne." *Rosenholmeren: Notiitser og Meddelelser fra Renaessancestudier ved Aarhus Universitet* 6/7 (October 1999): 1–4.

———."Lady Margaret Clifford's Alchemical Receipt Book and the John Dee Circle," *Ambix* (November 2005): 271–84

———. "Women's Alchemical Literature 1560–1616 in Italy, France, the Swiss Cantons and England, and its Diffusion to 1660." Unpublished PhD thesis, University of Warwick, 2003.

Beer, Gillian. "*Square Rounds* and Other Awkward Fits: Chemistry as Theatre." *Ambix* 41.1 (March 1994): 33–44.

Beier, Lucinda McCray. *Sufferers and Healers: The Experience of Illness in Seventeenth-Century England.* London: Routledge and Kegan Paul, 1987.

Bernheimer, Richard. *Wild Men in the Middle Ages: A Study in Art, Sentiment, and Demonology*. New York, Octagon Books, 1970.

Berriot-Salvadore, Evelyne. *Un Corps, un Destin: la femme dans la médecine de la Renaissance*. Paris: Champion, 1993.

———. "Marie Le Gendre et Marie de Gournay: A la manière de…" *Le Lecteur, l'auteur et l'écrivain: Montaigne 1492, 1592, 1992, Actes du colloque international de Haïfa, Avril-Mai 1992*. Paris: Champion, 1993. pp. 237–51.

Berthelot, Marcelin. *Collection des Alchemistes Grecs*. 3 volumes. Paris: Steinheil, 1887–8.

Bicks, Caroline. *Midwiving Subjects in Shakespeare's England.* Hampshire, England: Ashgate, 2003.

Blake, John B. "The Complete Housewife." *Bulletin of the History of Medicine* 49.1 (1975): 30–42.

Boase, A. *The Fortunes of Montaigne*. New York: Octagon Books, 1970.

Bonnefon, P. *Montaigne et ses amis*. Geneva: Slatkine Reprints, 1969 (1898).

Bouce, Paul-Gabriel. "Imagination, Pregnant Women, and Monsters, in Eighteenth Century England and France." In *Sexual Underworlds of the Enlightenment*. Eds G.S. Rousseau and Roy Porter. Chapel Hill: North Carolina University Press, 1988.

Bouswma, William J. *Concordia Mundi: The career and thought of Guillaume Postel* (1510–1581). Cambridge, MA: Harvard University Press, 1957.

Bowerbank, Sylvia. "The Spider's Delight: Margaret Cavendish and the 'Female' Imagination." *English Literary Renaissance* 14.3 (Autumn 1984): 392–408.

Braun, Lucien. *Paracelse*. Paris: A. Michel, 1980.

Breisach, Ernst. *Caterina Sforza: A Renaissance Virago*. Chicago: University of Chicago Press, 1967.

Brockliss, Laurence and Colin Jones. *The Medical World of Early Modern France*. Oxford: Clarendon Press, 1997.

Broomhall, Susan. *Women's Medical Work in Early Modern France*. Manchester: Manchester University Press, 2004.

Bucher, Bernadette. *Icon and Conquest: A Structural Analysis of the Illustrations of de Bry's Great Voyages*. Trans. Basia Miller Gulati. Chicago: University of Chicago Press, 1981.

Burke, James F. "Metamorphosis and the Imagery of Alchemy in *la Celestina*," *Revista Canadiense de Estudios Hispánicos* 1.2 (1977): 129–52.

Cacho Blecua, Juan Manuel. *Amadís: heroísmo mítico cortesano*. Madrid: Cupsa Editorial, 1979.

Campo, Victoria. "La historia y la política a través de las relaciones en verso en pliegos sueltos." *Les* Relaciones de sucesos *(canards) en Espagne (1500–1750). Actes du premier colloque international (Alcalá de Henares, 8, 9 et 10 juin 1995)* Alcalá: Universidad de Alcalá de Henares/Publications de la Sorbonne, 1996. pp 19–32.

Canning, Kathleen. *Gender History in Practice: Historical Perspectives on Bodies, Class and Citizenship*. Ithaca: Cornell University Press, 2006.

Caputo, John. *The Prayers and Tears of Jacques Derrida*. Bloomington: Indiana University Press, 1997.

Carr, Helen. *Inventing the American Primitive: Politics, Gender and the Representation of Native American Literary Traditions, 1789–1936*. New York: New York University Press, 1996.

Cassirer, Ernst. *The Individual and the Cosmos in Renaissance Philosophy*. Trans. Mario Domandi. Mineola, NY: Dover Publications, 2000.

Chéreau, Achille. *Esquisse historique sur Louise Bourgeois Dite Boursier, sage-femme de la Reine Marie de Médicis*. Paris: L'Union Médicale, 1852.

Cholakian, Patricia F. "The Identity of the Reader in Marie de Gournay's 'Le Proumenoir de Monsieur de Montaigne' [1594]." *Seeking the Woman in Late Medieval and Renaissance Writings*. Sheila Fisher and Janet E. Halley, eds. Knoxville: University of Tennessee Press, 1989. pp. 207–32.

Ciasca, Raffaele. *L'arte dei medici e speziali nella storia e nel commercio fiorentino dal secolo XII al XV*. Florence: Olschki, 1927.

Clough, Cecil H. "The Sources for the Biography of Caterina Sforza and for the History of Her State During Her Rule, With Some Hitherto Unpublished Letters Illustrative of Her Chancery Archives." *Atti e Memorie, Deputazione di storia patria per le provincie di Romagna,* vv. 15–6 (1963): 57–143.

Cody, Lisa Forman. "The Politics of Reproduction: From Midwives' Alternative Public Sphere to the Public Spectacle of Man Midwifery." *Eighteenth-Century Studies* 32, 4 (1999): 477–795.

Cohen, Jeffrey Jerome, ed. *Monster Theory*. Minneapolis: University of Minnesota Press, 1996.

———. *Of Giants. Sex, Monsters and the Middle Ages*. Minneapolis: University of Minnesota Press, 1999.

Comelli, Giovanni. *Ricettario di bellezza di Eustachio Celebrino, medico e incisore del Cinquecento*. Florence: Sansoni, 1960.

Conrad, Lawrence I. et al. *The Western Medical Tradition: 800 B.C. to A.D. 1800*. Cambridge: Cambridge University Press, 1995.

Copenhaver, Brian P. and Charles B. Schmitt. *Renaissance Philosophy. A History of Western Philosophy: 3*. New York and Oxford: Oxford University Press, 1992.

Coudert, Alison. *Alchemy: The Philosopher's Stone*. Boulder: Shambhala, 1980.

Cox, Virginia. *Women's Writing in Italy, 1400–1650*. Baltimore: Johns Hopkins University Press, 2008.

Daly, Mary. *Gyn/Ecology*. Boston: Beacon Press, 1978.

Darmon, P. *Mythologie de la femme dans l'Ancienne France*. Paris: Seuil, 1983.

Daston, Lorraine. "Marvelous Facts and Miraculous Evidence in Early Modern Europe." *Critical Inquiry* 18 (Fall, 1991): 93–124.

——— and Katharine Park. "The Hermaphrodite and the Orders of Nature: Sexual Ambiguity in Early Modern France." *Gay and Lesbian Quarterly* 1 (1995): 419–38.

——— and Katharine Park. *Wonders and the Order of Nature 1150–1750*. New York: Zone, 1998.

Davies, Norman. *Europe: A History*. Oxford; New York: Oxford University Press, 1996.

Davis, Lennard. "Constructing Normalcy: The Bell Curve, the Novel, and the Invention of the Disabled Body in the Nineteenth Century." *The Disability Studies Reader*. New York: Routledge, 2006. pp. 3–16.

de Riquer, Martin. "Agora lo veredes, dixo Agrajes." *Estudios sobre el Amadís de Gaula*. Barcelona: Sirmio, 1987. pp. 7–54.

Debus, Allen. *The Chemical Philosophy: Paracelsian Science and Medicine in the Sixteenth and Seventeenth Centuries*. 2 vols. New York: Science History Publications, 1977; revised edition, Mineola, NY: Dover Publications, 2002.

———. *Chemistry, Alchemy and the New Philosophy, 1550–1700: Studies in the History of Science and Medicine*. New York: Variorum Reprints, 1987.

———. *The French Paracelsians: The Chemical Challenge to Medical and Scientific Tradition in Early Modern France*. Cambridge: Cambridge University Press, 1991.

The Defiant Muse: French Feminist Poems from the Middle Ages to the Present. Donna Stanton, ed. New York: Feminist Press, 1986.

Derrida, Jacques. *L'animal que donc je suis*. Paris: Galilée, 2006.

Desan, Philippe. "The Book, the Friend, the Woman: Montaigne's Circular Exchanges." In *Contending Kingdoms*, Marie-Rose Logan and Peter Rudnytsky, ed. Detroit, MI: Wayne State University Press, 1991. pp. 225–62.

DeVries, Joyce. "Casting Her Widowhood: The Contemporary and Posthumous Portraits of Caterina Sforza." *Widowhood and Visual Culture in Early Modern Europe*. Allison Levy, ed. Aldershot, UK: Ashgate, 2003. pp. 77–92.

———. "Caterina Sforza's Portrait Medals: Power, Gender, and Representation in the Italian Renaissance Court." *Women's Art Journal* 24.1 (2003): 23–28, 24.

DeVun, Leah. "The Jesus Hermaphrodite: Science and Sex Difference in Premodern Europe." *Journal of the History of Ideas*, 69, 2 (April 2008): 193–218

———. *Prophecy, Alchemy, and the End of Time: John of Rupescissa in the Late Middle Ages*. New York: Columbia University Press, 2009.

Deyermond, A. "El hombre salvaje en la novela sentimental." *Actas del Segundo Congreso Internacional de Hispanistas*. Nijmeigen: University of Nijmeigen, 1967. pp. 265–72.

Dickson, Donald R. "The Alchemistical Wife: The Identity of Thomas Vaughan's 'Rebecca.'" *The Seventeenth Century* 13 (1998): 34–46.

Dictionnaire de Biographie Française. Roman d'Amat and R. Limouzin-Lamothe, ed., 11th vol. Paris: Librairie Letouzey et Ane, 1967.

Dobbie, B.M. Wilmott. "An Attempt to Estimate the True Rate of Maternal Mortality, Sixteenth to Eighteenth Centuries." *Medical History* 26 (1982): 79–90.

Dobbs, Betty Jo Teeter. *The Founding of Newton's Alchemy or "The Hunting of the Green Lyon."* Cambridge: Cambridge University Press, 1975.

Dodds, E.R. *Pagan and Christian in an Age of Anxiety*. Cambridge: Cambridge University Press, 1965.

Donnison, Jean. *Midwives and Medical Men: A History of Inter-professional Rivalries and Women's Rights*. New York: Schocken Books, 1977.

Dreger, Alice. *One of Us: Conjoined Twins and the Future of Normal*. Cambridge, MA: Harvard University Press, 2005.

DuMaître, Paule. "Autour d'Ambroise Paré: Ses Élèves, Ses Amis." *Histoire des Sciences Médicales* XXX, 3 (1996): 354.

Dupebe, Jean. "Poursuites contre Postel en 1553." *Guillaume Postel, 1581–1981: actes du colloque international d'Avranches, 5–9 septembre 1981*. Paris: Editions de la Maisnie, 1985. pp. 29–39.

Dusinberre, Juliet. *Virginia Woolf's Renaissance: Woman Reader or Common Reader?* Basingstoke: Macmillan, 1997.

Eamon, William. *Science and the Secrets of Nature: Books of Secrets in Medieval and Early Modern Culture*. Princeton, NJ: Princeton University Press, 1994.

——— and Françoise Peheau. "The Accademia Segreta of Girolamo Ruscelli. A Sixteenth-Century Italian Scientific Society." *Isis* 75 (1984): 327–42.

Earenfight, Theresa ed. *Queenship and Political Power in Medieval and Early Modern Spain*. Burlington, VT: Ashgate, 2005.

Ehrenreich, Barbara and Deirdre English. *Witches, Midwives, and Nurses: A History of Women Healers*. New York: The Feminist Press, 1973.

Eliade, Mircea. *Forgerons et alchimistes*. Paris: Flammarion, 1977.

Evans, R.J.W. and Alexander Marr, eds. *Curiosity and Wonder From the Renaissance to the Enlightenment*. Aldershot, UK: Ashgate, 2006.

Ezell, Margaret J.M. *The Patriarch's Wife: Literary Evidence and the History of the Family*. London: The University of North Carolina Press, 1987.

———. *Writing Women's Literary History*. Baltimore: Johns Hopkins University Press, 2003.

Fairchild, Hoxie Neale. *The Noble Savage: A Study in Romantic Naturalism*. New York: Columbia University Press, 1928.

Farmer, Stephen Alan. *Syncretism in the West: Pico's 900 Theses (1486): The Evolution of Traditional, Religious, and Philosophical Systems, with Text, Translation, and Commentary*. Tempe, AZ: Medieval and Renaissance Texts and Studies, 1998.

Fernández Valladares, Mercedes "Historia y política en las relaciones góticas de la Colección Medinaceli (Descripciones: segunda parte)." *Les* Relaciones de sucesos *(canards) en Espagne (1500–1750). Actes du premier colloque international (Alcalá de Henares, 8, 9 et 10 juin 1995)* Alcalá: Universidad de Alcalá de Henares/Publications de la Sorbonne, 1996. pp. 133–56.

Findlen, Paula. "Two Cultures of Scholarship?" *Isis* 96 (2005): 230–37.

Fogel, Michèle. *Marie de Gournay. Itinéraires d'une femme savante*. Paris: Fayard, 2004.

Frame, Donald. *Montaigne: A Biography*. New York: Harcourt, Brace and World, 1965.

Freccero, John. "Medusa and the Madonna of Forli: Political Sexuality in Machiavelli." *Machiavelli and the Discourse of Literature*. Albert Russell Ascoli and Victoria Kahn, ed. Ithaca: Cornell University Press, 1993. pp. 161–78.

French, Peter. *John Dee: The World of an Elizabethan Magus*. New York: Dorset Press, 1972/1989.

French, Roger. *Medicine Before Science: The Business of Medicine from the Middle Ages to the Enlightenment*. Cambridge: Cambridge University Press, 2003.

García-Rojas, Axayácatl Campos. "'Ser muy bien hablado en diuersas lenguas': el poliglotismo como arma cortesana en los libros de caballerías (Claribalte)." *Actas del Congreso Internacional X Jornadas Medievales* (México del 20 al 24 de septiembre del 2004), ed. Concepción Company, Aurelio González Pérez and Lillian von der Walde Moheno, eds. Mexico City: UNAM/ El Colegio de México/ UAM-Iztapalapa. pp. 17–30.

Gatens, Moira. *Imaginary Bodies: Ethics, Power, and Corporeality*. London: Routledge, 1996.

Gelbart, Nina Rattner. *The King's Midwife: A History and Mystery of Madame du Coudray*. Berkeley: University of California Press, 1998.

Gélis, Jacques. *L'arbre et le Fruit. La naissance dans l'occident moderne, XVIe—XIXe siècles*. Paris: Fayard, 1984.

———. *History of Childbirth: Fertility, Pregnancy, and Birth in Early Modern Europe*. Rosemary Morris, trans. Boston: Northeastern University Press, 1991.

———. *La sage-femme ou le médecin: une nouvelle conception de la vie*. Paris: Fayard, 1988.

Gélis, Jacques, Mireille Laget, and Marie-France Morel. *Entrer dans la vie*. Paris: Gallimard, 1978.

Ginzburg, Carlo. "Micro-History: Two or Three Things that I know about it," *Critical Inquiry*, 20 (1993): 10–35.

Goldberg, Harriet. "The Several Faces of Ugliness in Medieval Castilian Literature." *La Corónica* 7 (1979): 80–92.

Góngora, Mar Martinez. "Poesía, Melancolía y Subjetividad Femenina: La Humanista Luisa Sigea. " *Neophilologus*: Springer Netherlands, 90.3 (July 2006): 423–43.

González, Javier Roberto. *Patagonia-patagones: orígenes novelescos del nombre*. Rawson, Argentina: Subsecretaría de cultura de la Provincia del Chubut, 1999.

———. "Libros de caballerás en América." *Amadís de Gaula 1508: Quinientos años de libros de caballerías*. Madrid: Biblioteca Nacional de España/Sociedad estatal de conmemoraciones culturales, 2008. pp. 369–82.

Gowing, Laura. *Domestic Dangers: Women, Words, and Sex in Early Modern London*. Oxford: Clarendon Press, 1996.

Gracia, Paloma. "El 'Palacio Tornante' y el bizantinismo del *Amadís de Gaula*." In *Medioevo y literatura*, ed. Juan Paredes. 4 vols. Granada: Universidad de Granada, 1995. Vol. 2. pp. 443–55.

Grafton, Anthony. *Cardano's Cosmos: The Worlds and Works of a Renaissance Astrologer*. Cambridge, MA: Harvard University Press, 1999.

——— and Nancy Siraisi, eds. *Natural Particulars: Nature and the Disciplines in Renaissance Europe*. Cambridge, MA: MIT Press, 1999.

Grassi, Ernesto. *Renaissance Humanism: Studies in Philosophy and Poetics*. Binghamton, NY: Medieval & Renaissance Texts & Studies, vol. 51, 1988.

Green, Arthur. *A guide to the Zohar*. Stanford: Stanford University Press, 2004.

Green, Miranda. *Celtic Goddesses, Warriors, Virgins and Mothers*. London: British Museum, 1995.

———. *The Gods of the Celts*. Gloucester: Alan Sutton, 1986.

Green, Monica H. *Women's Healthcare in the Medieval West*. Aldershot, UK: Ashgate, 2000.

Greenblatt, Stephen. *Marvelous Possessions: The Wonder of the New World*. Chicago: Chicago University Press, 1991.

Grell, Ole Peter, ed. *Paracelsus*. Leiden; Boston; Koln: Brill, 1998.

Gubar, Susan. "'The Blank Page' and the Issues of Female Creativity" in Elizabeth Abel (ed.), *Writing and Sexual Difference* (Chicago, 1982), pp. 73–93.

Haeffner, Mark. *The Dictionary of Alchemy*. London: Aquarian Press, 1991.

Hairston, Julia. "Out of the Archive: Four Newly-Identified Figures in Tullia d'Aragona's *Rime della Signora Tullia di Aragona et di diversi a lei* (1547)." *MLN* 118 (2003): 257–63.

———. "Skirting the Issue: Machiavelli's Caterina Sforza." *Renaissance Quarterly* 53.3 (2000): 687–712.

Hannaway, Owen. "Laboratory Design and the Aim of Science: Andreas Libavius Versus Tycho Brahe." *Isis* 77: 585–610.

Hannay, Margaret P. "'How I These Studies Prize': The Countess of Pembroke and Elizabethan Science." *Women, Science and Medicine, 1500–1700*. Ed. Lynette Hunter and Sarah Hutton. Stroud: Sutton Publishing, 1997.

Hartsock, Nancy C.M. "The Feminist Standpoint: Developing the Ground for a Specifically Feminist Historical Materialism." *The Feminist Standpoint Theory Reader: Intellectual and Political Controversies*, ed. Sandra Harding. New York: Routledge, 2004. pp. 35–54.

Heitsch, Dorothea. "From Dialogue to Conversation: The Place of Marie de Gournay." *Printed Voices: The Renaissance Culture of Dialogue*. Dorothea Heitsch and Jean-François Vallée, eds. Toronto: University of Toronto Press, 2004. pp. 113–33.

Heusch, Carlos and Jesús Rodríguez Velasco, eds. *La caballería castellana. Textos y contextos*. Montpellier: Equipe d'études ibériques, latinoaméricaines et du monde lusophone, Université de Montpellier III, 2000.

Hirst, Desirée. *Hidden Riches: Traditional Symbolism from the Renaissance to Blake*. London: Eyre and Spottiswoode, 1964.

Holmyard, Eric J., *Alchemy*, New York: Dover Publications, 1990 (1957).

Huet, Marie-Hélène. *Monstrous Imagination*. Cambridge, MA: Harvard University Press, 1993.

Hunter, Lynette. *Seventeenth-Century English Recipe Books: Cooking, Physic and Chirurgery in the Works of Elizabeth Talbot Grey and Aletheia Talbot Howard*. Elizabeth Spiller, ed. Aldershot: Ashgate, 2008.

———. and Sarah Hutton, eds. *Women, Science and Medicine 1500–1700: Mothers and Sisters of the Royal Society*. Thrupp, Stroud, Gloucestershire: Sutton Publishing, 1997.

Hunter, Michael, ed. *Robert Boyle Reconsidered*. Michael Hunter, ed. Cambridge: Cambridge University Press, 1994.

Hutin, Serge. *L'alchimie*. Paris: Presses Universitaires de France, 1999.

Idel, Moshe. *Kabbalah: New Perspectives*. New Haven and London: Yale University Press, 1988.

———. *Language, Torah, and Hermeneutics in Abraham Abulafia*. Trans. Menahem Kallus. Albany: State University of New York Press, 1989.

Ilsley, M. *A Daughter of the Renaissance. Marie le Jars de Gournay*. The Hague: Mouton, 1963.

Izquierdo, Juan Carlos. "El Luteranismo en las relaciones de sucesos del siglo XVI." *Les* Relaciones de sucesos *(canards) en Espagne (1500–1750). Actes du premier colloque international (Alcalá de Henares, 8, 9 et 10 juin 1995)* Alcalá: Universidad de Alcalá de Henares/Publications de la Sorbonne, 1996. pp. 217–26.

Jansen, Sharon L. *The Monstrous Regiment of Women. Female Rulers in Early Modern Europe*. New York: Palgrave, 2002.

Johnson, Francis R. *Astronomical Thought in Renaissance England: A Study of English Scientific Writings from 1500–1645*. Baltimore: Johns Hopkins Press, 1963.

Joly, B. *La Rationalité de l'Alchimie au XVIIe siècle*. Paris: Vrin, 1992.

Jong, H.M.E. de. *Michael Maier's Atalanta Fugiens: Sources of an Alchemical Book of Emblems*. Leiden: E.J. Brill, 1969.

Jung, C.G. *Psychology and Alchemy*. Trans. R.F.C. Hull. Princeton: Princeton University Press, 1968.

———. *The Archetypes and the Collective Unconscious. The Complete Works of C.G. Jung*, vol. 9. Trans. R.F.C. Hull, Bollingen Foundation. Princeton: Princeton University Press, 1981.

Kahn, Didier. *Alchimie et Paracelsisme en France* (1567–1625). Geneva: Droz, 2007.

———. "Cinquante-neuf thèses de Paracelse censurées par la faculté de théologie de Paris, le 9 octobre 1578," *Documents oubliés sur l'alchimie, la kabbale et Guillaume Postel*, edited by Sylvain Matton, Geneva: Droz, 2001, 161–78.

———. "Jean d'Espagnet," *Dictionary of Seventeenth-Century French Philosophers*, edited by Luc Foisneau, London, New York: Thoemmes Continuum, 2008. pp. 438–41.

Kappler, Claude-Claire. *Monstres, démons et merveilles à la fin du Moyen Age*. Paris: Payot, 1999 [1980].

Kassell, Lauren. *Magic and Medicine in Elizabethan London: Simon Forman, Astrologer, Alchemist, and Physician*. Oxford: Oxford University Press, 2005.

Kavey, Allison. *Books of Secrets: Natural Philosophy in England 1550–1600*. Urbana: University of Illinois Press, 2007.

Keefer, M.H. "Agrippa's Dilemma: Hermetic 'Rebirth' and the Ambivalence of *De Vanitate* and *De Occulta Philosophia*." *Renaissance Quarterly,* 41(1988): 614–53.

Keller, Eve. "Producing Petty Gods: Margaret Cavendish's Critique of Experimental Science." *English Literary History*, 64.2 (Summer 1997): 447–71.

King, Helen. "Agnodike and the Profession of Medicine." *Proceedings of the Cambridge Philological Society*, 32 (1986): 53–77.

Klossowski de Rola, Stanislas. *The Golden Game*. London: Thames and Hudson, 1988.

Kristeller, Paul O. *The Philosophy of Marsilio Ficino*. Trans. Virginia Conant. New York: Columbia University Press, 1943.

Kristeva, Julia. *Powers of Horror: An Essay on Abjection*. Trans. Leon S. Roudiez. New York: Columbia University Press, 1982.

Kritzman, Lawrence. "Of Ashes Born: Montaigne's Surrogate Daughter." *The Journal of Medieval and Renaissance Studies* 1995 Fall (25:3): 419–31.

Kuntz, Marion L. *Guillaume Postel: Prophet of the Restitution of all Things, His Life and Thought*. London: Martinus Nijhoff, 1981.

Laget, Mireille. "Childbirth in Seventeenth- and Eighteenth-Century France: Obstetrical Practice and Collective Attitudes." In *Medicine and Society in France: Selections from the Annales: E.S.C.,* 6. R. Forster and O. Ranum, ed. Baltimore: Johns Hopkins University Press, 1980. pp. 137–76.

———. *Naissances: L'accouchement avant l'âge de la clinique*. Paris: Ed. du Seuil, 1982.

Larsen, Anne R. *Madeleine and Catherine des Roches: From Mother and Daughter*. Chicago, 2006.

Lebrun, François. *Se soigner autrefois: Médecins, saints et sorciers aux XVIIe et XVIIIe siècles*. Paris: Éditions du Seuil, 1995.

Lee, R.W. *Ut Pictura Poesis: the Humanist Theory of Painting*. New York: Norton & Company, 1912.

Lehoux, Françoise. *Le Cadre de vie des médecins Parisiens aux XVIe et XVIIe Siècles*. Paris: Éditions A. & J. Picard, 1976.

Leong, Elaine and Sara Pennell. "Recipe Collections and the Currency of Medical Knowledge in the Early Modern 'Medical Marketplace'." *Medicine and the Marketplace in England and Its Colonies c. 1450-c. 1850.* Ed. Mark Jenner and Patrick Wallis. Basingstoke: Palgrave Macmillian, 2007. pp. 133–52.

Lesage, Claire. "La litterature des 'secrets' e 'I secreti d'Isabella Cortese.'" *Chroniques italiennes* 36 (1993): 145–78.

Lestringant, Frank. *Cannibals: The Discovery and Representation of the Cannibal from Columbus to Jules Verne*. Trans. Rosemary Morris. Berkeley: California University Press, 1997.

———. *Mapping the Renaissance World: The Geographical Imagination in the Age of Discovery*. Trans. David Fausett. Berkeley: California University Press, 1994.

Lilley, Kate. "Blazing Worlds: Seventeenth Century Women's Utopian Writing." *Women, Texts & Histories*. Clare Brant and Diane Purkiss, ed.. London: Routledge, 1992, pp. 101–32

Lindemann, Mary. *Medicine and Society in Early Modern Europe*. Cambridge: Cambridge University Press, 1999.

Linden, Stanton J. *Darke Hierogliphicks: Alchemy in English Literature from Chaucer to the Restoration*. Lexington: University Press of Kentucky, 1996.

Lindsay, Jack. *The Origins of Alchemy in Graeco-Roman Egypt*. London: Frederick Muller, 1970.

Lingo, Alison Klairmont. "Empirics and Charlatans in Early Modern France: The Genesis of the Classification of the 'Other' in Medical Practice." *Journal of Social History* 19, 4 (1986): 583–603.

———. "Print's Role in the Politics of Women's Health Care in Early Modern France." In *Culture and Identity in Early Modern Europe (1500–1800): Essays in Honor of Natalie Zemon Davis*. Barbara Diefendorf and Carla Hesse, ed. Ann Arbor: University of Michigan Press, 1993. pp. 203–21.

Livet, C. *Précieux et précieuses. Caractères et moeurs littéraires du XVIIe siècle*. Paris: H. Welter, 1895 (3 edn).

Long, Kathleen P. *Hermaphrodites in Renaissance Europe*. Aldershot, UK: Ashgate, 2006.

———. "Salomon Trismosin and Clovis Hesteau de Nuysement: The Sexual Politics of Alchemy in Early Modern France." *L'Esprit créateur*, XXXV (Summer 1995): 9–21.

———. "The Chemical Wedding in the Works of Clovis Hesteau de Nuysement." *Dalhousie French Studies*, 56 (2001): 27–35.

Long, Pamela O. *Openness, Secrecy, Authorship: Technical Arts and the Culture of Knowledge From Antiquity to the Renaissance*. Baltimore: Johns Hopkins, 2001.

López-Ríos, Santiago. *Salvajes y razas monstruosas en la literatura castellana medieval*. Madrid: Fundación Universitaria Española, 1999.

Lorant, Stefan, ed. *The New World: The First Pictures of America*. New York: Duell, Sloan and Pierce, 1965.

Lorber, Judith. *Paradoxes of Gender*. New Haven: Yale University Press, 1994.

Mandosio, Jean-Marc. "L'Alchimie dans les classifications des sciences et des arts à la Renaissance." *Alchimie et philosophie à la Renaissance*. Jean-Claude Margolin and Sylvain Matton, eds. Paris: J. Vrin, 1993. pp. 11–41.

Marín Pina, María Carmen."Aproximación al tema de la virgo bellatrix en los libros de caballerías españoles," *Criticón* 45 (1989): 81–94

———. "Los monstruos híbridos en los libros de caballerías españoles." In *Actas do IV Congresso da Associaçao Hispanica de Literatura Medieval* (Lisboa, 1–5 Outubro 1991), vol. IV. Lisboa: Cosmos, 1993: 27–33.

———. "Don Quijote, las mujeres y los libros de caballerías." Kurt Reichenberger, ed. and prologue and Darío Fernández-Morera, ed. *Cervantes y su mundo II*. Kassel, Germany: Reichenberger, 2005. pp. 309–40.

Maulde-La-Clavière, René and George Herbert Ely. *The Women of the Renaissance: A Study of Feminism*. London: Swan Sonnenschein & Co., Ltd., 1900.

McClive, Cathy. "The Hidden Truths of the Belly: The Uncertainties of Pregnancy in Early Modern Europe." *The Society for the Social History of Medicine* 15, 2 (2002): 209–27.

McLean, I. *Woman Triumphant, Feminism in French Literature 1610–1652*. Oxford Clarendon Press, 1977.

McTavish, Lianne. *Childbirth and the Display of Authority in Early Modern France*. Aldershot, UK: Ashgate, 2005.

Meinel, Christopher, ed. *Die Alchemie in der europäischen Kultur- und Wissenschaftsgeschichte*. Weisbaden: Harrassowitz, Wolfbütteler Forschungen Band 32, 1986.

Mérida, Rafael. "Tres gigantas sin piedad: Gromadaça, Andandona y Bandaguida." In *Literatura de caballerías y orígenes de la novela*, ed. Rafael Beltrán. Valencia: Universitat de València, 1998. pp. 219–33.

Michel, Pierre. "La chatte de Montaigne." *BSIAM*, no. 29 (1964): 14–8.

Moran, Bruce T. *The Alchemical World of the German Court: Occult Philosophy and Chemical Medicine in the Circle of Moritz of Hessen* (1572–1632). Stuttgart: F. Steiner, 1991.

———. *Distilling Knowledge: Alchemy, Chemistry, and the Scientific Revolution*. Cambridge, MA: Harvard University Press, 2005.

Morgan, Erica. "Rhetorical Technique in the Persuasion of Melibea," *Celestinesca* 3.2 (1979): 7–18.

Morison, Stanley. *Eustachio Celebrino da Udene Calligrapher, Engraver, and Writer for the Venetian Printing Press*. Paris: Pegasus Press, 1929.

Multhauf, Robert. "The Significance of Distillation in Renaissance Medical Chemistry." *Bulletin of the History of Medicine* 30 (1956): 329–46.

Murphy, James M. "Antonio de Nebrija in the European Rhetorical Tradition." *Antonio de Nebrija: Edad Media y Rencimiento*. Ed. Carmen Codoñer and Juan Antonio González Iglesias. Salamanca: Universidad de Salamanca, 1944. pp. 447–56.

Murphy, Joseph. *The Power of Your Subconscious Mind.* New York: Prentice-Hall, Inc., 1987.

Nagy, Doreen F. *Popular Medicine in Seventeenth-Century England*. Bowling Green, OH: Bowling Green State University Press, 1988.

Naissance, enfance et éducation dans la France Méridionale du XVIe au XXe siècles: Hommage à Mireille Laget. Roland Andréani, Henri Michel, and Elie Pélaquier, ed. Montpellier: Université Paul-Valéry Montpellier III, 1999.

Nauert, Charles G. *Agrippa and the Crisis of the Renaissance*. Urbana: University of Illinois Press, 1965.

Newman, William R. *Gehennical Fire: The Lives of George Starkey, an American Alchemist in the Scientific Revolution*. Cambridge, MA: Harvard University Press, 1994.

———. *Promethean Ambitions: Alchemy and the Quest to Perfect Nature*. Chicago: The University of Chicago Press, 2004.

——— and Anthony Grafton, ed. *Secrets of Nature: Astrology and Alchemy in Early Modern Europe*. Cambridge, MA: MIT Press, 2001.

Noble, David. *A World Without Women: The Christian Clerical Culture of Western Science*. New York: Alfred A Knopf, 1992.

Notestein, Wallace. *A History of Witchcraft in England: From 1558–1718*. New York: Thomas Y. Crowell Co., 1968.

Nummedal, Tara. "Alchemical Reproduction and the Career of Anna Maria Zieglerin." *Ambix* 49 (2001): 56–68

———. *Alchemy and Authority in the Holy Roman Empire*. Chicago: University of Chicago Press, 2007.

Obrist, Barbara. *Les Débuts de l'imagerie alchimique (XIVe–XVe siècles)*. Paris: Le Sycomore, 1982.

Ogrinc, Will. "Western Society and Alchemy from 1200 to 1500." *Journal of Medieval History*. 6 (1980): 103–32.

Packard, Francis R. *Life and Times of Ambroise Paré [1510–1590]: With a New Translation of his Apology and an Account of his Journeys in Divers Places*. New York: Benjamin Blom, Inc., 1971.

Pagel, Walter. *Paracelsus*. Basel, New York: Karger, 1958.

———. "The Eightness of Adam and Related 'Gnostic' Ideas in the Paracelsian Corpus." *Religion and Neoplatonism in Renaissance medicine*. London: Variorum Reprints, 1985. pp. 119–39.

———. *Paracelsus: An Introduction to Philosophical Medicine in the Era of the Renaissance*. London: Karger, 1982.

Park, Katharine. *Secrets of Women: Gender, Generation, and the Origins of Human Dissection*. New York: Zone Books, 2006.

Pasolini, Pier Desiderio. *Caterina Sforza*. Rome: Loescher, 1893.

Patai, Raphael. "Maria the Jewess – Founding Mother of Alchemy." *Ambix*, 29 (1982): 177–97.

———. *The Jewish Alchemists: A History and Source Book*. Princeton, NJ: Princeton University Press, 1994.

Pelling, Margaret."Defensive Tactics: Networking by Female Medical Practitioners in Early Modern London."*Communities in Early Modern England: Networks,*

Places, Rhetoric. Alexandra Shepherd and Phil Withington, ed. Manchester: Manchester University Press, 2000.

———. *Medical Conflicts in Early Modern London: Patronage, Physicians, and Irregular Practitioners 1550–1640*. Oxford: Oxford University Press, 2003.

Pennell, Sara. "Perfecting Practice?: Women, Manuscript Recipes and Knowledge in Early Modern England." In *Early Modern Women's Manuscript Writing: Selected Papers from the Trinity/Trent Colloquium*. Victoria Burke and Jonathan Gibson, ed. Aldershot, UK: Ashgate, 2004. pp. 237–58.

Percheron, J. *Le livre d'Or de l'alchimie*. Villeselve: Ramuel, 1998.

Perkins, Wendy. *Midwifery and Medicine in Early Modern France: Louise Bourgeois*. Exeter: University of Exeter Press, 1996.

Petrelli, Richard. "The Regulation of French Midwifery during the *Ancien Régime*." *Journal of the History of Medicine and Allied Sciences* XXVI (1971): 276–92.

Petry, Yvonne. *Gender, Kabbalah and the Reformation: The Mystical Theology of Guillaume Postel (1510–1581)*. Leiden: Koninklijke Brill, 2004.

Pinet, S. "Babel historiada: un episodio del *Libro de Alexandre*." In *Literatura y conocimiento medieval. Actas de las VIII Jornadas Medievales*. Lillian von der Walde, Concepción Company, Aurelio González, eds. México: Universidad Nacional Autónoma de México, Universidad Autónoma Metropolitana, El Colegio de México, 2003. pp. 371–89.

———. *Archipelagoes*. Minneapolis: University of Minnesota Press, 2010.

Place, E.B. "El *Amadís* de Montalvo como manual de cortesanía en Francia." *Revista de Filología Española* 38 (1954): 151–69.

Plantié, J. *La Mode du portrait littéraire en France (1641–1681)*. Paris: Champion, 1994.

Platt, Peter G., ed. *Wonders, Marvels, and Monsters in Early Modern Culture*. Newark: University of Delaware Press, 1999.

Pollock, Linda. *With Faith and Physic: The Life of a Tudor Gentlewoman Lady Grace Mildmay 1552–1620*. London: Collins and Brown, 1993.

Portilla, Miguel León. *Cartografía y crónicas de la antigua California*. Mexico City: Universidad Nacional Autónoma de México, 2001.

Poulain, François. "La Vie et L'Oeuvre de Deux Chirurgiens: Jacques Guillemeau (1550–1613) et Charles Guillemeau (1588–1656)." Thesis, Université de Montpellier, 1993.

Principe, Lawrence M. *The Aspiring Adept: Robert Boyle and His Alchemical Quest*. Princeton, NJ: Princeton University Press, 1998.

Principe, Lawrence M., ed. *Chymists and Chymistry: Studies in the History of Alchemy and Early Modern Chemistry*. Sagamore Beach, MA: Science History Publications, 2007.

Principe, Lawrence M. and William R. Newman. "Some Problems with the Historiography of Alchemy." In *Secrets of Nature: Astrology and Alchemy in Early Modern Europe*, William R. Newman and Anthony Grafton, eds. Cambridge, MA: MIT Press, 2001. pp. 385–431.

Pulz, Waltraud. “Aux origines de l’obstétrique moderne en Allemagne (XVIe-XVIIIe Siécle): Accoucheurs contre matrones?” *Revue d’histoire modern et contemporaine,* Mathilde LeMiére trans., Marie-France Morel, ed. 43, 4 (1996): 593–617.

Ramos, Rafael.“El *Amadís* de Juan de Dueñas: ‘La ínsola del Ploro’.” *Actas del III Congreso de la Asociación Hispánica de Literatura Medieval*, ed. María Isabel Toro Pascua. Salmanca: Biblioteca Española del siglo XV. Departamento de Literatura Española e Hispanoamericana, vol. II, 1994. pp. 843–52.

Randall Coats, Catharine. “A Surplus of Significance: Hermaphrodites in Early Modern France.” *French Forum* 19 (1994): 17–35.

Rankin, Alisha. “The Practice of Pharmacology and Laywomen.” *Encyclopedia of Women in the Renaissance: Italy, France, and England.* Diana Robin, Anne R. Larsen, and Carole Levin, eds. Santa Barbara, CA: ABC-CLIO Inc., 2007.

Rattansi, Piyo and Antonio Clericuzio, eds. *Alchemy and Chemistry in the Sixteenth and Seventeenth Centuries*. Dodrecht: Kluwer, 1994.

Ray, Meredith. *Writing Gender in Women’s Letter Collections of the Italian Renaissance.* Toronto: University of Toronto Press, 2009.

Read, Malcolm K. “The Rhetoric of Social Encounter: *La Celestina* and the Renaissance Philosophy of Language.” *The Birth and Death of Language: Spanish Literature and Linguistics. 1300–1700*. Potomac: Studia Humanitatis, 1983.

Redondo, Augustin. “Los prodigios en las relaciones de sucesos de los siglos XVI y XVII.” *Les* Relaciones de sucesos *(canards) en Espagne (1500–1750). Actes du premier colloque international (Alcalá de Henares, 8, 9 et 10 juin 1995)* Alcalá: Universidad de Alcalá de Henares/Publications de la Sorbonne, 1996. pp. 287–304.

Redpath, Peter A. “The nature of woman and her role in religion according to Guillaume Postel. ” *Guillaume Postel, 1581–1981: actes du colloque international d’Avranches, 5–9 septembre 1981.* Paris: Editions de la Maisnie, 1985. pp. 137–49.

Reynolds, Winston A. “Los caballeros soberbiosos del Amadís.” *In Cuadernos Hispanoamericanos: Revista Mensual de Cultura Hispánica*, 350 (1979): 387–96.

Rico, Francisco. “Brujería y literatura.” *Brujología: Ponencias y comunicaciones del primer congreso español de brujología celebrado en San Sebastián, septiembre de 1972*. Madrid: Seminarios, 1975.

Rigall, Juan Casas. “Las razas monstruosas según Nebrija.” *Fantasía y literatura en la Edad Media y los Siglos de Oro*. Ed. Nicasio Salvador Miguel, Santiago López Ríos, and Esther Borrego Gutiérrez. Madrid: Iberoamericana/Vervuert, 2004. pp. 121–44.

Río Parra, Elena del. *Una era de monstruos. Representaciones de lo deforme en el Siglo de Oro español*. Madrid: Iberoamericana/Vervuert, 2003.

Roberts, Gareth. *The Mirror of Alchemy: Alchemical Ideas and Images in Manuscripts and Books From Antiquity to the Seventeenth Century*. London: The British Library, 1994.

Rodilla, María José. "La caballería de las damas: Un acercamiento a la mujer en el 'Amadís.'" Serafín González and Lillian von der Walde, ed. and preface. *Palabra crítica: Estudios en homenaje a José Amezcua*. Mexico City: Universidad Autónoma Metropolitana, Unidad Iztapalapa--Fondo de Cultura Económica, 1997. pp. 285–94.

Rodríguez Velasco, Jesús. "Teoría de la fábula caballeresca." *Libros de caballerías (de "Amadís" al "Quijote".)* Salamanca: SEMYR, 2002. pp. 343–58.

Roelker, Nancy L. "The Appeal of Calvinism to French Noblewomen in the Sixteenth Century." *Journal of Interdisciplinary History,* 2 (1972): 391–418.

Rothstein, Marian. "Mutations of the Androgyne: Its Functions in Early Modern French Literature." *Sixteenth Century Journal* 34, 2 (2003): 409–37.

Roubaud-Bénichou, Sylvia. "Corps en beauté, corps à l'épreuve: le héros du roman de chevalerie." In *Le Corps dans la societé espagnole des XVIè et XVIIè siècles*. A. Redondo, ed. Paris: Publications de la Sorbonne, 1990. pp. 253–66.

Roy, Bruno (ed.). *Devinettes françaises du moyen âge*. Montréal: Bellarmin, Paris: Vrin, 1977.

Ruland, Martin *A Lexicon of Alchemy*. A.E. Waite, trans. London: John M. Watkins, 1964.

Rummel, Erika. *The Case Against Johann Reuchlin: Religious and Social Controversy in Sixteenth-Century Germany*. Toronto and London: University of Toronto Press, 2002.

Russell, P. "El descubrimiento de las canarias y el debate medieval acerca de los derechos de los príncipes y pueblos paganos." *Revista de Historia Canaria* 36, 171(1978): 9–32.

Sainte-Beuve, Charles Augustin. *Nouveaux Lundis*. Paris: C. Lévy, 1876.

Salisbury. Joyce E. *The Beast Within: Animals in the Middle Ages*. New York: Routledge, 1994.

Sankovitch, Tilde. *French Women Writers and the Book. Myths of Access and Desire*. Syracuse, NY: Syracuse University Press, 1988.

Sarduy, Severo. *Ensayos generales sobre el Barroco*. México: Fondo de Cultura Económica, 1987.

Sawday, Jonathan . *The Body Emblazoned: Dissection and the Human Body in Renaissance Culture*. London and New York: Routledge, 1995.

Sayre, Gordon M. *Les Sauvages Américains: Representations of Native Americans in French and English Colonial Literature*. Chapel Hill: North Carolina University Press, 1997.

Schachter, Marc. *Voluntary Servitude and the Erotics of Friendship. From Classical Antiquity to Early Modern France*. Aldershot, UK: Ashgate, 2008.

Schiebinger, Londa L. *The Mind Has No Sex? Women in the Origins of Modern Science*. Cambridge, MA: Harvard University Press, 1989.

———. *Nature's Body: Sexual Politics and the Making of Modern Science*. London: Pandora, 1994.

Schofield, Roger. "Did the Mothers Really Die? Three Centuries of Maternal Mortality in 'The World We Have Lost.'" *The World We Have Gained: Histories of Population and Social Structure* . Ed. Lloyd Bonfield, Richard Smith, and Keith Wrightson. New York: Blackwell Publishers, 1986, pp. 231–60.

Scholem, Gershom. *Elements of the Kabbalah and Its Symbolism*. Jerusalem: Keter Publishing, 1976.

———. *Kabbalah*. New York: New York Times Book Co., 1974/1987.

———. *Major Trends in Jewish Mysticism*. New York: Schocken Books, 1961.

Scholem, Gershom Gerhard. *On the Kabbalah and Its Symbolism*. New York: Schocken Books, 1996.

Scott, Daniel. "Recent Discoveries in the Muniment Rooms of Appleby Castle and Skipton Castle." *Transactions of the Cumberland and Westmoreland Antiquarian and Archaeological Society* 18 (1918): 189–210.

Scott, Joan. *Gender and the Politics of History*. New York: Columbia University Press, 1988.

Secret, François. "Mlle de Gournay, alchimiste." *BHR* XXXV (1973): 526–31.

Shapin, Steven. *A Social History of Truth: Civility and Science in Seventeenth-Century England.* Chicago: University of Chicago Press, 1994.

Sheridan, Bridgette. "Childbirth, Midwifery, and Science: The Life and Work of the French Royal Midwife Louise Bourgeois." PhD dissertation, Boston College, 2002.

Sherwood Taylor, Frank. *The Alchemists, founders of modern chemistry*. London: W. Heinemann, 1951.

———. "The Origins of Greek Alchemy," *Ambix*, 1 (1937): 30–47.

Simons, Patricia and Monique Kornell. "Annibal Caro's After-Dinner Speech (1536) and the Question of Titian as Vesalius's Illustrator." *Renaissance Quarterly,* 61, 4 (2008): 1069–97.

Simonton, O. Carl, Stephanie Matthews-Simonton, and James L. Creighton. *Getting Well Again.* New York: Bantam Books, 1978/1980.

Siraisi, Nancy G. *Medieval and Early Renaissance Medicine: An Introduction to Knowledge and Practice*. Chicago: The University of Chicago Press, 1990.

Smith, Pamela H. *The Business of Alchemy: Science and Culture in the Holy Roman Empire*. Princeton, NJ: Princeton University Press, 1997.

Smith, Paul Julian. *The Body Hispanic: Gender and Sexuality in Spanish and Spanish American literature*. Oxford and New York: Clarendon Press/Oxford University Press, 1989.

Stern, Menahem. *Greek and Latin Authors on Jews and Judaism*. In two volumes. Jerusalem: Israel Academy of Sciences and Humanities, 1980.

Stone, Lawrence. *The Family, Sex, and Marriage in England 1500–1800*. New York: Harper & Row, 1977.

Strocchia, Sharon. *Nuns and Nunneries in Renaissance Florence*. Baltimore: Johns Hopkins University Press, 2009.

Tatlock, Lynne. "Speculum Feminarum: Gendered Perspectives on Obstetrics and Gynecology in Early Modern Germany." *Signs: Journal of Women in Culture and Society* 17, 4 (1992): 725–60.

Tester, S.J. *A History of Western Astrology*. Suffolk, UK: The Boydell Press, 1987, reprint 1999.

Thomas, Keith. *Religion and the Decline of Magic*. Hammondsworth: Penguin Books, 1971/1973.

Thompson, John Lee. *John Calvin and the Daughters of Sarah: Women in Regular and Exceptional Roles in the Exegesis of Calvin, his Predecessors, and his Contemporaries*. Geneva: Droz, 1992.

Thorndike, Lynn. *A History of Magic and Experimental Science*. New York: Columbia University Press, 1947–58. Vol. 5: *The Sixteenth Century*.

Tilton, Hereward. *The Quest for the Phoenix: Spiritual Alchemy and Rosicrucianism in the Work of Count Michael Maier (1569–1622)*. Christoph Markschies and Gerhard Mueller, eds. *Arbeiten zur Kirchesgeschichte 88*. Berlin: Walter de Gruyter, 2003.

Todorov, Tzvetan. *The Conquest of America: The Question of the Other*. Trans. Richard Howard. New York: Harper, 1994.

Tosi, Lucia. "Marie Meurdrac: Paracelsian Chemist and Feminist." *Ambix* 48.2 (2001): 69–82.

Toro Pascua, María Isabel. "*Amadís de Gaula* y la tradición apocalíptica medieval." *Amadís de Gaula: quinientos años después. Estudios en homenaje a Juan Manuel Cacho Blecua*. Alcalá de Henares: Centro de estudios cervantinos, 2008. pp. 285–94

Trevor-Roper, H. "The Court Physician and Paracelsianism." In *Medicine at the Courts of Europe, 1500–1837*. V. Nutton, ed. New York, London: Routledge, 1990, 79–94.

Trexler, Richard. *Sex and Conquest: Gendered Violence, Political Order, and the European Conquest of the Americas*. Ithaca, NY: Cornell University Press, 1995.

Trollope, T. Adolphus *A Decade of Italian Women*. London: Chapman & Hall, 1859.

Uildriks, Anne. *Les Idées littéraires de Mlle de Gournay*. Groningen: Kleine, 1962.

Velasco, Sherry "Marimachos, hombrunas, barbudas: The Masculine Woman in Cervantes," *Cervantes: Bulletin of the Cervantes Society of America* 20.1 (2000): 69–78.

———. *Male Delivery: Reproduction, Effeminacy, and Pregnant Men in Early Modern Spain*. Nashville, TN: Vanderbilt University Press, 2006.

Villey, Pierre. *Montaigne devant la postérité*. Paris: Boivin, 1935.

Walker, Daniel P. *Spiritual and Demonic Magic, from Ficino to Campanella*. University Park: Pennsylvania State University Press, 1958. Reprint with introduction by Brian P. Copenhaver, 2003.

Walsh, John K. "The chivalric dragon: hagiographic parallels in early Spanish romances." *Bulletin of Hispanic Studies* 54 (1977): 189–98.

Warlick, M.E. "The Domestic Alchemist: Women as Housewives in Alchemical Emblems." *Emblems and Alchemy*. Alison Adams and Stanton J. Linden, ed. Glasgow: Glasgow Emblem Studies, 1998. pp. 25–47.

Webster, Charles. *From Paracelsus to Newton: Magic and the Making of Modern Science*. Cambridge: Cambridge University Press, 1982.

———. *Health, Medicine and Mortality in the Sixteenth Century*. Cambridge: Cambridge University Press, 1979.

Weiss, Roberto. *The Renaissance Discovery of Classical Antiquity*. Oxford: Oxford University Press, 1969.

Weissberger, Barbara *Isabel Rules. Constructing Queenship, Wielding Power*. Minneapolis: University of Minnesota Press, 2004.

Williams, David. *Deformed Discourse: the Functions of the Monster in Medieval Thought and Literature*. Montreal: McGill-Queen's University Press, 1996.

Wilson, Adrian. *The Making of Man-midwifery: Childbirth in England, 1660–1770*. Cambridge, MA: Harvard University Press, 1995.

Woolley, Benjamin. *The Queen's Conjuror: The Science and Magic of Dr Dee*. London: Flamingo, 2002.

Yates, Frances A. *Giordano Bruno and the Hermetic Tradition*. London: Routledge and Kegan Paul, 1964.

Index

Page numbers in *italics* denote titles of books, or illustrations. Page numbers in italics with a *t* indicate tables.